Student Resources

Online Student Resources are **included** with this textbook.
Visit **http://nursing.pearsonhighered.com** for the following assets and activities:

- Learning Outcomes
- Chapter Review Questions
- Case Studies

- Application Activities
- Additional content updates
- Weblinks

- Links to additional nursing resources

Additional resources available. For more information and purchasing options visit **nursing.pearsonhighered.com**

CLASSROOM

Dosage Calculation Online Application

- A unique online interface guides the user through examples of chapter topics, provides practice questions, chapter challenge tests, and a comprehensive final test.

CLINICAL

Pearson's Nurse's Drug Guide

- Published annually to be your current, comprehensive, and clinically relevant source for drug information

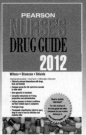

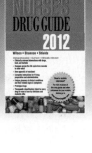
• Your complete mobile solution!

Real Nursing Skills

- Video demonstrations of over 200 clinical nursing skills
- Each skill includes Purpose, Preparation, Procedure, Post-Procedure, Expected and Unexpected Outcomes, Documentation and References and Resources

NCLEX®

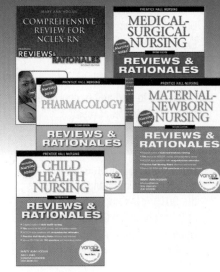

- Concentrated review of core content
- Thousands of practice questions with comprehensive rationales

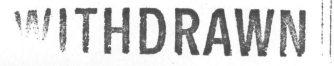

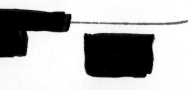
PEARSON

ALWAYS LEARNING

PEARSON NURSING CLASS PREPARATION RESOURCES

New and Unique!

- Use this preparation tool to find animations, videos, images, and other media resources that cross the nursing curriculum! Organized by topic and fully searchable by resource type and key word, this easy-to-use platform allows you to:
  - Search through the media library of assets
  - Upload your own resources
  - Export to PowerPoint™ or HTML pages

Use this tool to find and review other unique instructor resources:

Correlation Guide to Nursing Standards

- Links learning outcomes of core textbooks to nursing standards such as the 2010 ANA Scope and Standards of Practice, QSEN Competencies, National Patient Safety Goals, AACN, Essentials of Baccalaureate Education and more!

Pearson Nursing Lecture Series

- Highly visual, fully narrated and animated, these short lectures focus on topics that are traditionally difficult to teach and difficult for students to grasp
- All lectures accompanied by case studies and classroom response questions for greater interactivity within even the largest classroom
- Use as lecture tools, remediation material, homework assignments and more!

MYTEST AND ONLINE TESTING

- Test questions even **more accessible** now with both pencil and paper (MyTest) and online delivery options (Online Testing)
- **NCLEX®-style** questions

BOOK-SPECIFIC RESOURCES
Also available to instructors:

- **Instructor's Manual and Resource Guide** organized by learning outcome
- Comprehensive **PowerPoint™** presentations integrating lecture notes and images
- **Image library**
- **Classroom Response Questions**
- **Online course management systems** complete with instructor tools and student activities

DOSAGE CALCULATION ONLINE APPLICATION

- A unique online interface guides the user through examples of chapter topics, provides practice questions, chapter challenge tests, and a comprehensive final test.

REAL NURSING SIMULATIONS

- 25 simulation scenarios that span the nursing curriculum
- Consistent format includes learning objectives, case flow, set-up instructions, debriefing questions and more!
- Companion online course cartridge with student pre- and post-simulation activities, videos, skill checklists and reflective discussion questions

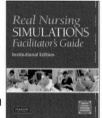

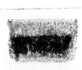

PEARSON   ALWAYS LEARNING

Dosage Calculations

A Multi-Method Approach

Anthony Patrick Giangrasso, PhD
Professor of Mathematics
LaGuardia Community College
Long Island City, NY

Dolores M. Shrimpton, MA, RN
Professor Emerita of Nursing
Department of Nursing
Kingsborough Community College
Brooklyn, NY

PEARSON

Boston   Columbus   Indianapolis   New York   San Francisco   Upper Saddle River
Amsterdam   Cape Town   Dubai   London   Madrid   Milan   Munich   Paris   Montréal   Toronto
Delhi   Mexico City   São Paulo   Sydney   Hong Kong   Seoul   Singapore   Taipei   Tokyo

Publisher: Julie Levin Alexander
Publisher's Assistant: Regina Bruno
Senior Acquisitions Editor: Kelly Trakalo
Assistant Editor: Lauren Sweeney
Development Editor: Michael Giacobbe
Managing Editor, Production: Patrick Walsh
Production Liason: Yagnesh Jani
Director of Marketing: David Gesell
Senior Marketing Manager: Phoenix Harvey

Marketing Coordinator: Michael Sirinides
Manufacturing Manager/Buyer: Ilene Sanford
Senior Art Director: Maria Guglielmo
Cover Designer: Diane Ernsberger
Media Project Manager: Rachel Collett/Leslie Brado
Composition and Production: Integra
Printer/Binder: Quebecor World Color–Versailles
Cover Printer: Lehigh-Phoenix Color/Hagerstown

10 9 8 7 6 5 4 3 2 1

Library of Congress Cataloging-in-Publication Data

Giangrasso, Anthony Patrick.
  Dosage calculations : a multi-method approach / Anthony Patrick Giangrasso,
Dolores M. Shrimpton.
    p. ; cm.
  Includes index.
  ISBN-13: 978-0-13-215862-6
  ISBN-10: 0-13-215862-0
  I. Shrimpton, Dolores M.   II. Title.
  [DNLM: 1. Drug Dosage Calculations—Nurses' Instruction.   2. Drug Dosage Calculations—Problems
and Exercises.   3. Pharmaceutical Preparations—administration & dosage—Nurses' Instruction.
4. Pharmaceutical Preparations—administration & dosage—Problems and Exercises. QV 18.2]
  LC Classification not assigned
  615.1'9—dc23
                                                        2011045320

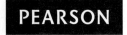

www.pearsonhighered.com

ISBN 10:   0-13-215862-0
ISBN 13: 978-0-13-215862-6

About the Authors

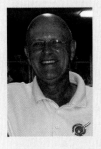

ANTHONY GIANGRASSO was born and raised in Maspeth, NY. He attended Rice High School on a scholarship and in his senior year was named in a citywide contest by the *New York Journal-American* newspaper as New York City's most outstanding high school scholar-athlete. He was also awarded a full-tuition scholarship to Iona College, from which he obtained a BA in mathematics, magna cum laude, with a ranking of sixth in his graduating class.

Anthony began his teaching career as a fifth-grade teacher in Manhattan as a member of the Christian Brothers of Ireland, and taught high school mathematics and physics in Harlem and Newark, NJ. He holds an MS and Ph.D. in from New York University, and has taught at all levels from elementary school through graduate school. He is currently teaching at Adelphi University and LaGuardia Community College, where he was chairman of the mathematics department. He has authored nine college textbooks through twenty-three editions.

Anthony's community service has included membership on the boards of directors of the Polish-American Museum Foundation, Catholic Adoptive Parents Association, and Family Focus Adoptive Services. He was the president of the Italian-American Faculty Association of the City University of New York, and the founding chairman of the board of the Italian-American Legal Defense and Higher Education Fund, Inc. He and his wife, Susan, are proud parents of three children Anthony, Michael, and Jennifer. He enjoys tennis, and in 2007 for the second time was ranked #1 for his age group in the Eastern Section by the United States Tennis Association.

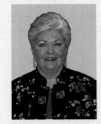

DOLORES M. SHRIMPTON is a Professor of Nursing at Kingsborough Community College (CUNY) where she was Chairperson of the department for thirteen years. She received a diploma in nursing from Kings County Hospital Center School of Nursing, a BS from C.W. Post College, an MA in nursing administration from New York University, and a post-Master's certificate in nursing education from Adelphi University. She is a member of the Upsilon and Mu Upilson Chapters of Sigma Theta Tau. She has taught a wide variety of courses in practical nursing, diploma, and associate degree nursing programs.

Dolores has held many leadership positions in nursing, including Board Member, Vice-President, and President of the NYS Associate Degree Nursing Council. She was the Co-Chair of the CUNY Nursing Discipline Council, and Member of the Board of Directors and Co-President of the Brooklyn Nursing Partnership. She has served on a number of Advisory Boards of LPN, associate degree, and baccalaureate degree nursing programs. She is a recipient of the Presidential Award in Nursing Leadership from the Nurses Association of Long Island (NACLI), the Mu Upsilon award for Excellence in Nursing Education, and Excellence in Nursing Leadership. She has also been recognized for her commitment to nursing by the Brooklyn Nursing Partnership.

Dolores lives in Brooklyn NY, and especially enjoys cooking, and spending time with her grandchildren, Brooke Elizabeth, Paige Dolores, Jack Paul, and their parents, Kim and Shawn. She also enjoys traveling and spending time with friends and family in Harwich Port, Cape Cod Massachusetts.

Dedication
To June Looby Olsen, RN, MS, our friend, mentor, and the person who brought each of us into the field of writing medical dosage calculation textbooks.

—Anthony P. Giangrasso and Dolores M. Shrimpton

Preface

In 1995, the Institute of Medicine issued its landmark report, "To Err Is Human: Building a Safer Health System," which claimed that nearly 100,000 people died annually due to medical errors. Since that report, greater emphasis has been placed on improving safety in medication administration. One aspect of that safety is accuracy in drug calculations. *Dosage Calculations* is not merely a textbook about math skills; it is also an introduction to the professional context of safe drug administration. Calculation skills and the rationales behind them are emphasized throughout.

This book offers all the standard methods of drug dosage calculation (Dimensional Analysis, Ratio & Proportion, and Formula). Explanations and illustrations of each method are provided. Alternative methods for a given problem are offered in a side-by-side format for easy comparison.

The student is urged to examine each of the methods illustrated, and to initially try them all. After a period of time the student will usually choose which methods fits his or her learning style best, and will use that method exclusively.

The book allows instructors to teach their own preferred method or to illustrate multiple methods to their students. This flexibility is an asset in departments where faculty have varied opinions of which approach should be used.

Dosage Calculations is a combined text and workbook. Its consistent focus on safety, accuracy, and professionalism make it a valuable part of a course for nursing or allied health programs. It is also highly effective for independent study and may be used as a refresher for dosage calculation skills and as a professional reference.

Dosage Calculations is arranged into four basic learning units:

Unit 1: Basic Calculation Skills and Introduction to Medication Administration
Chapter 1 includes a diagnostic test of arithmetic and reviews the necessary basic mathematics skills. Chapter 2 introduces the student to the essentials of the medication administration process. Chapter 3 introduces the dimensional analysis and ratio & proportion methods in small increments using a simple, step-by-step, common sense approach.

Unit 2: Systems of Measurement
Chapters 4 and 5 present the metric and household systems of measurement that nurses and other allied health professionals must understand in order to interpret medication orders and calculate dosages. Students learn to convert measurements between and within measurement systems.

Unit 3: Oral and Parenteral Medications
This unit prepares students to calculate oral and parenteral dosages and introduce them to the essential equipment needed for administration and preparation of solutions. Chapter 6 introduces oral drug dosage calculations using a third approach, the Formula method. It also includes dosages based on patient size. Chapter 7 discusses syringes and insulin. Chapter 8 deals with solutions, and Chapter 9 introduces parenteral medications and heparin.

Unit 4: Infusions and Pediatric Dosages

Chapters 10 and 11 provide a solid foundation for calculating intravenous and enteral dosage rates and flow rates and include titrating IV medications. Pediatric dosages and daily fluid maintenance needs are discussed in Chapter 12.

Features and Benefits of *Dosage Calculations*

- Keystroke Sequences in chapter one. This enables students to check their calculations and ensure safety.
- Updated and revised drug labels and drug examples throughout the text that contain both trade and generic drug names.
- Increased emphasis on the safety in medication administration following the Joint Commission National Patient Safety Goals.
- *MyNursingLab* for *Dosage Calculations* provides diagnostic testing and student remediation with hundreds of additional practice questions.
- Information on insulin administration and calculations.
- Information on heparin administration and calculations.
- Titration tables and a section on IV push are included.
- Throughout the textbook there are worked out solutions to all illustrated examples. Care is taken to show each step in the process. Many examples are solved using two different methods set up side-by-side for easy comparison.
- Constant skill reinforcement through frequent practice opportunities.
- More than 1,000 problems for students to solve.
- Actual drug labels, syringes, drug package inserts, prescriptions, and medication administration records (MARs) are illustrated throughout the text.
- Ample work space on every page for note taking and problem solving.
- Answers to practice exercises are found in the textbook in Appendix A.

Acknowledgments

Our special thanks to the nursing and mathematics faculty and the students at LaGuardia Community College and Kingsborough Community College. Also, a special thank you to our editor, Kelly Trakalo, and development editor, Michael Giacobbe, and to the production and marketing teams at Pearson.

Thank you also to the following manufacturers for supplying labels and art for this textbook:

Abbott Laboratories; Astra Zeneca; Baxter; Eli Lilly and Company; Forrest Pharmaceuticals, Inc.; Merck and Company, Inc.; Novartis Pharmaceuticals; Pfizer, Inc.; Purdue Pharma; Roxane Laboratories; Teva Pharmaceutical Industries Ltd.

Accuracy Reviewers for *Dosage Calculations*

Charlene M. Chapman BSN, RN
Pennsylvania Institute of Technology
Philadelphia, PA

Dr. Jim Hodge
Mountain State University
Beckley, WV

Carol A. Penrosa, RN, MSN
Southeast Community College
Lincoln, NE

Mary G. Tan, PhD, MSN, RN
South University
Savannah, GA

Dr. Mandyam Tirumalachar
Austin Community College
Austin, TX

Linda Walter, RN. MSN
Northwest Michigan College
Traverse City, MI

Learn to Calculate Dosages Safely and Accurately!

The Ease of Learning Dosage Calculations

Dosage Calculations provides the ease of learning the dimensional analysis, ratio & proportion, and formula methods of calculation with a building block approach of the basics.

Name: _____   Date: _____

Diagnostic Test of Arithmetic

The following Diagnostic Test illustrates *all* the arithmetic skills needed to do the computations in this textbook. Take the test and compare your answers with the answers found in Appendix A. If you discover areas of weakness, carefully review the relevant review materials in this chapter so that you will be mathematically prepared for the rest of the textbook.

1. Write 0.375 as a fraction in lowest terms. _____

2. Write $\frac{28,500}{100,000}$ as a decimal number. _____

3. Round off 6.492 to the nearest tenth. _____

4. Write $\frac{5}{6}$ as a decimal number rounded off to the nearest hundredth. _____

5. Simplify $\frac{0.63}{0.2}$ to a decimal number rounded off to the nearest tenth. _____

6. $0.038 \times 100 = $ _____

7. $4.26 \times 0.015 = $ _____

8. $55 \div 0.11 = $ _____

9. $90 \times \frac{1}{300} \times \frac{20}{3} = $ _____

10. Write $5\frac{3}{4} \div 23$ as a fraction and as a decimal number. _____

11. Write $\frac{7}{100} \div \frac{3}{100}$ as a mixed number. _____

12. Write $\frac{\frac{4}{5}}{20}$ as a simple fraction in lowest terms. _____

The Diagnostic Test of Arithmetic helps students rediscover their understanding of basic math concepts and guides them in identifying areas for review.

Learn by Example. Each chapter unfolds basic concepts and skills through completely worked out questions with solutions.

EXAMPLE 9.5

The prescriber ordered *Tigan (trimethobenzamide hydrochloride) 200 mg IM stat*. You have a 20 mL multidose vial, and the label indicates that the strength is 100 mg/mL. How many milliliters of this antiemetic drug will you prepare?

Begin by determining how many milliliters of the solution in the vial contain the prescribed quantity of the medication. That is, you want to convert 200 mg to an equivalent in milliliters.

DIMENSIONAL ANALYSIS

$$200 \text{ mg} = ? \text{ mL}$$

You cancel the milligrams and obtain the equivalent quantity in milliliters.

$$200 \text{ mg} \times \frac{? \text{ mL}}{? \text{ mg}} = ? \text{ mL}$$

The label indicates that there are 100 mg per milliliter.

So, the unit fraction is $\frac{1 \text{ mL}}{100 \text{ mg}}$.

$$200 \text{ mg} \times \frac{1 \text{ mL}}{100 \text{ mg}} = 2 \text{ mL}$$

RATIO & PROPORTION

$$200 \text{ mg} = x \text{ mL} \quad \text{(dose)}$$
$$100 \text{ mg} = 1 \text{ mL} \quad \text{(strength)}$$
$$\frac{200 \text{ mg}}{x \text{ mL}} \diagdown \frac{100 \text{ mg}}{1 \text{ mL}}$$
$$100x = 200$$
$$x = \frac{200}{100}$$
$$x = 2$$

So, you would give the patient 2 mL.

EXAMPLE 6.1

The order reads *Cymbalta (duloxetine HCl) 60 mg PO daily*.

Read the drug label shown in • **Figure 6.1**. How many capsules of this antidepressant drug will you administer to the patient?

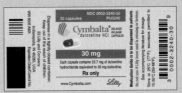

• Figure 6.1
Drug label for Cymbalta.

Safe and Accurate Dosage Calculation

Safe and accurate dosage calculation comes from practice and critical thinking.

Try These for Practice, Exercises, and
Additional Exercises, found in every chapter,
test your comprehension of material.

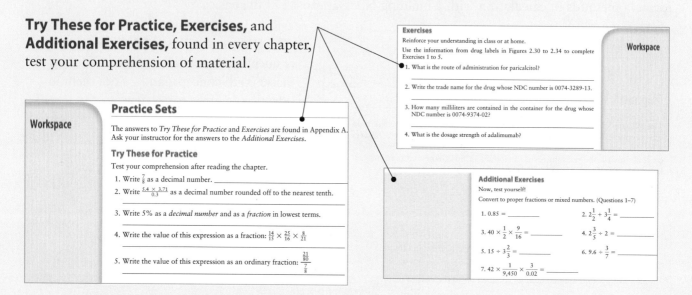

Exercises

Reinforce your understanding in class or at home.
Use the information from drug labels in Figures 2.30 to 2.34 to complete
Exercises 1 to 5.

Workspace

1. What is the route of administration for paricalcitol?

2. Write the trade name for the drug whose NDC number is 0074-3289-13.

3. How many milliliters are contained in the container for the drug whose NDC number is 0074-9374-02?

4. What is the dosage strength of adalimumab?

Workspace

Practice Sets

The answers to *Try These for Practice* and *Exercises* are found in Appendix A. Ask your instructor for the answers to the *Additional Exercises.*

Try These for Practice

Test your comprehension after reading the chapter.

1. Write $\frac{7}{8}$ as a decimal number. _____

2. Write $\frac{5.4 \times 3.71}{0.3}$ as a decimal number rounded off to the nearest tenth.

3. Write 5% as a *decimal number* and as a *fraction* in lowest terms.

4. Write the value of this expression as a fraction: $\frac{14}{15} \times \frac{25}{16} \times \frac{8}{21}$

5. Write the value of this expression as an ordinary fraction: $\frac{\frac{21}{80}}{\frac{7}{8}}$

Additional Exercises

Now, test yourself!

Convert to proper fractions or mixed numbers. (Questions 1–7)

1. $0.85 =$ _____   2. $2\frac{1}{2} + 3\frac{1}{4} =$ _____

3. $40 \times \frac{1}{2} \times \frac{9}{16} =$ _____   4. $2\frac{3}{5} \div 2 =$ _____

5. $15 \div 3\frac{2}{3} =$ _____   6. $9.6 \div \frac{3}{7} =$ _____

7. $42 \times \frac{1}{9,450} \times \frac{3}{0.02} =$ _____

Cumulative Review Exercises begin in
Chapter 4 and review mastery of earlier chapters.

Case Studies. Clinical case scenarios provide
opportunities for critical thinking as you apply
concepts and techniques presented in the text.

Cumulative Review Exercises

Reinforce your mastery of previous chapters.

Workspace

1. $1.3 \text{ g} =$ _____ mg
2. $24 \text{ oz} =$ _____ cups
3. $4.2 \text{ L} =$ _____ mL
4. $9 \text{ T} =$ _____ t
5. $900 \text{ mL} =$ _____ L
6. $1\frac{1}{2} \text{ pt} =$ _____ cups
7. Convert 560 mg to grams.
8. How many ounces are contained in 12 teaspoons?
9. Order: *Motrin (ibuprofen) 200 mg po q4h prn back pain.* What is the maximum number of milligrams of Motrin that the patient could receive in any 6-hour period?
10. Order: *ampicillin 250 mg t.i.d.* What is missing from this order?
11. If a patient receives a drug *40 mg po b.i.d.*, how many mg would be administered in a 24-hour period?
12. If a patient receives a drug *40 mg po q12h*, how many mg would be administered in a 24-hour period?
13. If a patient receives a drug *40 mg po daily in two divided doses*, how many mg would be administered in a 24-hour period?

Case Study 6.1

Read the case study and answer the questions. Answers can be found in Appendix A.

A 58 year old male who has a history of angina, type II diabetes mellitus, hypertension, and hyperlipidemia has had a cardiac catheterization. He is 6 feet tall and weighs 325 pounds, and has a very stressful job in the financial business. His vital signs are stable, there is no bleeding from the catheterization site, and he is awaiting his discharge. Review his discharge orders, and use the labels to answer the questions if required.

Discharge Orders

- 2,200 calorie ADA diet
- Follow-up with PMD in one week
- Janumet (sitagliptin/metformin HCl) 50/1,000 mg PO B.I.D.
- lansoprazole 30 mg PO daily before breakfast
- Xanax (alprazolam) 2 mg PO prn anxiety
- Lipitor (atorvastatin calcium) 40 mg PO daily
- Lovaza (omega-3-acid ethyl esters) 2 g PO B.I.D.
- lisinopril/hydrochlorothiazide 20/12.5 mg PO daily

- Coreg (carvedilol) 12.5 mg PO B.I.D.
- Sumaycin (tetracycline HCl) 500 mg PO B.I.D.

1. Select the appropriate label and calculate how many tablets of sitagliptin/metformin the patient must take for each dose.
2. How many capsules of omega-3-acid ethyl esters contain the dose?
3. How many tablets of atorvastatin will the patient take each day?
4. Calculate the number of tablets of carvedilol the patient will take per day.
5. How many tablets of alprazolam may the patient take per dose?
6. What is the dose of clopidogrel in grams?
7. How many tablets of fenofibrate will the patient take in four weeks?
8. The strength of the glimepiride is 1 mg/tab. How many tablets contain the dose?
9. How many capsules of lansoprazole contain the dose?

ALERT

The calibrations on the 1 mL syringe are very small and close together. Use caution when drawing up medication in this syringe.

Notes and **Alerts** highlight concepts and principles for safe medication calculation and administration.

NOTE

If your calculations indicate a large number of tablets (or capsules) per dose, you should verify your calculations with another health professional. Also check the usual dosage of the medication with a pharmacist and/or a drug reference.

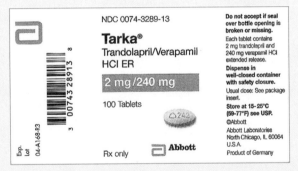

NDC 0074-3289-13

Tarka®
Trandolapril/Verapamil HCl ER

2 mg/240 mg

100 Tablets

△242

Rx only

Ⱥ **Abbott**

Do not accept if seal over bottle opening is broken or missing.

Each tablet contains 2 mg trandolapril and 240 mg verapamil HCl extended release.

Dispense in well-closed container with safety closure.

Usual dose: See package insert.

Store at 15-25°C (59-77°F) see USP.

©Abbott
Abbott Laboratories
North Chicago, IL 60064
U.S.A.
Product of Germany

Exp.
Lot
04-A168-R3

Realistic Illustrations. Real drug labels and realistic syringes aid in identifying and practicing with what you will encounter in actual clinical settings.

Additional Student Resources!
Go to http://nursing.pearsonhighered.com for animated examples, additional practice questions, and more!

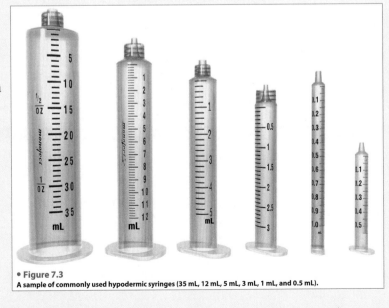

• Figure 7.3
A sample of commonly used hypodermic syringes (35 mL, 12 mL, 5 mL, 3 mL, 1 mL, and 0.5 mL).

Contents

Chapter 3   ## Dimensional Analysis and Ratio & Proportion   75

Chapter 7   ## Syringes   204

Chapter 8   ## Solutions   242

Unit 1

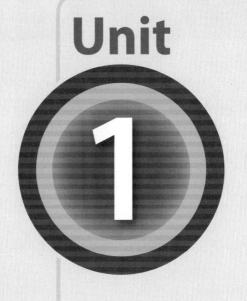

Basic Calculation Skills and Introduction to Medication Administration

CHAPTER 1

Review of Arithmetic for Dosage Calculations

CHAPTER 2

Safe and Accurate Drug Administration

CHAPTER 3

Dimensional Analysis and Ratio & Proportion

Review of Arithmetic for Dosage Calculations

Learning Outcomes

$$5\tfrac{3}{4} \div 23$$

After completing this chapter, you will be able to

1. Reduce and build fractions into equivalent forms.
2. Add, subtract, multiply, and divide fractions.
3. Simplify complex fractions.
4. Convert between decimal numbers and fractions.
5. Add, subtract, multiply, and divide decimal numbers.
6. Round decimal numbers to a desired number of decimal places.
7. Write percentages as decimal numbers and fractions.
8. Find a percent of a number and the percent of change.
9. Estimate answers.
10. Use a calculator to verify answers.

Medical dosage calculations can involve whole numbers, fractions, decimal numbers, and percentages. Your results on the *Diagnostic Test of Arithmetic*, found on the next page, will identify your areas of strength and weakness. You can use this chapter to improve your math skills or simply to review the kinds of calculations you will encounter in this text.

Diagnostic Test of Arithmetic

The following Diagnostic Test illustrates *all* the arithmetic skills needed to do the computations in this textbook. Take the test and compare your answers with the answers found in Appendix A. If you discover areas of weakness, carefully review the relevant review materials in this chapter so that you will be mathematically prepared for the rest of the textbook.

1. Write 0.375 as a fraction in lowest terms. _____

2. Write $\frac{28,500}{100,000}$ as a decimal number. _____

3. Round off 6.492 to the nearest tenth. _____

4. Write $\frac{5}{6}$ as a decimal number rounded off to the nearest hundredth.

_____

5. Simplify $\frac{0.63}{0.2}$ to a decimal number rounded off to the nearest tenth.

_____

6. $0.038 \times 100 =$ _____

7. $4.26 \times 0.015 =$ _____

8. $55 \div 0.11 =$ _____

9. $90 \times \frac{1}{300} \times \frac{20}{3} =$ _____

10. Write $5\frac{3}{4} \div 23$ as a fraction and as a decimal number. _____

11. Write $\frac{7}{100} \div \frac{3}{100}$ as a mixed number. _____

12. Write $\frac{\frac{4}{5}}{20}$ as a simple fraction in lowest terms. _____

13. Write 45% as a fraction in lowest terms. _____

14. Write $2\frac{1}{2}\%$ as a decimal number. _____

15. Write $2\frac{4}{7}$ as an improper fraction. _____

16. 30% of 40 = _____

17. $4.1 + 0.5 + 3 =$ _____

18. $\dfrac{3}{4} = \dfrac{?}{8}$ _____

19. Which is larger, 0.4 or 0.21? _____

20. Express the ratio *15 to 20* as a fraction in lowest terms. _____

Workspace

Changing Decimal Numbers and Whole Numbers to Fractions

A decimal number represents a fraction with a denominator of 10; 100; 1,000; and so on. Each decimal number has three parts: the whole-number part, the decimal point, and the fraction part. Table 1.1 shows the names of the decimal positions.

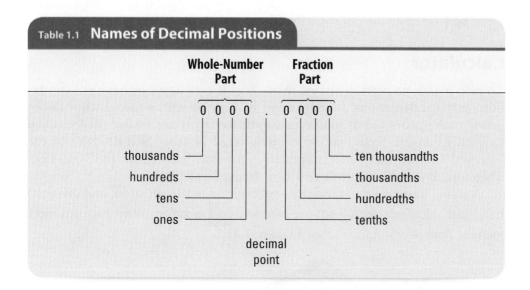

| Table 1.1 **Names of Decimal Positions** |

Reading a decimal number will help you write it as a fraction.

Decimal Number	⟶	Read	⟶	Fraction
4.1	⟶	four and one tenth	⟶	$4\dfrac{1}{10}$
0.3	⟶	three tenths	⟶	$\dfrac{3}{10}$
6.07	⟶	six and seven hundredths	⟶	$6\dfrac{7}{100}$
0.231	⟶	two hundred thirty-one thousandths	⟶	$\dfrac{231}{1,000}$
0.0025	⟶	twenty-five ten thousandths	⟶	$\dfrac{25}{10,000}$

> **NOTE**
>
> A decimal number that is less than 1 is written with a leading zero, for example, 0.3 and 0.0025.

A number can be written in different forms. A decimal number *less than 1*, such as 0.9, is read as *nine tenths* and can also be written as the *proper fraction* $\frac{9}{10}$. In a **proper fraction,** the **numerator** (the number on the top) of the fraction is smaller than its **denominator** (the number on the bottom).

A decimal number *greater than 1*, such as 3.5, is read as *three and five tenths* and can also be written as the *mixed number* $3\frac{5}{10}$ or reduced to lowest terms as $3\frac{1}{2}$. A **mixed number** combines a whole number and a proper fraction. The *mixed number* $3\frac{1}{2}$, can be changed to an *improper fraction* as follows:

$$3\frac{1}{2} = \frac{3 \times 2 + 1}{2} = \frac{7}{2}$$

The numerator (top number) of an **improper fraction** is larger than or equal to its denominator (bottom number).

Any number can be written as a fraction by writing it over 1. For example, 9 can be written as the improper fraction $\frac{9}{1}$.

Calculator

To help avoid medication errors, many health care agencies have policies requiring that calculations done by hand be verified with a calculator. "Drop-down" calculators are available to candidates who are taking the National Council Licensure Examination for Registered Nurses (NCLEX-RN) or the National Council Licensure Examination for Practical Nurses (NCLEX-PN). Therefore, it is important to know how to use a calculator.

A basic, four-function (addition, subtraction, multiplication, and division) handheld calculator with a square-root key $\sqrt{}$ is sufficient to perform most medical dosage calculations. See • **Figure 1.1.**

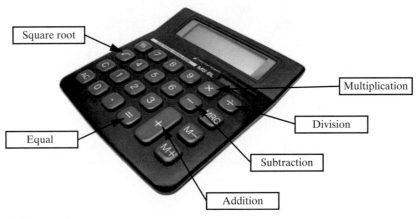

• **Figure 1.1**
Basic Handheld Calculator.

Some students might prefer a calculator that also has a percent key %, a fraction key $a^b/_c$, and parentheses keys (and).

To change the improper fraction $\frac{7}{2}$ to a decimal number with a calculator:

First press   7
Then press   ÷
Then press   2
Then press   =
The display shows   3.5

This keystroke sequence will be abbreviated as 7 ÷ 2 = 3.5

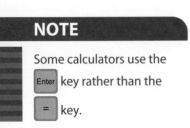

NOTE

Some calculators use the Enter key rather than the = key.

If the calculator has a fraction key, the mixed-number form of $\frac{7}{2}$ will be obtained by the following keystroke sequence:

$$7 \;\boxed{a^{b/c}}\; 2 \;\boxed{=}\; \boxed{3\tfrac{1}{2}}$$

Throughout this chapter, keystroke sequences will be shown for selected examples. The calculator icon, , will indicate where this occurs.

NOTE

The keystroke sequences presented in this chapter apply to many calculators. But not all calculators work the same way. If you have a problem, consult the user's manual for your calculator.

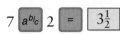 **Keystroke Sequence for Example 1.1:**

To obtain the simplified mixed number, enter the following keystroke sequence.

$$2 \;\boxed{a^{b/c}}\; 25 \;\boxed{a^{b/c}}\; 100 \;\boxed{=}$$
$$\boxed{2\tfrac{1}{4}}$$

EXAMPLE 1.1

Write 2.25 as a mixed number and as an improper fraction.

The number 2.25 is read *two and twenty-five hundredths* and is written $2\frac{25}{100}$. You can simplify:

$$2\frac{25}{100} = 2\frac{\overset{1}{\cancel{25}}}{\underset{4}{\cancel{100}}} = 2\frac{1}{4} = \frac{2 \times 4 + 1}{4} = \frac{9}{4}$$

So, 2.25 can be written as the mixed number $2\frac{1}{4}$ or as the improper fraction $\frac{9}{4}$.

Ratios

A **ratio** is a comparison of two numbers.

The ratio of *5 to 10* can also be written as *5:10* or in fractional form as $\frac{5}{10}$. This fraction may be *reduced by cancelling* by a number that evenly divides both the numerator and the denominator. Because 5 evenly divides both 5 and 10, divide as follows:

$$\frac{5}{10} = \frac{5 \div 5}{10 \div 5} = \frac{1}{2}$$

The fraction $\frac{5}{10}$ is *reduced to lowest terms* as $\frac{1}{2}$.

So, the ratio of *5 to 10* can also be written as the ratio of *1 to 2* or *1:2*.

 Keystroke Sequence for Example 1.2:

$$6 \;\boxed{a^{b/c}}\; 18 = \boxed{\tfrac{1}{3}}$$

EXAMPLE 1.2

Express 6:18 as an equivalent fraction in lowest terms.

The ratio *6:18*, also written as *6 to 18*, can be written in fractional form as $\frac{6}{18}$. This fraction may be *reduced by cancelling* by a number that evenly divides both the numerator and the denominator. Because 6 divides both 6 and 18, divide as follows:

$$\frac{6}{18} = \frac{6 \div 6}{18 \div 6} = \frac{1}{3}$$

So, the ratio 6 to 18 equals the fraction $\frac{1}{3}$.

Keystroke Sequence for Example 1.3:

To check the answer use

$12 \; \boxed{a^{b/c}} \; 120 = \boxed{\tfrac{1}{10}}$

NOTE

When *reducing* a fraction, you *divide* both numerator and denominator by the same number. This process is called *cancelling*.

When *building* a fraction, you *multiply* both numerator and denominator by the same number.

EXAMPLE 1.3

Write the ratio 1:10 as an equivalent fraction with 120 in the denominator.

Because 1:10 as a fraction is $\frac{1}{10}$, you need to write this fraction with the larger denominator of 120. Such processes are called **building fractions**.

$$\frac{1}{10} = \frac{?}{120}$$

$\frac{1}{10}$ may be built up by *multiplying numerator and denominator of the fraction by the same number* (12 in this case) as follows:

$$\frac{1}{10} = \frac{1 \times 12}{10 \times 12} = \frac{12}{120}$$

So, 1:10 is equivalent to $\frac{12}{120}$

Changing Fractions to Decimal Numbers

To change a fraction to a decimal number, think of the fraction as a division problem. For example:

$$\frac{2}{5} \quad \text{means} \quad 2 \div 5 \quad \text{or} \quad 5\overline{)2}$$

Here are the steps for this division.

Step 1 Replace 2 with 2.0 and then place a decimal point directly above the decimal point in 2.0

$$5\overline{)2.0}^{\,\cdot}$$

Step 2 Perform the division.

$$\begin{array}{r} 0.4 \\ 5\overline{)2.0} \\ \underline{2\,0} \\ 0 \end{array}$$

Keystroke sequence:

$2 \; \boxed{\div} \; 5 = \boxed{0.4}$

So, $\dfrac{2}{5} = 0.4$

EXAMPLE 1.4

Write $\frac{5}{2}$ as a decimal number.

$$\frac{5}{2} \quad \text{means} \quad 5 \div 2 \quad \text{or} \quad 2\overline{)5}$$

Step 1 $2\overline{)5.0}$

Step 2 $\begin{array}{r} 2.5 \\ 2\overline{)5.0} \\ \underline{4} \\ 1\,0 \\ \underline{1\,0} \end{array}$

So, $\dfrac{5}{2} = 2.5$

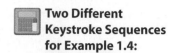

Two Different Keystroke Sequences for Example 1.4:

• 5 ÷ 2 = 2.5

If your calculator has a fraction key, you can also use the keystroke sequence:

• 5 $a^{b}/_{c}$ 2 = $2\frac{1}{2}$

EXAMPLE 1.5

Write $\dfrac{193}{10}$ as a decimal number.

$$\dfrac{193}{10} \quad \text{means} \quad 193 \div 10 \quad \text{or} \quad 10\overline{)193}$$

Step 1 $10\overline{)193.0}$

Step 2 $\begin{array}{r} 19.3 \\ 10\overline{)193.0} \\ \underline{10} \\ 93 \\ \underline{90} \\ 30 \\ \underline{30} \\ 0 \end{array}$

So, $\dfrac{193}{10} = 19.3$

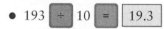

Two Different Keystroke Sequences for Example 1.5:

• 193 ÷ 10 = 19.3

If your calculator has a fraction key, you can also use:

• 193 $a^{b}/_{c}$ 10 = $19\frac{3}{10}$

There is a quicker way to do Example 1.5. To divide a *decimal number by 10,* you *move* the decimal point in the number *one place to the left.* Notice that there is one zero in 10.

$$\dfrac{193}{10} = \dfrac{193.}{10} = 193. = 19.3$$

To *divide a number by 100, move* the decimal point in the number *two places to the left* because there are two zeros in 100. So, the quick way to divide by 10; 100; 1,000; and so on is to count the zeros and then move the decimal point to the left the same number of places; the answer should always be a *smaller* number than the original number. Check your answer to be sure.

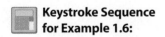

**Keystroke Sequence
for Example 1.6:**

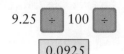

9.25 ÷ 100 ÷

0.0925

EXAMPLE 1.6

Write $\frac{9.25}{100}$ as a decimal number.

This fraction means 9.25 ÷ 100. There are two zeros in 100, so move the decimal point in 9.25 two places to the left, and fill the empty position with a zero.

$$\frac{9.25}{100} = \underset{\smile\smile}{}9.25 = 0.0925$$

Rounding Decimal Numbers

Sometimes it is convenient to round an answer—that is, to use an approximate answer rather than an exact one.

Rounding Off

To round off 1.267 to the *nearest tenth*—that is, to round off the number to one decimal place—do the following:

Look at the digit after the tenths place (the hundredths place digit). Because this digit (6) is 5 or more, round off 1.267 by adding 1 to the tenths place digit. Finally, drop all the digits after the tenths place.

So, 1.267 is approximated by 1.3 when rounded off to the nearest tenth.

To round off 0.8345 to the *nearest hundredth*—that is, to round off the number to two decimal places—do the following:

Look at the digit after the hundredths place (the thousandths place digit). Because this digit (4) is less than 5, round off 0.8345 by leaving the hundredths digit alone. Finally, drop all the digits after the hundredths place.

So, 0.8345 is approximated by 0.83 when rounded off to the nearest hundredth.

EXAMPLE 1.7

Round off 4.8075 to the nearest hundredth, tenth, and whole number.

4.8075 rounded off to the nearest: hundredth → 4.81

tenth → 4.8

whole number → 5

Rounding *off* numbers produces results that can be either larger or smaller than the given numbers. When numbers are rounded *down*, however, the results cannot be larger than the given numbers.

NOTE

Rounding down is also referred to as *truncating*, which means "cutting off" digits.

Rounding Down

Pediatric dosages are sometimes *rounded down* rather than *rounded off*. Rounding down is simple to do: part of the number is merely deleted (truncated).

To round down 1.267 to the tenths place—that is, to round down 1.267 to one decimal place—do the following:

> *Locate the digit in the tenths place. Delete all the digits after the tenths-place digit.*   1. 2̲ 6̶ 7̶
>
> *So, 1.267 is approximated by 1.2 when rounded down to the tenths place.*

To round down 0.83452 to the hundredths place—that is, to round down 0.83452 to two decimal places—do the following:

> *Locate the digit in the hundredths place. Delete all the digits after the hundredths-place digit.*   0 . 8 3̲ 4̶ 5̶ 2̶
>
> *So, 0.83452 is approximated by 0.83 when rounded down to the hundredths place.*

EXAMPLE 1.8

Round down 4.8075 to hundredth, tenth, and whole number.

4.8075 rounded *down* to   hundredth → 4.80

tenth → 4.8

whole number → 4

Adding Decimal Numbers

When adding decimal numbers, write the numbers in a column with the *decimal points lined up under each other*.

EXAMPLE 1.9

$$3.4 + 0.07 + 6 = ?$$

Write the numbers in a column with the decimal points lined up. *Trailing zeros* may be included to give each number the same amount of decimal places. Therefore, write 6 as 6.00 [Think: $6 is equivalent to $6.00].

$$
\begin{array}{r}
3.40 \\
0.07 \\
+\ 6.00 \\
\hline
9.47
\end{array}
$$

So, the sum of 3.4, 0.07, and 6 is 9.47

Subtracting Decimal Numbers

When adding or subtracting decimal numbers, write the numbers in a column with the *decimal points lined up under each other*.

NOTE

Unless otherwise specified, quantities *less than 1* will generally be rounded to the *nearest hundredth*, whereas quantities *greater than 1* will generally be rounded to the *nearest tenth*. For the sake of uniformity, when rounding numbers in this book, rounding *off* will be used rather than rounding *down*. However, in Chapter 12 *all pediatric dosages will be rounded down*.

ALERT

The danger of an overdose must always be guarded against. Therefore, the amount of medication to be administered is often rounded *down* instead of rounded *off*. This rounding down is sometimes done in pediatrics and when administering high-alert drugs to adults.

Keystroke Sequence for Example 1.9:

3.4 $+$ .07 $+$ 6 $=$

9.47

Keystroke Sequence for Example 1.10:

5 .45 4.55

ALERT

Be careful: the *subtraction* (minus) key looks like $\boxed{-}$, whereas the *negative* key looks like $\boxed{(-)}$ or $\boxed{+/-}$.

EXAMPLE 1.10

$$5 - 0.45 = ?$$

Write the numbers in a column with the decimal points lined up. Include *trailing zeros* to give each number the same amount of decimal places.

$$
\begin{array}{r}
5.00 \\
- \ 0.45 \\
\hline
4.55
\end{array}
$$

So, the difference between 5 and 0.45 is 4.55

Multiplying Decimal Numbers

To multiply two decimal numbers, multiply first, ignoring the decimal points. Then count the total number of decimal places (digits to the right of the decimal point) in the original two numbers. That sum equals the number of decimal places in the answer.

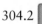 **Keystroke Sequence for Example 1.11:**

304.2 .16

48.672

You need not press the leading zero when entering 0.16

EXAMPLE 1.11

$$304.2 \times 0.16 = ?$$

$$
\begin{array}{r}
304.2 \quad \leftarrow 1 \text{ decimal place} \\
\times \ 0.16 \quad \leftarrow 2 \text{ decimal places} \\
\hline
18252 \\
3042 \quad \\
\hline
48.672
\end{array}
$$

Total of 3 decimal places

There are 3 decimal places in the answer. Place the decimal point here.

So, $304.2 \times 0.16 = 48.672$

 Keystroke Sequence for Example 1.12:

304.25 10 =

3042.5

EXAMPLE 1.12

$$304.25 \times 10 = ?$$

$$
\begin{array}{r}
304.25 \quad \leftarrow 2 \text{ decimal places} \\
\times \quad \ \ 10 \quad \leftarrow 0 \text{ decimal places} \\
\hline
3\,042.50
\end{array}
$$

Total of 2 decimal places

There are 2 decimal places in the answer. Place the decimal point here.

So, $304.25 \times 10 = 3{,}042.50$ or $3{,}042.5$

There is a quicker way to do Example 1.12. To *multiply any decimal number by 10, move* the decimal point in the number being multiplied *one place to the right*. Notice that there is one zero in 10.

$$304.25 \times 10 = 304{,}25 \quad \text{or} \quad 3{,}042.5$$

To *multiply a number by 100, move* the decimal point in the number *two places to the right* because there are two zeros in 100. So, the quick way to multiply by 10, 100, 1,000, and so on is to count the zeros and then move the decimal point to the right the same number of places. The answer should always be a *larger* number than the original. Check your answer to be sure.

EXAMPLE 1.13

$$23.597 \times 1,000 = ?$$

There are three zeros in 1,000, so move the decimal point in 23.597 three places to the right.

$$23.597 \times 1,000 = 23.5\,9\,7 \quad \text{or} \quad 23,597$$

So, $23.597 \times 1,000 = 23,597$

Keystroke Sequence for Example 1.13:

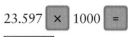

23.597 ☒ 1000 ☐
23597

Dividing Decimal Numbers

When dividing with decimal numbers, be sure that you are careful where you place the decimal point in the answer.

EXAMPLE 1.14

Write the fraction $\frac{106.8}{15}$ as a decimal number rounded off to the nearest tenth; that is, round off the answer to one decimal place.

Treat this fraction as a division problem.

$$\frac{106.8}{15} \quad \text{means} \quad 15\overline{)106.8}$$

Step 1 $15\overline{)106.8}$

Step 2   Because you want the answer to the nearest tenth (one decimal place), do the division to two decimal places and then round off the answer.

$$
\begin{array}{r}
7.12 \\
15\overline{)106.80} \\
\underline{105} \\
1\,8 \\
\underline{1\,5} \\
30 \\
\underline{30} \\
0
\end{array}
$$

Because the hundredths place digit in the answer is *less than 5*, leave the tenths place digit alone. Finally, drop the digit in the hundredths place. So, $\frac{106.8}{15}$ is approximated by the decimal number 7.1 to the nearest tenth.

Keystroke Sequence for Example 1.14:

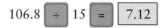

106.8 ☐ 15 ☐ 7.12

≈ 7.1 after rounding off. The symbol "≈" means "is approximately equal to."

Keystroke Sequence for Example 1.15:

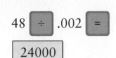

48 ÷ .002 =

24000

EXAMPLE 1.15

Simplify $\frac{48}{0.002}$

Think of this fraction as a division problem. Because there are three decimal places in 0.002, move the decimal points in both numbers three places to the right.

$$\frac{48}{0.002} \quad \text{means} \quad 0.002\overline{)48.} \quad \text{or} \quad 0.0\,0\,2\,\overline{)48.0\,0\,0}$$

$$\begin{array}{r} 24{,}000. \\ 2\overline{)48{,}000.} \\ \underline{4} \\ 08 \\ \underline{8} \\ 0 \end{array}$$

So, $\dfrac{48}{0.002} = 24{,}000$

Estimating Answers

When you use a calculator, errors in the keystroke sequence may lead to dangerously high or dangerously low dosages. To help avoid such mistakes:

1. *Carefully* enter the keystroke sequence. A calculator that shows both your entries and the answer in the display is desirable.

2. Think: *Is the answer reasonable*? For example, an oral dosage of 50 tablets is not reasonable!

3. Use rounding to *estimate* the size of the answer. The product of 498 and 49 can be estimated by rounding the numbers off to 500 and 50, respectively. 500 × 50 = 25,000. Because each factor was made larger, the product of 498 and 49 is a little less than 25,000. Sometimes it is useful to know whether an answer will be larger or smaller than a given number.

Keystroke Sequence for Example 1.16:

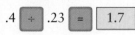

.4 ÷ .23 = 1.7

Because 1.7 is larger than 1, the first number entered (0.4) is larger than the second (0.23).

EXAMPLE 1.16

Which is larger, 0.4 or 0.23?

Write the numbers in a column with the decimal points lined up, and include trailing zeros to give each number the same amount of decimal places.

0.40

0.23

Because 40 hundredths is larger than 23 hundredths, 0.4 is larger than 0.23

When one number is divided by a second number, if the answer is larger than 1, the first number is the larger. If the answer is less than 1, the second number is larger.

EXAMPLE 1.17

Is $\frac{0.5}{0.4}$ smaller or larger than 1?

Because the value in the numerator 0.5 is larger than the value in the denominator 0.4, the fraction represents a quantity larger than 1.

Keystroke Sequence for Example 1.17:

0.5 ÷ 0.4 = 1.25

EXAMPLE 1.18

Estimate the value of $\frac{200}{2.2}$

Because the denominator is approximately equal to 2, the given fraction will be close in value to $\frac{200}{2}$ or 100. In this case, by making the denominator smaller (2 instead of 2.2), you made the value of the entire fraction larger. Therefore, 100 is too large (an overestimate). So, the actual value of $\frac{200}{2.2}$ is a number somewhat less than 100.

Keystroke Sequence for Example 1.18:

200 ÷ 2.2 =

90.9090... ≈ 91

Multiplying Fractions

To *multiply fractions*, multiply the numerators to get the new numerator and multiply the denominators to get the new denominator.

EXAMPLE 1.19

$$\frac{3}{5} \times 6 \times \frac{1}{5} = ?$$

A whole number can be written as a fraction with 1 in the denominator. So, in this example, write 6 as $\frac{6}{1}$ to make all the numbers fractions.

$$\frac{3}{5} \times \frac{6}{1} \times \frac{1}{5} = \frac{3 \times 6 \times 1}{5 \times 1 \times 5} = \frac{18}{25}$$

Three Different Keystroke Sequences for Example 1.19:

- Using parentheses:

  (3 × 6) ÷
  (5 × 5) =
  0.72

- Multiply the numerators, and then divide by each of the denominators:

  3 × 6 ÷ 5 ÷ 5
  = 0.72

- Using the fraction key:

  3 $a^{b}/_{c}$ 5 × 6 × 1
  $a^{b}/_{c}$ 5 = $\frac{18}{25}$

EXAMPLE 1.20

$$\frac{4}{5} \times \frac{3}{10} \times \frac{20}{7} = ?$$

It is often convenient to cancel before you multiply.

$$\frac{4}{5} \times \frac{3}{\cancel{10}_1} \times \frac{\cancel{20}^2}{7} = \frac{24}{35}$$

Keystroke Sequence for Example 1.20:

Multiply the numerators and divide by each of the denominators:

4 × 3 × 20 ÷

5 ÷ 10 ÷ 7 =

0.6857...

Do not verify the answer to Example 1.20 on the calculator by using the cancelled numbers 4 × 3 × 2

÷ 5 ÷ 7 = 0.686...

because the calculator will not uncover previous cancellation errors. Therefore, use the original numbers as shown in the keystroke sequences.

Keystroke Sequence for Example 1.21:

21 × 15 ÷ 7 =

45

Keystroke Sequence for Example 1.22:

1 $a^b/_c$ 2 $a^b/_c$ 5 ÷

7 $a^b/_c$ 9 = 1$\frac{4}{5}$

NOTE

Avoid cancelling decimal numbers. It is a possible source of error.

Keystroke Sequence for Example 1.23:

60 ÷ 300 ÷ .4

= 0.5

EXAMPLE 1.21

Simplify $\frac{21 \times 15}{7}$

Method 1: Multiply the numbers in the numerator, which yields $\frac{315}{7}$, and then divide 315 by 7, which yields 45

Method 2: First cancel by 7, then multiply

$$\frac{\overset{3}{\cancel{21}} \times 15}{\underset{1}{\cancel{7}}} = \frac{3 \times 15}{1} = \frac{45}{1} = 45$$

So, $\frac{21 \times 15}{7} = 45$

Dividing Fractions

To *divide fractions*, change the division problem to an equivalent multiplication problem by inverting the second fraction.

EXAMPLE 1.22

$$1\frac{2}{5} \div \frac{7}{9} = ?$$

Write $1\frac{2}{5}$ as the improper fraction $\frac{7}{5}$.

The *division* problem

$$\frac{7}{5} \div \frac{7}{9}$$

Becomes the *multiplication* problem by inverting the second fraction.

$$\frac{7}{5} \times \frac{9}{7}$$

$$\frac{\overset{1}{\cancel{7}}}{5} \times \frac{9}{\underset{1}{\cancel{7}}} = \frac{9}{5} = 1\frac{4}{5}$$

Sometimes you must deal with whole numbers, fractions, and decimal numbers in the same multiplication and division problems.

EXAMPLE 1.23

Give the answer to the following problem in simplified fractional form.

$$\frac{1}{300} \times 60 \times \frac{1}{0.4} = ?$$

Write 60 as a fraction and cancel.

$$\frac{1}{\underset{5}{\cancel{300}}} \times \frac{\overset{1}{\cancel{60}}}{1} \times \frac{1}{0.4} = \frac{1}{5 \times 0.4} = \frac{1}{2}$$

Sometimes you will need to simplify *fractions that contain decimal numbers.*

EXAMPLE 1.24

Give the answer to the following problem in simplified fractional form.

$$0.35 \times \frac{1}{60} = ?$$

Write 0.35 as the fraction $\frac{0.35}{1}$.

$$\frac{0.35}{1} \times \frac{1}{60} = \frac{0.35}{60}$$

The numerator of this fraction is 0.35, a decimal number. You can write an equivalent form of the fraction by multiplying the numerator and denominator by 100.

$$\frac{0.35}{60} \times \frac{100}{100} = \frac{0.35}{60.00} = \frac{35}{6,000} = \frac{7}{1,200}$$

Two Different Keystroke Sequences for Example 1.24:

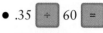
- .35 ÷ 60 =

  0.0058...

- If you think of 0.35 as $\frac{35}{100}$, then use the fraction key:

  35 $a^{b}/_{c}$ 100 × 1 $a^{b}/_{c}$

  60 = $\frac{7}{1,200}$

EXAMPLE 1.25

Give the answer to the following problem in simplified fractional form.

$$0.88 \times \frac{1}{2.2} = ?$$

$$\frac{0.88}{1} \times \frac{1}{2.2} = \frac{0.88}{2.2}$$

Multiply the numerator and the denominator of this fraction by 100 to eliminate both decimal numbers.

$$\frac{0.88}{2.2} \times \frac{100}{100} = \frac{0.88}{2.2} = \frac{88}{220} = \frac{2}{5}$$

You can simplify $\frac{0.88}{2.2}$ a different way by dividing 0.88 by 2.2

$$2.2\overline{)0.88} \quad \overset{0.4}{} \quad \text{and} \quad 0.4 = \frac{4}{10} \quad \text{or} \quad \frac{2}{5}$$

Keystroke Sequence for Example 1.25:

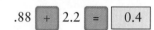
.88 ÷ 2.2 = 0.4

To change 0.4 to a fraction in lowest terms:

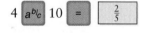
4 $a^{b}/_{c}$ 10 = $\frac{2}{5}$

Complex Fractions

Fractions that have numerators or denominators that are themselves fractions are called *complex fractions.*

The longest line in the complex fraction separates the numerator (top) from the denominator (bottom) of the complex fraction. As with any fraction, you can write the complex fraction as a division problem [*Top ÷ Bottom*].

In the complex fraction $\frac{1}{\frac{2}{5}}$, the numerator is 1 and the denominator is $\frac{2}{5}$.

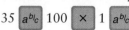

You can simplify this complex fraction as follows:

$$\frac{1}{\frac{2}{5}} \quad \text{means} \quad 1 \div \frac{2}{5} \quad \text{or} \quad 1 \times \frac{5}{2}, \quad \text{which is} \quad \frac{5}{2}$$

In the complex fraction $\dfrac{\frac{1}{2}}{5}$, the numerator is $\frac{1}{2}$ and the denominator is 5. You can simplify this complex fraction as follows:

$$\frac{\frac{1}{2}}{5} \quad \text{means} \quad \frac{1}{2} \div 5 \quad \text{or} \quad \frac{1}{2} \times \frac{1}{5}, \quad \text{which is} \quad \frac{1}{10}$$

In the complex fraction $\dfrac{\frac{3}{5}}{\frac{2}{5}}$, the numerator is $\frac{3}{5}$ and the denominator is $\frac{2}{5}$.

You can simplify this complex fraction as follows:

$$\frac{\frac{3}{5}}{\frac{2}{5}} \quad \text{means} \quad \frac{3}{5} \div \frac{2}{5} \quad \text{or} \quad \frac{3}{\overset{}{\underset{1}{5}}} \times \frac{\overset{1}{5}}{2}, \quad \text{which is} \quad \frac{3}{2}$$

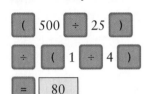

Keystroke Sequence for Example 1.26:

(500 ÷ 25)

÷ (1 ÷ 4)

= 80

EXAMPLE 1.26

$$\frac{\dfrac{1}{25} \times 500}{\dfrac{1}{4}} = ?$$

In this complex fraction, the numerator is $\left(\frac{1}{25} \times 500\right)$ and the denominator is $\frac{1}{4}$. So, you can write the following:

$$\frac{1}{25} \times \frac{500}{1} \div \frac{1}{4} = ?$$

$$\frac{1}{\underset{1}{25}} \times \frac{\overset{20}{\cancel{500}}}{1} \times \frac{4}{1} = 80$$

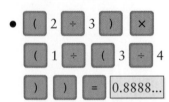

Two Different Keystroke Sequences for Example 1.27:

- (2 ÷ 3) ×

(1 ÷ (3 ÷ 4

)) = 0.8888...

- To obtain the fractional form:

2 $a^{b/c}$ 3 × (1 $a^{b/c}$

(3 $a^{b/c}$ 4))

= $\frac{8}{9}$

EXAMPLE 1.27

$$\frac{\dfrac{2}{3} \times \dfrac{1}{3}}{\dfrac{3}{4}} = ?$$

You can multiply the numerators to get the new numerator and multiply the denominators to get the new denominator, as follows:

$$\frac{2}{3} \times \frac{1}{\dfrac{3}{4}} = \frac{2 \times 1}{3 \times \dfrac{3}{4}} = \frac{2}{\dfrac{9}{4}}$$

Now, the numerator is 2 and the denominator is $\frac{9}{4}$, so you get

$$\frac{2}{1} \div \frac{9}{4}$$

which becomes
$$\frac{2}{1} \times \frac{4}{9} = \frac{8}{9}$$

This problem could have been done another way by simplifying $\dfrac{1}{\frac{3}{4}}$ first.

You can write $\dfrac{1}{\frac{3}{4}}$ as $1 \div \dfrac{3}{4}$ as $1 \times \dfrac{4}{3}$ or $\dfrac{4}{3}$

Then
$$\frac{2}{3} \times \frac{4}{3} = \frac{8}{9}$$

Addition and Subtraction of Fractions

Addition and subtraction of fractions in this textbook generally involves fractions with denominators of 2 or 4.

Same Denominators

When adding or subtracting fractions that have the *same denominators, add or subtract the numerators and keep the common denominator.*

Add $\frac{1}{2}$ and $\frac{1}{2}$

$$\frac{1}{2} + \frac{1}{2} = \frac{1+1}{2} = \frac{2}{2}, \text{ which equals 1}$$

From $\frac{11}{4}$ subtract $\frac{5}{4}$

$$\frac{11}{4} - \frac{5}{4} = \frac{11-5}{4} = \frac{6}{4}, \text{ which can be reduced to } \frac{3}{2} \text{ or } 1\frac{1}{2}$$

For *mixed numbers* add (or subtract) the whole number and fraction parts separately.

Add $3\frac{1}{4}$ and $2\frac{1}{4}$

$$
\begin{array}{r}
3 \quad \dfrac{1}{4} \\[2mm]
+ \quad 2 \quad \dfrac{1}{4} \\[1mm]
\hline
5 \quad \dfrac{1+1}{4} = 5\dfrac{2}{4}, \text{ which equals } 5\dfrac{1}{2}
\end{array}
$$

From $10\frac{3}{4}$, *subtract* $6\frac{1}{4}$

$$
\begin{array}{r}
10 \quad \dfrac{3}{4} \\[2mm]
-\ 6 \quad \dfrac{1}{4} \\[1mm]
\hline
4 \quad \dfrac{3-1}{4} = 4\dfrac{2}{4}, \text{ which equals } 4\dfrac{1}{2}
\end{array}
$$

Different Denominators

When adding or subtracting fractions that have *different denominators*, build the fraction(s) so that the denominators are the same (have a common denominator), and proceed as before.

Add $\frac{1}{2}$ and $\frac{1}{4}$

This problem has fractions with different denominators. Recall that $\frac{1}{2} = \frac{2}{4}$. Then the problem becomes

$$\frac{2}{4} + \frac{1}{4} = \frac{2+1}{4} = \frac{3}{4}$$

From $\frac{3}{4}$ subtract $\frac{1}{2}$

Recall that $\frac{1}{2} = \frac{2}{4}$. Then the problem becomes

$$\frac{3}{4} - \frac{2}{4} = \frac{3-2}{4} = \frac{1}{4}$$

For *mixed numbers* add (or subtract) the whole number and fraction parts separately.

Add $9\frac{3}{4}$ and $6\frac{1}{2}$

To make the denominators the same, use $\frac{1}{2} = \frac{2}{4}$

$$
\begin{array}{rcl}
9 \quad \dfrac{3}{4} &=& 9 \quad \dfrac{3}{4} \\[2mm]
+\ 6 \quad \dfrac{1}{2} &=& 6 \quad \dfrac{2}{4} \\[1mm]
\hline
&& 15 \quad \dfrac{3+2}{4} = 15\dfrac{5}{4}, \text{which equals } 16\dfrac{1}{4}
\end{array}
$$

From $9\frac{3}{4}$ subtract $6\frac{1}{2}$

To make the denominators the same, use $\frac{1}{2} = \frac{2}{4}$

$$
\begin{array}{rcl}
9 \quad \dfrac{3}{4} &=& 9 \quad \dfrac{3}{4} \\[2mm]
-\ 6 \quad \dfrac{1}{2} &=& 6 \quad \dfrac{2}{4} \\[1mm]
\hline
&& 3 \quad \dfrac{3-2}{4} = 3\dfrac{1}{4}
\end{array}
$$

From $6\frac{1}{4}$ subtract $4\frac{3}{4}$

Method 1: Use borrowing (renaming).

Because $\frac{3}{4}$ is larger than $\frac{1}{4}$, subtraction of the fractions is not possible. Therefore, you may rename $6\frac{1}{4}$ as follows: Borrow 1 from the whole number part (6), and add the 1 to the fractional part ($\frac{1}{4}$). This results in $6\frac{1}{4} = (6-1) + (1+\frac{1}{4})$ or $5\frac{5}{4}$.

$$
\begin{array}{rcl}
6\ \dfrac{1}{4} &=& 5\ \dfrac{5}{4}\\[2mm]
-\ 6\ \dfrac{3}{4} &=& 4\ \dfrac{3}{4}\\[2mm]
\hline
1\ \dfrac{5-3}{4} &=& 1\dfrac{2}{4}\ \text{or}\ 1\dfrac{1}{2}
\end{array}
$$

Method 2: Change the mixed numbers to improper fractions.

$$
\begin{array}{rcl}
6\dfrac{1}{4} &=& \dfrac{25}{4}\\[2mm]
-4\dfrac{3}{4} &=& \dfrac{19}{4}\\[2mm]
\hline
& & \dfrac{25-19}{4} = \dfrac{6}{4}\ \text{which also equals}\ 1\dfrac{1}{2}
\end{array}
$$

EXAMPLE 1.28

Add $4\frac{1}{2} + 5\frac{1}{2}$.

$$
\begin{array}{r}
4\ \dfrac{1}{2}\\[2mm]
+\ 5\ \dfrac{1}{2}\\[2mm]
\hline
9\ \dfrac{1+1}{2} = 9\dfrac{2}{2},\ \text{which equals}\ 9+1\ \text{or}\ 10
\end{array}
$$

Keystroke Sequence for Example 1.28:

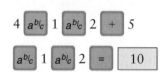

Percentages

Percent (%) means *parts per 100* or *divided by 100*. Thus 50% means 50 *parts per hundred* or 50 *divided by 100*, which can also be written as the fraction $\frac{50}{100}$. The fraction $\frac{50}{100}$ can be changed to the decimal numbers 0.50 and 0.5 or reduced to the fraction $\frac{1}{2}$.

13%	means	$\dfrac{13}{100}$	or	0.13
100%	means	$\dfrac{100}{100}$	or	1
12.3%	means	$\dfrac{12.3}{100}$	or	0.123
$\dfrac{1}{2}\%$	means	6.5%	or $\dfrac{6.5}{100}$	or 0.065

ALERT

Calculating with numbers in percent form can be difficult, so percentages should be converted to either fractional or decimal form before performing any calculations.

EXAMPLE 1.29

Write 0.5% as a fraction in lowest terms and as a decimal number.

$$0.5\% = \frac{0.5}{100} = \frac{5}{1,000} = \frac{1}{200}$$

There is another way to get the answer. Because you understand that $0.5 = \frac{1}{2}$, then

$$0.5\% = \frac{1}{2}\% = \frac{1}{2} \div 100 = \frac{1}{2} \div \frac{100}{1} = \frac{1}{2} \times \frac{1}{100} = \frac{1}{200}$$

To obtain a decimal number, write

$$0.5\% = \frac{0.5}{100} = 0.5 = 0.005$$

EXAMPLE 1.30

Write $\frac{3}{4}$ as a decimal number and as a percent.

$$\frac{3}{4} = 3 \div 4 = 0.75$$

To change the decimal number 0.75 to a percent, move the decimal point two places to the right and add the percent sign.

$$0.75 = 75\%$$

To find a *percent of a number* or a *fraction of a number*, translate the word "of" as "multiplication," as illustrated in Examples 1.31 and 1.32.

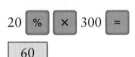

Keystroke Sequence for Example 1.31:

20 [%] [×] 300 [=]

[60]

EXAMPLE 1.31

What is 20% of 300?

To find a percent of a number, translate the "of" as multiplication.

$$20\% \text{ of } 300 \quad \text{means} \quad 20\% \times 300 \text{ or}$$
$$0.20 \times 300 = 60$$

So, 20% of 300 is 60.

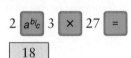

Keystroke Sequence for Example 1.32:

2 [a^b/c] 3 [×] 27 [=]

[18]

EXAMPLE 1.32

What is two-thirds of 27?

To find a fraction of a number, translate the "of" as multiplication.

$$\frac{2}{3} \text{ of } 27 \quad \text{means} \quad \frac{2}{3} \times 27 = 18$$

So, two-thirds of 27 is 18.

Percent of Change

It is often useful to determine a *percent of change* (increase or decrease). For example, you might want to know if a 20-pound weight loss for a patient is significant. For an adult patient who was 200 pounds, a 20-pound loss would be a decrease in weight of 10%. However, for a child who was 50 pounds, a 20-pound loss would be a decrease in weight of 40%, which is far more significant than a 10% loss.

To obtain the fraction of change, you may use the formula:

$$\text{Fraction of Change} = \frac{Change}{Original}$$

Then change the fraction to a percent to obtain the percent of change.

EXAMPLE 1.33

A daily dosage increases from 4 tablets to 5 tablets. What is the fraction of change and percent of change in daily dosage?

$$\text{Fraction of Change} = \frac{Change}{Original}$$

Because the original dosage is 4 tablets, and the new dosage is 5 tablets, then the change in dosage is

$$\text{Change} = 5\,\text{tablets} - 4\,\text{tablets} = 1\,\text{tablet}.$$

$$\text{Fraction of Change} = \frac{Change}{Original} = \frac{1}{4} \text{ or } 25\%.$$

So, the dosage has increased by $\frac{1}{4}$ or 25%.

EXAMPLE 1.34

A person was drinking 40 ounces of fluid per day, but this was reduced to 10 ounces of fluid per day. What is the percent of change in fluid intake?

$$\text{Fraction of Change} = \frac{Change}{Original}$$

Because the original amount is 40 ounces, and the new amount is 10 ounces, the change is

$$\text{Change} = 40 - 10 = 30\,\text{ounces}.$$

$$\text{Fraction of Change} = \frac{Change}{Original} = \frac{30}{40} = \frac{3}{4} \text{ or } 75\%.$$

So, this is a 75% decrease in fluid intake.

Summary

In this chapter, all the essential mathematical skills that are needed for dosage calculation were reviewed.

When working with fractions:
- Proper fractions have smaller numbers in the numerator than in the denominator.
- Improper fractions have numerators that are larger than or equal to their denominators.
- Improper fractions can be changed to mixed numbers, and vice versa.
- Any number can be changed into a fraction by writing the number over 1.
- Cancel first when you multiply fractions.
- Change a fraction to a decimal number by dividing the numerator by the denominator.
- A ratio may be written as a fraction.
- Simplify complex fractions by dividing the numerator by the denominator.

When working with decimals:
- Line up the decimal points when adding or subtracting.
- Move the decimal point three places to the right when multiplying a decimal number by 1,000.
- Move the decimal point three places to the left when dividing a decimal number by 1,000.
- Count the total number of places in the numbers you are multiplying to determine the number of decimal places in the answer.
- Avoid cancelling with decimal numbers.

When working with percentages:
- Change to fractions or decimal numbers before doing any calculations.
- "Of" means multiply when calculating a percent of a number.
- Fraction of Change $= \dfrac{Change}{Original}$

Workspace

Practice Sets

The answers to *Try These for Practice* and *Exercises* are found in Appendix A. Ask your instructor for the answers to the *Additional Exercises*.

Try These for Practice

Test your comprehension after reading the chapter.

1. Write $\frac{7}{8}$ as a decimal number. _____

2. Write $\frac{5.4 \times 3.71}{0.3}$ as a decimal number rounded off to the nearest tenth.

   _____

3. Write 5% as a *decimal number* and as a *fraction* in lowest terms.

   _____

4. Write the value of this expression as a fraction: $\frac{14}{15} \times \frac{25}{16} \times \frac{8}{21}$

   _____

5. Write the value of this expression as an ordinary fraction: $\dfrac{\frac{21}{80}}{\frac{7}{8}}$

   _____

Exercises

Reinforce your understanding in class or at home.

Convert to whole numbers, proper fractions, or mixed numbers (Questions 1–7).

1. $0.65 =$ _____

2. $3\frac{1}{4} + 4\frac{1}{4} =$ _____

3. $50 \times \frac{3}{5} \times \frac{1}{30} =$ _____

4. $6\frac{3}{5} \div 11 =$ _____

5. $60 \div \dfrac{13}{5} =$ _____

6. $6.3 \div \dfrac{3}{4} =$ _____

7. $52 \times \dfrac{5}{8,400} \times \dfrac{21}{0.13} =$ _____

Convert to decimal numbers (Questions 8–19)

8. $\dfrac{3}{8} =$ _____ (round down to the hundredths place)

9. $\dfrac{16}{25} =$ _____

10. $6\dfrac{7}{10} =$ _____

11. $\dfrac{3}{200} =$ _____

12. $\dfrac{5}{24} =$ _____ (round off to the hundredths place)

13. $\dfrac{457}{1,000} =$ _____

14. $\dfrac{4.56}{200} =$ _____

15. $\dfrac{20}{7} =$ _____ (round down to the tenths place)

16. $\dfrac{0.72}{0.9} =$ _____

17. $\dfrac{0.072}{0.08} =$ _____

18. $6\dfrac{1}{4}\% =$ _____

19. $0.9\% =$ _____

Simplify and write the answer in decimal form (Questions 20–24).

20. $0.24 \times 6.23 =$ _____ (round off to the nearest hundredth)

21. $0.0047 \times 100 =$ _____

22. $0.0047 \times 1,000 =$ _____

23. $0.77 \div 0.3 =$ _____ (round off to the nearest tenth)

24. $7 \div 0.13 =$ _____ (round down to the hundredths place)

Simplify and write the answer in fractional form and in decimal form rounded off to the nearest tenth (Questions 25–30).

25. $0.56 \div \dfrac{1}{0.9} =$ _____

26. $\dfrac{13}{\frac{3}{4}} =$ _____

27. $\dfrac{\frac{5}{7}}{100} \times \dfrac{200}{7} =$ _____

28. $\dfrac{15 \times \frac{3}{8}}{\frac{7}{8}} =$ _____

29. $12.5\% =$ _____

30. $37\dfrac{1}{2}\% =$ _____

31. Express the ratio 25:50 as a fraction in lowest terms.

_____

32. Express the ratio 24 to 36 as a fraction in lowest terms.

_____

Workspace

33. Find the numerator of the equivalent fraction with the given denominator.

$$\frac{3}{5} = \frac{?}{100}$$ _____

34. Find the numerator of the equivalent fraction with the given denominator.

$$\frac{3}{4} = \frac{?}{8} = $$ _____

35. Simplify $0.4 + 7 + 2.55$ _____

36. Simplify $2.06 - 1.222$ _____

37. Which is larger 0.7 or 0.24? _____

38. What is 20% of 80? _____

39. The number of patients in the hospital has increased from 160 to 200. What is the percent of change? _____

40. A patient weighed 400 pounds before a diet program. After the program she weighed 280 pounds. What was the percent of change in the patient's weight? _____

Additional Exercises

Now, test yourself!

Convert to proper fractions or mixed numbers. (Questions 1–7)

1. $0.85 = $ _____

2. $2\frac{1}{2} + 3\frac{1}{4} = $ _____

3. $40 \times \frac{1}{2} \times \frac{9}{16} = $ _____

4. $2\frac{3}{5} \div 2 = $ _____

5. $15 \div 3\frac{2}{3} = $ _____

6. $9.6 \div \frac{3}{7} = $ _____

7. $42 \times \frac{1}{9,450} \times \frac{3}{0.02} = $ _____

Convert to decimal numbers. (Questions 8–19)

8. $\frac{1}{8} = $ _____ (round down to the hundredths place)

9. $\frac{14}{25} = $ _____

10. $5\frac{3}{10} = $ _____

11. $\frac{1}{200} = $ _____

12. $\frac{1}{75} = $ _____ (round off to the nearest hundredth)

13. $\frac{870}{1,000} = $ _____

14. $\frac{2.73}{100} = $ _____

15. $\frac{14.36}{7} = $ _____ (round down to the tenths place)

16. $\dfrac{0.63}{0.9} =$ _____

17. $\dfrac{0.063}{0.09} =$ _____

18. $5\dfrac{1}{2}\% =$ _____

19. $55\% =$ _____

Workspace

Simplify and write the answer in decimal form. (Questions 20–24)

20. $4.63 \times 6.21 =$ _____
(round off to the nearest hundredth)

21. $0.004 \times 100 =$ _____

22. $2.3456 \times 1{,}000 =$ _____

23. $0.85 \div 0.03 =$ _____
(round off to the nearest tenth)

24. $8.5 \div 0.12 =$ _____ (round down to the hundredths place)

Simplify and write the answer in fractional form and in decimal form rounded off to the nearest tenth. (Questions 25–30)

25. $0.72 \times \dfrac{1}{0.7} =$ _____

26. $\dfrac{\frac{2}{3}}{8} =$ _____

27. $\dfrac{\frac{2}{5}}{100} \times \dfrac{500}{6} =$ _____

28. $\dfrac{26 \times \frac{5}{13}}{\frac{9}{100}} =$ _____

29. $10.3\% =$ _____

30. $99.5\% =$ _____

31. Express the ratio 25:40 as a fraction in lowest terms. _____

32. Express the ratio 60 to 90 as a fraction in lowest terms. _____

33. Find the numerator of the equivalent fraction with the given denominator. $\dfrac{3}{7} = \dfrac{?}{21}$ _____

34. Find the numerator of the equivalent fraction with the given denominator. $\dfrac{6}{11} = \dfrac{?}{55}$

_____

35. Simplify $0.3 + 2 + 2.55$

_____

36. Simplify $2.56 - 1.93$

_____

37. Which is larger, 0.37 or 0.244?

_____

38. What is 30% of 500?

_____

39. The number of nurses on the night shift has increased from 4 to 5. What is the percent of change? _____

40. A patient was 300 pounds before a diet program. Now she is 240 pounds. What is the percent of change in the patient's weight?

_____

nursing.pearsonhighered.com
Prepare for success with animated examples, practice questions, challenge tests, and interactive assignments.

Chapter

2 Safe and Accurate Drug Administration

Learning Outcomes

After completing this chapter, you will be able to

1. Describe the six "rights" of safe medication administration.
2. Explain the legal implications of medication administration.
3. Describe the routes of medication administration.
4. Identify common abbreviations used in medication administration.
5. Compare the trade name and generic name of drugs.
6. Describe the forms in which medications are supplied.
7. Identify and interpret the components of a Drug Prescription, Physician's Order, and Medication Administration Record.
8. Interpret information found on drug labels and in prescribing information.

This chapter introduces the process of safe and accurate medication administration. Patient safety is a primary goal for all healthcare providers. Safety in medication administration involves more than merely calculating accurate dosages. Patient rights, knowledge of potential sources of error, critical thinking, and attention to detail are all important in ensuring patient safety. The responsibilities of the people involved in the administration of medication are described.

The various forms and routes of drugs are presented, as well as abbreviations used in prescribing and documenting the administration of medications. You will learn how to interpret information found in drug labels, Web site "prescribing information," the *Physician's Desk Reference (PDR)*, package inserts, and drug guide books.

The Drug Administration Process

Drug administration is a process involving a chain of healthcare professionals. The **prescriber writes** the drug order, the **pharmacist fills** the order, and the **nurse administers** the drug to the patient; each is responsible for the accuracy of the order. To ensure patient safety, each must understand how a patient's drugs act and interact.

Drugs can be life-saving or life-threatening. Every year, thousands of deaths occur because of medication errors. Errors can occur at any point in the medication process.

Physicians, medical doctors (MD), osteopathic doctors (DO), podiatrists (DPM), and dentists (DDS) can legally prescribe medications. In many states, *physician's assistants, certified nurse midwives,* and *nurse practitioners* can also prescribe a range of medications related to their areas of practice.

Although prescribers may administer drugs to patients, the *registered professional nurse (RN), licensed practical nurse (LPN),* and *licensed vocational nurse (LVN)* are usually responsible for administering drugs ordered by the prescriber.

Preventing Medication Errors

Personnel who administer medications must be familiar with and follow applicable laws, policies, and procedures relative to the administration of medications, and they have a legal and ethical responsibility to report medication errors. When an error occurs, it must be reported immediately, the patient assessed for any adverse drug events (ADEs), and an incident report prepared. The reason for the error must be determined and corrective policies or procedures must be instituted. Best practices for preventing ADEs begin with a review of the patient's current drug regimen, allergies, and diagnosis. The healthcare professional must be knowledgeable of the drugs' expected benefits, actions, adverse reactions, interactions, and the appropriateness for the patient's diagnosis.

The Joint Commission requires "accurate and complete *Medication Reconciliation* across all healthcare settings, including: ambulatory, emergency and urgent care, long term care, home care, and inpatient services." The Medication Reconciliation helps to prevent medication errors, such as omissions, duplications, dosing errors, or drug interactions. It must be done at every transition of care, including changes in setting, service, practitioner, or level of care. The process includes developing a list of all current medications that a patient is taking, a list of medications to be prescribed, comparing the two lists, making clinical decisions based on the comparison, and communicating the new list to appropriate caregivers and to the patient.

NOTE

For additional information about Medication Reconciliation, refer to the Joint Commission's National Patient Safety Goals (www.JointCommission.org) and the Institute for Healthcare Improvement (IHI)(www.IHI.org).

Six Rights of Medication Administration

To prepare and administer drugs safely, it is imperative that you understand and follow the **Six Rights of Medication Administration:**

- Right drug
- Right dose
- Right route

ALERT

The person who administers the drug has the last opportunity to identify an error before a patient might be injured.

- Right time
- Right patient
- Right documentation

These six "rights" should be checked before administering any medications. Failure to achieve any of these rights constitutes a medication error.

Some institutions recognize additional rights, such as the *right to know* and the *right to refuse*. Patients need to be educated about their medications, and if a patient refuses a medication, the reason must be documented and reported.

The Right Drug

A drug is a chemical substance that acts on the physiological processes in the human body. For example, the drug insulin is given to patients whose bodies do not manufacture sufficient insulin. Some drugs have more than one action. Aspirin, for example, is an antipyretic (fever-reducing), analgesic (pain-relieving), and anti-inflammatory drug that also has anticoagulant properties (keeps the blood from clotting). A drug may be taken for one, some, or all its therapeutic properties.

The **generic** name is the official accepted name of a drug, as listed in the United States Pharmacopeia (USP). The designation of USP after a drug name indicates that the drug meets government standards. A drug has only one generic name, but can have many trade names. By law, generic names must be identified on all drug labels.

Many companies may manufacture the same drug using different **trade** (patented, brand, or proprietary) names. The drug's trade name is prominently displayed and followed by the trademark symbol™ or the registration symbol®. For example, **ZyPREXA** is the trade name and olanzapine is the generic name for the drug shown in • **Figure 2.1.**

NOTE

A generic drug may be manufactured by different companies under different trade names. For example, the generic drug ibuprofen is manufactured by McNeil PPC under the trade name Motrin, and by Wyeth pharmaceuticals under the trade name Advil. The active ingredients in Motrin and Advil are the same, but the size, shape, color, or fillers may be different. Be aware that patients may become confused and worried about receiving a medication that has a different name or appears to be dissimilar from their usual medication. State and federal governments now permit, encourage, and in some states mandate that the consumer be given the generic form when buying prescription drugs.

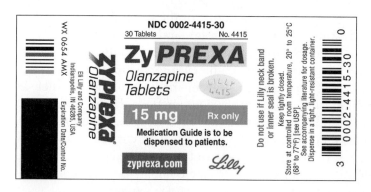

• Figure 2.1
Drug label for ZyPREXA.

Dosage strength indicates the amount of drug in a specific unit of measurement. The dosage strength of ZyPREXA is 15 mg per tablet.

Each drug has a unique identification number. This number is called the **National Drug Code (NDC) number.** The NDC number for ZyPREXA is 0002-4415-30. It is printed in two places on the label and is also encoded in the bar code. The *Food and Drug Administration (FDA)* regulates the manufacturing, sale, and effectiveness of all medications sold in the United States. Legislatures and other governmental agencies also regulate the administration of medications. The FDA estimates that the bar coding of prescription drugs reduces medication errors by as much as 50 percent.

To help avoid errors, drugs should be prescribed using only the generic name or by using both the generic and trade names. Many drugs have names that sound alike, or have names or packaging that look alike. To avoid medication errors the *FDA, Institute for Safe Medication Practice (ISMP), Joint Commission,* and *National Board of Pharmacy* recommend the use of TALL MAN Lettering in drug names. TALL MAN letters are uppercase letters used within a drug name to highlight its primary dissimilarities with look-alike drug names (ISMP Nov, 2010). For example, in Figure 2.1 the drug name ZyPREXA uses tall man lettering to help distinguish it from the drug ZyrTEC.

To meet the National Patient Safety Goals of the Joint Commission, a healthcare organization must develop its own list of look-alike/sound-alike drugs that it stores, dispenses, or administers. Table 2.1 includes a sample list of drugs whose names may be confused. See Appendix B for more complete FDA and ISMP Lists of Look-Alike Drug Names with Recommended Tall Man letters. See www.ismp.org for the ISMP'S List of *Confused Drug* Names.

Table 2.1 **Look-Alike/Sound-Alike Drugs with Tall Man Lettering**	
Drug Name	**Confused with**
acetaZOLAMIDE	acetoHEXAMIDE
buPROPion	busPIRone
chloroproMAZINE	chloroproPAMIDE
DAUNOrubicin	DOXOrubicin
DOBUTamine	DOPamine
EPINEPHrine	ePHEDrine
fentaNYL	SUFentanil
glipiZIDE	glyBURIDE
hydrALAZINE	hydrOXYzine
HumaLOG	HumuLIN
niCARdipine	NIFEdipine
prednisoLONE	prednisone
TOLAZamide	TOLBUTamide
vinBLAStine	vinCRIStine

The Right Dose

A person prescribing or administering medications has the *legal responsibility* of knowing the correct dose. Calculations may be necessary, and appropriate equipment must be used to measure the dose. Because no two people are exactly alike, and no drug affects every human body in exactly the same way, drug doses must be individualized. Responses to drug actions may differ according to the gender, race, genetics, nutritional and health status, age and weight of the patient (especially children and the elderly), as well as the route and time of administration.

The **standard adult dosage** for each drug is determined by its manufacturer. A standard adult dosage is recommended based on the requirements of an average-weight adult and may be stated either as a *set dose* (20 mg) or as a *range* (150–300 mg). In the latter case, the minimum and maximum recommended dosages given are referred to as the **safe dosage range.** Recommended dosage may be found in many sources, including the package insert, the Hospital Formulary, and the manufacturer's Web site.

Body surface area (BSA) is an estimate of the total skin area of a person measured in meters squared (m^2). Body surface area is determined by formulas based on height and weight (see Chapter 6). Many drug doses administered to children or used for cancer therapy are calculated based on BSA.

Carefully read the drug label to determine the *dosage strength*. Perform and *check calculations* and pay special attention to decimal points. When giving an intravenous drug to a pediatric patient or giving a high-alert drug (one that has a high risk of causing injury), always *double check the dosage and pump settings*, and confirm these with a colleague. Be sure to check for the recommended *safe dosage range* based on the patient's age, BSA, or weight. After you have calculated the dose, be certain to use a standard measuring device, such as a calibrated medicine dropper, syringe, or cup to administer the drug.

Medications may be prepared by the pharmacist or drug manufacturer in unit-dose packaging or multiple-dose packaging. **Unit-dose** medications may be in the forms of single tablets, capsules, or a liquid dosage sealed in an individual package. Unit-dose medications may be packaged in vials, bottles, prefilled syringes, or ampules, each of which contains only one dosage of a medication. When more than one dose is contained in a package, this is referred to as **multidose** packaging. See • **Figures 2.2 and 2.3.**

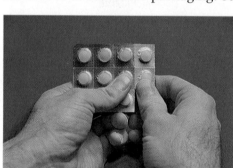
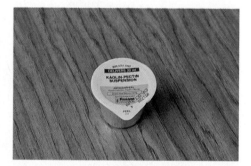

• **Figure 2.2**
Unit-dose packages.

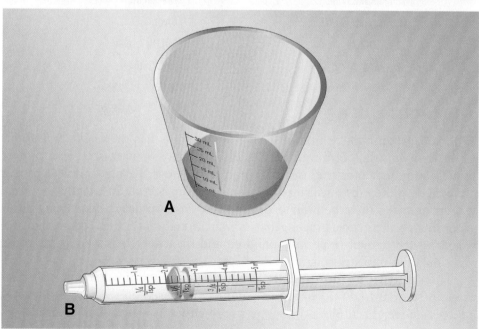

• **Figure 2.3**
Liquid medication in a
a. medication cup
b. oral syringe

The Right Route

Medications must be administered *in the form* and *via the route specified by the prescriber*. Medications are manufactured in the **form** of tablets, capsules, liquids, suppositories, creams, patches, or injectable medications (which are supplied in solution or in a powdered form to be reconstituted). The form (preparation) of a drug affects its speed of onset, intensity of action, and route of administration. The **route** indicates the site of the body and method of drug delivery.

Oral Medications. Oral medications are administered **by mouth** (PO) and are supplied in both solid and liquid form. The most common solid forms are *tablets* (tab), *capsules* (cap), and *caplets* (• **Figure 2.4**).

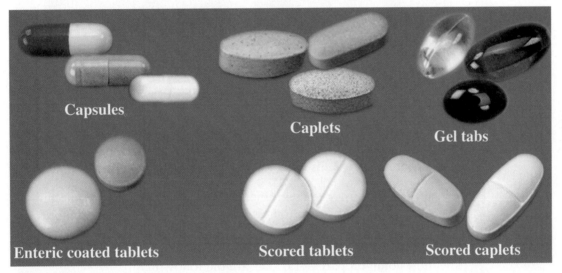

• **Figure 2.4**
Forms of oral medications.

Scored tablets have a groove down the center so that the tablet can be easily broken in half. To avoid an incorrect dose, unscored tablets should never be broken.

Enteric-coated tablets are meant to dissolve in the intestine rather than in the stomach. Therefore, they should be swallowed whole, and neither chewed nor crushed. A **capsule** is a gelatin case containing a powder, liquid, or granules (pulverized fragments of solid medication). When a patient cannot swallow, certain capsules may be opened and their contents mixed in a liquid or sprinkled on a food, such as apple sauce. Theo-dur Sprinkles is an example of such a medication.

Sustained-release (SR), extended-release (XL), or delayed-release (DR) tablets or capsules slowly release a controlled amount of medication into the body over a period of time. Therefore, these drugs *should not be opened, chewed, or crushed.*

Tablets for **buccal** administration are absorbed by the mucosa of the mouth (see • **Figure 2.5**). Tablets for **sublingual** (**SL**) administration are absorbed under the tongue (see • **Figure 2.6**). Tablets for buccal or sublingual administration should never be swallowed.

Oral drugs also come in liquid forms: *elixirs, syrups,* and *suspensions.* An **elixir** is an alcohol solution, a **syrup** is a medication dissolved in a sugar-and-water solution, and a **suspension** consists of an insoluble drug in a liquid base.

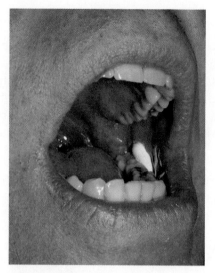

• Figure 2.5
Buccal route: Tablet between cheek and teeth.

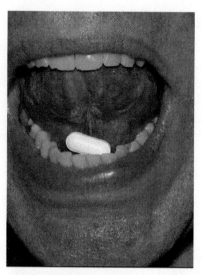

• Figure 2.6
Sublingual route: Tablet under tongue.

Liquid medications may also be administered **enterally** into the gastrointestinal tract via a specially placed tube, such as a *nasogastric (NG), gastrostomy (GT), or percutaneous endoscopic gastrostomy (PEG) tube* (see Chapter 10).

Parenteral Medications. Parenteral medications are those that are injected (via needle) into the body by various routes. They are absorbed faster and more completely than drugs given by other routes. Drug forms for parenteral use are sterile and must be administered using aseptic (sterile) technique. See Chapters 7 and 9.

The most common parenteral sites are the following:

- **Epidural:** into the epidural space (in the lumbar region of the spine)
- **Intramuscular (IM):** into the muscle
- **Subcutaneous (subcut):** into the subcutaneous tissue
- **Intravenous (IV):** into the vein
- **Intradermal (ID):** beneath the skin
- **Intracardiac (IC):** into the cardiac muscle
- **Intrathecal:** into the spinal column

Cutaneous Medications. Cutaneous medications are those that are administered through the skin or mucous membrane. Cutaneous routes include the following:

- **Topical:** administered *on the skin surface* and may provide a *local* or *systemic* effect. Those drugs applied for a **local** effect are absorbed very slowly, and amounts reaching the general circulation are minimal. Those administered for a **systemic** effect provide a slow release and absorption in the general circulation.
- **Transdermal:** contained *in a patch or disk and applied to the skin*. These are administered for their *systemic* effect. Patches allow constant, controlled amounts of drug to be released over 24 hours or more. Examples include nitroglycerin for angina or chest pain, nicotine to control the urge to smoke, and fentanyl for chronic pain. See **• Figure 2.7.**

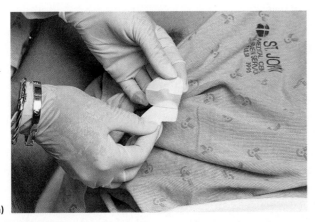

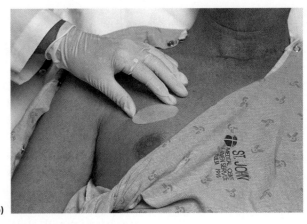

(a)   (b)

• **Figure 2.7**
Transdermal patch: (a) protective coating removed; (b) patch immediately applied to clean, dry, hairless skin and labeled with date, time, and initials.

- **Inhalation:** breathed into the respiratory tract through the nose or mouth. *Nebulizers, dry powder inhalers (DPI), and metered dose inhalers (MDI)* are types of devices used to administer drugs via inhalation. A **nebulizer** vaporizes a liquid medication into a fine mist that can then be inhaled using a face mask or handheld device. A **DPI** is a small device used for solid drugs. The device is activated by the process of inhalation, and a fine powder is inhaled. An **MDI** uses a propellant to deliver a measured dose of medication with each inhalation. See • **Figure 2.8.**

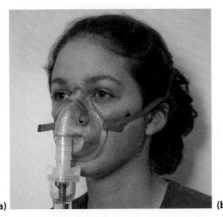

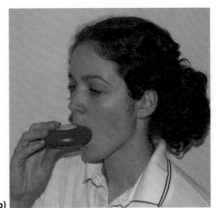

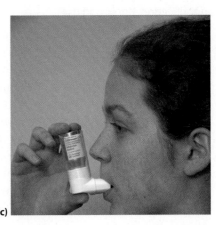

(a)   (b)   (c)

• **Figure 2.8**
Inhalation devices: (a) nebulizer with face mask; (b) dry powder inhaler; (c) metered dose inhaler.

- **Solutions and ointments:** applied to the mucosa of the eyes (optic), nose (nasal), ears (otic), or mouth
- **Suppositories:** are shaped for insertion into a body cavity (vagina, rectum, or urethra) and dissolve at body temperature

Some drugs are supplied in multiple forms and therefore can be administered by a variety of routes. For example, Tigan (trimethobenzamide HCl) is supplied as a capsule, suppository, or solution for injection.

The Right Time

The prescriber will indicate when and how often a medication should be administered. Oral medications can be given either before or after meals, depending on the action of the drug. Factors such as the purpose of the drug, drug interactions, absorption of the drug, and side effects must be considered when medication times are scheduled. Medications can be ordered *once a day* (daily), *twice a day* (b.i.d.), *three times a day* (t.i.d.), and *four times a day* (q.i.d). Most healthcare facilities designate specific times for these administrations. To maintain a more stable level of the drug in the patient, the period between administrations of the drug should be prescribed at regular intervals, such as q4h (every four hours), q6h, q8h, or q12h.

Incorrect interpretation of abbreviations related to medication administration times could result in drug errors. For example, *30 mg B.I.D.* (twice a day) is not necessarily the same as *30 mg q12h* (every twelve hours). Depending on the institution's drug delivery time schedule, *30 mg B.I.D.* may mean administer at 30 mg at 10:00 A.M. and 30 mg at 6:00 P.M., whereas *30 mg q12h* may mean administer at 30 mg at 10:00 A.M. and 30 mg at 10:00 P.M.

B.I.D. should also not be confused with "daily in two divided doses." For example, *30 mg B.I.D.* requires administering two doses of 30 mg each for a total daily dose of 60 mg. Whereas *30 mg daily in two divided doses* requires administering two doses of 15 mg each for a total daily dose of 30 mg.

The Right Patient

Before administering any medication, it is essential to determine the identity of the recipient. Administering a medication to a patient other than the one for whom it was ordered is one example of a medication error. The Joint Commission continues to include proper patient identification in its National Patient Safety Goals, and it requires the use of at least two forms of patient identification. Suggested identifiers include: the patient identification bracelet information, verbalization of the patient's name by the patient or parent, the patient's home telephone number, or the patient's hospital number.

After identifying the patient, match the drug order, patient's name, and age to the **Medication Administration Record (MAR)**. To help reduce errors many agencies now use computers at the bedside or use handheld devices (scanners) to read the bar code on a patient's identification bracelet and on the medication packages. See • **Figure 2.9.**

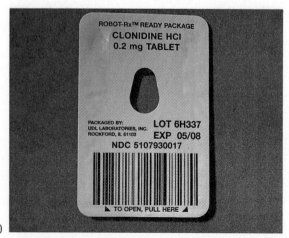

(a)

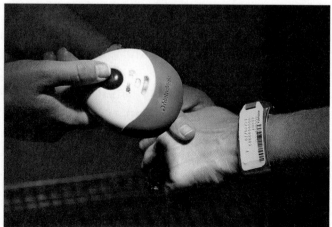

(b)

• **Figure 2.9**
Bar codes: (a) unit-dose drug; (b) scanner reading a patient's identification band.

The Right Documentation

Always document the name and dosage of the drug, as well as the route and time of administration on the MAR. Sign your initials *immediately after, but never before*, the dose is given. It is important to include any relevant information. For example, document patient allergies to medications, heart rate (when giving digoxin), and blood pressure (when giving antihypertensive drugs). All documentation must be legible. Remember the axiom, "If it's not documented, it's not done."

Anticipate side effects! A **side effect** is an undesired physiologic response to a drug. For example, codeine relieves pain, but its side effects include constipation, nausea, drowsiness, and itching. Be sure to record any observed side effects and discuss them with the prescriber.

Safe drug administration requires a knowledge of common abbreviations. For instance, when the prescriber writes **"Demerol 75 mg IM q4h prn pain,"** the person administering the drug reads this as "Administer the drug Demerol; the dose is seventy-five milligrams, the route is intramuscular, the time is every four hours, and it is to be given when the patient has pain." Be cautious with abbreviations because they can be a source of medication error. Only approved abbreviations should be used (Table 2.2).

Table 2.2 Common Abbreviations Used for Medication Administration

Abbreviation	Meaning	Abbreviation	Meaning
Route:		q12h	every twelve hours
GT	gastrostomy tube	Q.I.D. or q.i.d.	four times per day
ID	intradermal	Stat	immediately
IM	intramuscular	T.I.D. or t.i.d.	three times per day
IV	intravenous	**General:**	
IVP	intravenous push		
IVPB	intravenous piggyback	c	with
NGT	nasogastric tube	cap	capsule
PEG	percutaneous endoscopic gastrostomy	d.a.w.	dispense as written
		DR	delayed release
		ER	extended release
PO	by mouth	g	gram
PR	by rectum	gr	grain
SL	sublingual	gtt	drop
Supp	suppository	kg	kilogram
		L	liter
Frequency:		mcg	microgram
ac	before meals	mg	milligram
ad lib	as desired	mL	milliliter
B.I.D. or b.i.d.	two times a day	NKA	no known allergies
h, hr	hour	NPO	nothing by mouth
hs	at bedtime	s	without
pc	after meals	Sig	directions to patient
prn	whenever needed or necessary	Susp	suspension
		SR	sustained release
q	every	t or tsp	teaspoon
q2h	every two hours	T or tbs	tablespoon
q4h	every four hours	tab	tablet
q6h	every six hours	XL or XR	extended release
q8h	every eight hours		

The Joint Commission requires healthcare organizations to follow its official "*Do Not Use List*" that applies to all medication orders and all medication documentation. See Table 2.3.

Table 2.3	JCAHO Official "Do Not Use List"[1]	
Do Not Use	**Potential Problem**	**Use Instead**
U (for unit)	Mistaken for "0" (zero), the number "4" (four) or "cc"	Write "unit"
IU (International Unit)	Mistaken for IV (intravenous) or the number 10 (ten)	Write "International Unit"
Q.D., QD, q.d., qd (daily)	Mistaken for each other	Write "daily"
Q.O.D., QOD, q.o.d, qod (every other day)	Period after the Q mistaken for "I" and the "O" mistaken for "I"	Write "every other day"
Trailing zero (X.0 mg)[2]	Decimal point is missed	Write X mg
Lack of leading zero (.X mg)		Write 0.X mg
MS	Can mean morphine sulfate or magnesium sulfate	Write "morphine sulfate" Write "magnesium sulfate"
MSO_4 and $MgSO_4$	Confused for one another	

[1] Applies to all orders and all medication-related documentation that is handwritten (including free-text computer entry) or on preprinted forms.

[2] **Exception:** A "trailing zero" may be used only where required to demonstrate the level of precision of the value being reported, such as for laboratory results, imaging studies that report size of lesions, or catheter/tube sizes. It may not be used in medication orders or other medication-related documentation.

Additional Abbreviations, Acronyms, and Symbols
(For *possible* future inclusion in the Official "Do Not Use" List)

Do Not Use	**Potential Problem**	**Use Instead**
> (greater than)	Misinterpreted as the number	Write "greater than"
< (less than)	"7" (seven) or the letter "L" Confused for one another	Write "less than"
Abbreviations for drug names	Misinterpreted due to similar abbreviations for multiple drugs	Write drug names in full
Apothecary units	Unfamiliar to many practitioners Confused with metric units	Use metric units
@	Mistaken for the number "2" (two)	Write "at"
cc	Mistaken for U (units) when poorly written	Write "mL" or "milliliters"
μg	Mistaken for mg (milligrams) resulting in one thousand-fold overdose	Write "mcg" or "micrograms"

Drug Prescriptions

Before anyone can administer any medication, there must be a legal order or prescription for the medication.

A **drug prescription** is a directive to the pharmacist for a drug to be given to a patient who is being seen in a medical office or clinic or is being discharged from a healthcare facility. A prescription may be written, faxed, phoned, or emailed from a secure encrypted computer system to a pharmacist. There are many varieties of prescription forms. All prescriptions should contain the following:

- Prescriber's full name, address, telephone number, and (when the prescription is given for a controlled substance), the Drug Enforcement Administration (DEA) number
- Date the prescription is written
- Patient's full name, address, and age or date of birth
- Drug name (generic name should be included), dosage, route, frequency, and amount to be dispensed
- When only the trade name is written, the prescriber must indicate whether it is acceptable to substitute a generic form
- Directions to the patient that must appear on the drug container
- Number of refills permitted

Every state has a drug substitution law that either mandates or may permit a less-expensive generic drug substitution by the pharmacist. If the prescriber has an objection to a generic drug substitute, the prescriber will write "do not substitute," "dispense as written," "no generic substitution," or "medically necessary" (• Figure 2.10). Some states require bar codes on prescription forms.

Adam Smith, M.D.
100 Main Street
Utopia, New York 10000

Phone (212) 345-6789   License # 123456

Name: _Joan Soto_   Date: _November 24, 2013_

Address: _4205 Main Street_   Age/DOB: _04/20/48_
Utopia, NY 10000

℞   _Lipitor 10 mg tablets_
  Sig: _1 tablet PO, daily_

Dispense: _90_
Refills: _0_

THIS PRESCRIPTION WILL BE FILLED GENERICALLY UNLESS THE PRESCRIBER WRITES "d a w" IN THE BOX BELOW.

	_d a w_	
	Adam Smith MD	‖‖‖‖‖‖‖

• **Figure 2.10**
Drug prescription for Lipitor.

This prescription is interpreted as follows:

- Prescriber: Adam Smith, M.D.
- Prescriber address: 100 Main Street, Utopia, NY 10000
- Prescriber phone number: (212) 345-6789
- Date prescription written: November 24, 2013
- Patient's full name: Joan Soto
- Patient address: 4205 Main Street, Utopia NY 10000
- Patient date of birth: April 20, 1948
- Drug name: Lipitor (trade name)
- Dosage: 10 mg
- Route: by mouth (PO)
- Frequency: once a day
- Amount to be dispensed: 90 tablets
- Acceptable to substitute   no, the prescriber has written "d a w"
  a generic form?
- Directions to the patient: take 1 tablet by mouth daily
- Refill instructions: no refills permitted

EXAMPLE 2.1

Read the prescription in • Figure 2.11 and complete the following information.

Primary Care Associates
1234 Spring Street, Manhattan, Kansas 10001
(913) 999-5678

Name: *Mary Moral*   Date: *10/22/13*
Address: *124 Winding Lane*   Date of Birth: *4/29/52*
              Manhattan, Kansas 10001

Rx *doxycycline (Vibra-Tabs) 100 mg*
         Disp # 14
         Sig: Take 1 capsule PO b.i.d. for 7 days

Refills: *0*

Alicia Rodriguez, ARNP
Alicia Rodriguez, Adult Registered Nurse Practitioner

Substitution is mandatory
unless the words "no substitution" appear in the box above.

• Figure 2.11
Drug prescription for doxycycline.

- Date prescription written: _____
- Patient full name: _____
- Patient address: _____
- Patient date of birth: _____
- Generic drug name: _____
- Dosage: _____
- Route: _____
- Frequency: _____
- Amount to be dispensed: _____
- Acceptable to substitute a generic form? _____
- Directions to the patient: _____
- Refill instructions: _____

This is what you should have found:

• Date prescription written:	10/22/2013
• Patient full name:	Mary Moral
• Patient address:	124 Winding Lane, Manhattan, Kansas 10001
• Patient date of birth:	4/29/52
• Generic drug name:	doxycycline
• Dosage:	100 mg
• Route:	by mouth
• Frequency:	two times a day
• Amount to be dispensed:	14 capsules
• Acceptable to substitute a generic form?	yes
• Directions to the patient:	take one capsule twice a day for 7 days
• Refill instructions:	cannot be refilled

Medication Orders

Medication orders are directives to the pharmacist for the drugs prescribed in a hospital or other healthcare facility. The terms *medication orders, drug orders*, and *physician's orders* are used interchangeably, and the forms used will vary from agency to agency. No medication should be given without a medication order. Medication orders can be *written* or *verbal*. Each medication order should follow a specific sequence: drug name, dose, route, and frequency.

Written medication orders are documented in a special book for doctor's orders, on a physician's order sheet in the patient's chart, or in a computer.

A **verbal** order must contain the same components as a written order or else it is invalid. To provide for the safety of the patient, generally verbal orders may be taken only in an emergency. The verbal order must eventually be written and signed by the physician.

ALERT

If persons administering medications have difficulty understanding or interpreting the orders, it is their responsibility to clarify the orders with the prescribers.

Types of Medication Orders

The most common type of medication order is the **routine order**, which indicates that the ordered drug is administered until a discontinuation order is written or until a specified date is reached.

A **standing order** is prescribed in anticipation of sudden changes in a patient's condition. Standing orders are used frequently in critical care units, where a patient's condition may change rapidly, and immediate action would be required. Standing orders may also be used in long-term care facilities where a physician may not be readily available; for example, "*Tylenol (acetaminophen) 650 mg PO q4h for temperature of 101° F or higher.*" This is interpreted as "Administer the drug Tylenol (acetaminophen), a dose of six hundred fifty milligrams; the route is by mouth, the time is every four hours, and it is to be given whenever the patient's temperature is one hundred one degrees Fahrenheit or more."

A **prn order** is written by the prescriber for a drug to be given when a patient needs it; for example, "*morphine sulfate 5 mg subcut q4h prn mild-moderate pain.*" This is interpreted as "Administer the drug morphine sulfate, a dose of five milligrams; the route is subcutaneous, the time is every four hours, and it is to be given as needed when the patient has mild or moderate pain."

A **stat order** is an order that is to be administered immediately. Stat orders are usually written for emergencies or when a patient's condition suddenly changes; for example, "*Lasix (furosemide) 80 mg IV stat.*" This is interpreted as "Administer the drug Lasix (furosemide), a dose of eighty milligrams; the route is intravenous, and the drug is to be given immediately."

Components of a Medication Order

The essential components of a medication order are the following:

- **Patient's full name and date of birth:** Often this information is stamped or imprinted on the medication order form. Additional information may include the patient's admission number, religion, type of insurance, and physician's name.

- **Date and time the order was written:** This includes the month, day, year, and time of day. Many institutions use military time, which is based on a "24-hour clock" that does not use A.M. or P.M. (•**Figure 2.12**). Military times are written as four-digit numbers followed by the word "hours."

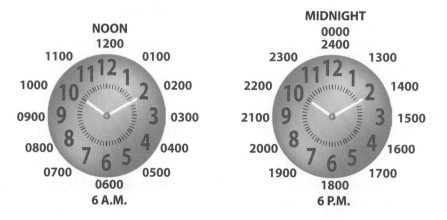

•**Figure 2.12**
Clocks Showing 10:10 A.M. (1010h) and 10:10 P.M. (2210h).

Thus, 2:00 A.M. in military time is 0200h (pronounced "Oh two hundred hours"), 12 noon is 1200h (pronounced twelve hundred hours), 2:00 P.M. is 1400h (pronounced *fourteen hundred hours*), and midnight is 2400h.

There is confusion between the meanings of 12 A.M. and 12 P.M. Twelve noon, for example, is literally neither A.M. (ante meridiem: before midday), nor is it P.M. (post meridiem: after midday). Noon *is* midday! Therefore, to avoid confusion when administering medications, for noon and midnight use *12 noon* and *12 midnight*, or use military time (*1200h* and *2400h*). The FDA recomends the use of military time.

- **Name of the medication:** The generic name is recommended. If a prescriber desires to prescribe a trade name drug, "no generic substitution" must be specified.
- **Dosage of the medication:** The amount of the drug.
- **Route of administration:** Only approved abbreviations may be used.
- **Time and frequency of administration:** When and how often the drug is to be given.
- **Signature of the prescriber:** The medication order is not legal without the signature of the prescriber.
- **Signature of the person transcribing the order:** This may be the responsibility of a nurse or others identified by agency policy.

The physician's order in • **Figure 2.13** can be interpreted as follows:

Name of patient: John Camden

Birth date: Feb. 11, 1955

Date of admission: Nov. 20, 2013

Admission number: 602412

Religion: Roman Catholic (RC)

Insurance: Blue Cross Blue Shield (BCBS)

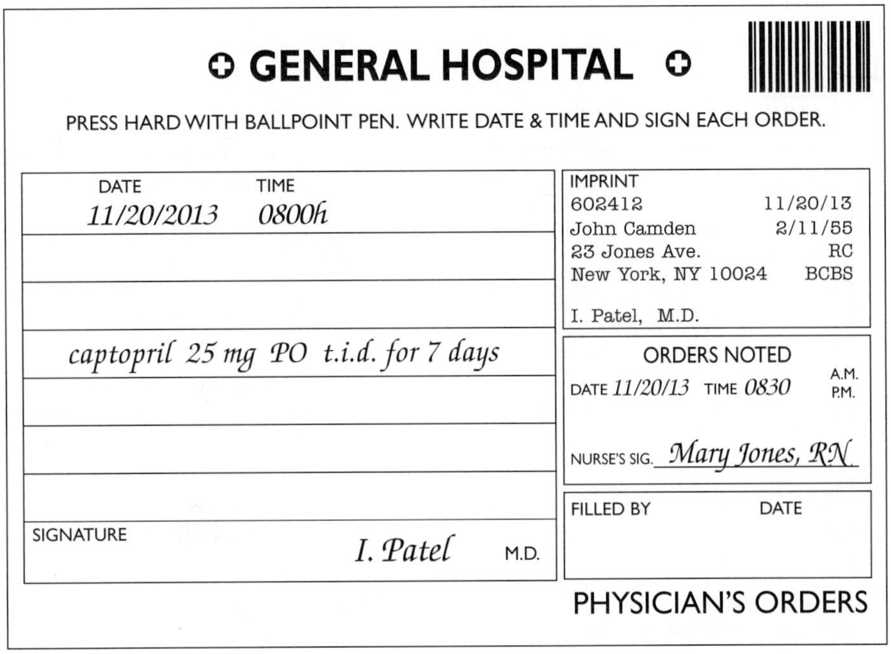

> **NOTE**
>
> When the dose includes a large number involving many zeros, use *words* instead of zeros. For example, write *500 thousand units* instead of *500,000 units*, and write *10 million units* instead of *10,000,000 units*.

> **NOTE**
>
> Drug orders follow a specific sequence: drug name, dosage, route, and frequency.

• **Figure 2.13**
Physician's order for captopril.

Date and time the order was written: 11/20/2013 at 0800h or 8:00 A.M.

Name of the medication: captopril

Dosage: 25 mg

Route of administration: PO (by mouth)

Frequency of administration: t.i.d., three times a day for 7 days

Signature of person writing the order: I. Patel, MD

Person who transcribed the order: Mary Jones, RN

EXAMPLE 2.2

Interpret the physician's order sheet shown in •Figure 2.14 and record the following information:

Date order written: _____

Time order written: _____

Name of drug: _____

Dosage: _____

Route of administration: _____

Frequency of administration: _____

Name of prescriber: _____

Name of patient: _____

Birth date: _____

Religion: _____

Type of insurance: _____

Person who transcribed the order: _____

✚ GENERAL HOSPITAL ✚

PRESS HARD WITH BALLPOINT PEN. WRITE DATE & TIME AND SIGN EACH ORDER.

DATE	TIME	IMPRINT
11/22/2013	1800h	422934 11/22/13
		Catherine Rodriguez 12/01/62
		40 Addison Avenue
		Rutlans, VT 06701 Prot
azithromycin 1% opthalmic solution		M. Ling, M.D. GHI-CBP
1 drop B.I.D. for 2 days, then daily		ORDERS NOTED
for 5 days		DATE 11/22/13 TIME 1830h A.M. P.M.
		NURSE'S SIG. Sara Gordon RN
SIGNATURE Mae Ling M.D.		FILLED BY DATE

PHYSICIAN'S ORDERS

• **Figure 2.14**
Physician's order for azithromycin.

This is what you should have found:

- Date order written: 11/22/2013
- Time order written: 1800h or 6:00 P.M.
- Name of drug: azithromycin 1% ophthalmic solution
- Dosage: 1 drop
- Route: topical
- Frequency of administration: 2 times a day for 2 days, then once a day for the next 5 days
- Name of prescriber: Mae Ling, M.D.
- Name of patient: Catherine Rodriguez
- Birth date: December 1, 1962
- Religion: Protestant
- Type of insurance: GHI-CBP
- Person who transcribed the order: Sara Gordon, RN

Medication Administration Records

A **Medication Administration Record (MAR)** is a form used by healthcare facilities to document all drugs administered to a patient. It is a legal document, part of the patient's medical record, and the format varies from agency to agency. Every agency develops policies related to using the *MAR* including: how to add new medications, discontinue medications, document one-time or stat medications, the process to follow if a medication is not administered or a patient refuses a medication, and how to correct an error on the *MAR*.

Routine, PRN, and STAT medications all may be written in separate locations on the MAR. PRN and STAT medications may also have a separate form. If a medication is to be given regularly, a complete schedule is written for all administration times. Each time a dose is administered, the healthcare worker initials the time of administration. The full name, title, and initials of the person who gave the medication must be recorded on the MAR.

After a prescriber's order has been verified, a nurse or other healthcare provider transcribes the order to the MAR. This record is used to check the medication order; prepare the correct medication dose; and record the date, time, and route of administration.

The essential components of the MAR include the following:

- **Patient information:** a stamp or printed label with patient identification (name, date of birth, medical record number).
- **Dates:** when the order was written, when to start the medication, and when to discontinue it.
- **Medication information:** full name of the drug, dose, route, and frequency of administration.
- **Time of administration:** frequency as stated in the prescriber's order; for example, t.i.d. Times for PRN and one-time doses are recorded *precisely* at the time they are administered.
- **Initials:** the initials and the signature of the person who administered the medication are recorded.
- **Special instructions:** instructions relating to the medication; for example, "Hold if systolic BP is less than 100."

ALERT

Before administering any medication, always compare the label on the medication with the information on the MAR. If there is a discrepancy, you must check the prescriber's original order.

EXAMPLE 2.3

Study the MAR in • Figure 2.15, then complete the following chart and answer the questions.

║║║║║║║║ UNIVERSITY
HOSPITAL

789652   9/11/2013
Wendy Kim   12/20/60
44 Chester Avenue   RC
New York, NY 10003   Medicaid

DAILY MEDICATION
ADMINISTRATION RECORD

Dr. Juan Rodriguez, M.D.

PATIENT NAME   _Wendy Kim_

ROOM #   _422_   IF ANOTHER RECORDS IS IN USE ☐

ALLERGIC TO (RECORD IN RED):   _tomato, codeine_

DATES GIVEN ⋮↓   DATE DISCHARGED:

RED CHECK INITIAL	ORDER DATE	INITIAL	EXP DATE	MEDICATION, DOSAGE, FREQUENCY AND ROUTE	HOURS	12	13	14	15										
	9/12	JY	9/19	ceftazidime 1 g	0600	/	MC	MC											
				IVPB q12h for 7 days begin at 1800h	1800	MJ	SG	SG											
	9/12	JY	9/18	digoxin 0.125 mg PO daily	0900	JY	JY	JY											
	9/12	JY	9/18	Lotensin (benazepril hydrochloride)	0900	JY	JY	JY											
				20 mg PO q12h	2100	MJ	SG	SG											
	9/12	JY	9/18	Plavix (clopidogrel bisulfate)	0900	JY	JY	JY											
				75 mg PO daily															
	9/12	JY	9/18	Tranxene (chlorazepate dipotassium)	2100	MJ	SG	SG											
				15 mg PO HS															

INT.	NURSES' FULL SIGNATURE AND TITLE	INT.	CODES FOR INJECTION SITES	
JY	Jim Young, RN		A- left anterior thigh	H- right anterior thigh
MC	Marie Colon, RN		B- left deltoid	I- right deltoid
MJ	Mary Jones, LPN		C- left gluteus medius	J- right gluteus medius
SG	Sara Gordon, RN		D- left lateral thigh	K- right lateral thigh
			E- left ventral gluteus	L- right ventral gluteus
			F- left lower quadrant	M- right lower quadrant
			G- left upper quadrant	N- right upper quadrant

• **Figure 2.15**
MAR for Wendy Kim.

Name of Drug	Dose	Route of Administration	Time of Administration

1. Identify the drugs and their doses administered at 9:00 A.M.

   _____

2. Identify the drugs and their doses administered at 9:00 P.M.

   _____

3. Who administered the clopidogrel bisulfate on 9/14?

   _____

4. What is the route of administration for ceftazidime?

   _____

5. What is the time of administration for benazepril hydrochloride?

   _____

This is what you should have found:

Name of Drug	Dose	Route of Administration	Time of Administration
ceftazidime	1 g	IVPB	0600h (6 A.M.) &1800h (6 P.M.)
digoxin	0.125 mg	PO	0900h (9 A.M.)
Lotensin (benazepril hydrochloride)	20 mg	PO	0900h (9 A.M.) & 2100h (9 P.M.)
Plavix (clopidogrel bisulfate)	75 mg	PO	0900h (9 A.M.)
Tranxene (chlorazepate dipotassium)	15 mg	PO	2100h (9 P.M.)

1. digoxin 0.125 mg; Lotensin (benazepril hydrochloride) 20 mg; Plavix (clopidogrel bisulfate) 75 mg
2. Lotensin (benazepril hydrochloride) 20 mg, and Tranxene (chlorazepate dipotassium) 15 mg
3. Jim Young, RN
4. Intravenous
5. 0900h (9:00 A.M.) and 2100h (9:00 P.M.)

EXAMPLE 2.4

Study the MAR in • Figures 2.16a and 2.16b, then fill in the following chart and answer the questions.

	UNIVERSITY HOSPITAL	659204 Mohammad Kamal 4103 Ely Avenue Bronx, NY 10466	11/20/2013 10/2/52 Musl GHI-CBP
	DAILY MEDICATION ADMINISTRATION RECORD	Dr. Indu Patel, M.D.	

PATIENT NAME __Mohammad Kamal__

ROOM # __302__   IF ANOTHER RECORDS IS IN USE ☐

ALLERGIC TO (RECORD IN RED): __sulfa, fish__

DATES GIVEN ⬇ MONTH/DAY   YEAR: __2013__

RED CHECK INITIAL	ORDER DATE	INITIAL	EXP DATE	MEDICATION, DOSAGE, FREQUENCY AND ROUTE	TIME	11/20	11/21	11/22	11/23	11/24	11/25	11/26
	11/20	MC	11/26	Coumadin (warfarin sodium) 10 mg	10AM		MC	MC	MC	MJ	MJ	JY
				PO daily								
	11/20	MC	11/26	Lotensin (benazepril HCL) 10 mg	10AM		MC	MC	MC	MJ	MJ	JY
				PO B.I.D.	BP		160/110	150/70	160/110	138/86	130/80	130/80
					6PM	MC	MC	MC	MC	MJ	MJ	JY
					BP	160/100	150/90	160/100	140/80	130/80	128/80	128/80
	11/20	MC	11/26	Lasix (furosemide) 20 mg PO daily	10AM		MC	MC	MC	MJ	MJ	JY
	11/20	SG	11/27	Maxipime (cefepime hydrochloride)	10AM		MC	MC	MC	MJ	MJ	JY
				1g IVPB q12hr for 7 days	10PM		SG	SG	SG	SG	SG	SG
	11/21	MC	11/27	Procrit (epoetin alfa) 3,000 units	10AM		MC		MC		MJ	
				subcutaneous, three times per week,								
				start on 11/21								
	11/21	MC	11/27	digoxin, 0.125 mg PO daily	10AM		MC	MC	MC	MJ	MJ	JY
					HR		72	70	96	76	80	80

INT.	NURSES' FULL SIGNATURE AND TITLE	INT.	NURSES' FULL SIGNATURE AND TITLE
MC	Marie Colon, RN		
SG	Sara Gordon, RN		
MJ	Mary Jones, LPN		
JY	Jim Young, RN		

• **Figure 2.16a**
MAR for Mohammad Kamal.

UNIVERSITY
HOSPITAL

659204   11/20/2013
Mohammad Kamal   10/2/52
4103 Ely Avenue   Musl
Bronx, NY 10466   GHI-CBP

DAILY MEDICATION
ADMINISTRATION RECORD

Dr. Indu Patel, M.D.

PATIENT NAME *Mohammad Kamal*

ROOM # *302*

	IF ANOTHER RECORDS IS IN USE ☐

ALLERGIC TO (RECORD IN RED): *sulfa, fish*

DATES GIVEN ⋮ MONTH/DAY   YEAR: *2013*

PRN MEDICATION

ORDER DATE	EXPIRATION DATE/TIME	MEDICATION, DOSAGE, FREQUENCY AND ROUTE		DOSES GIVEN						
11/20	11/27	*Tylenol (acetaminophen) 650 mg PO q 3-4 h prn pain*	DATE	11/20	11/20	11/20				
			TIME	6 PM	10 AM	6 PM				
			INIT	MJ	MC	6 PM				
11/20	11/27	*Robitussin DM 10 ml*	DATE	11/20	11/21					
			TIME	10 AM	10 PM					
			INIT	MJ	SG					
		PO q12h prn	DATE							
			TIME							
			INIT							
11/20	11/27	*Tylenol (acetaminophen) 325 mg PO q 3-4 h prn*	DATE							
			TIME							
			INIT							
		Temp above 101° F	DATE							
			TIME							
			INIT							

STAT-ONE DOSE-PRE-OPERATIVE MEDICATIONS

◯ **Check here if additional sheet in use.**

ORDER DATE	MEDICATION-DOSAGE ROUTE	DATE	TIME	INIT	ORDER DATE	MEDICATION-DOSAGE ROUTE	DATE	TIME	INIT
11/23	*Dilaudid (hydromorphone) 2 mg IV now*	11/23	10AM	MC					

INT.	NURSES' FULL SIGNATURE AND TITLE	INT.	NURSES' FULL SIGNATURE AND TITLE
MJ	*Mary Jones, RN*		
MC	*Marie Colon, RN*		
SG	*Sara Gordon, RN*		

• **Figure 2.16b**
MAR for Mohammad Kamal.

Name of Routine Drug	Dose	Route of Administration	Time of Administration

1. Which drugs were administered at 10:00 A.M. on 11/23?

   _____

2. Which drug was given stat and what was the route; date and time?

   _____

3. Who administered the benazapril at 6:00 P.M. on 11/21?

   _____

4. What is the route of administration for Procrit?

   _____

5. How many doses of Lotensin did the patient receive by 7:00 P.M. on 11/24?

   _____

Here is what you should have found:

Name of Routine Drug	Dose	Route of Administration	Time of Administration
Coumadin (warfarin sodium)	10 mg	PO	10:00 A.M.
Lotensin (benazepril HCl)	10 mg	PO	10:00 A.M. & 6:00 P.M.
Lasix (furosemide)	20 mg	PO	10:00 A.M.
Maxipime (cefepime hydrochloride)	1 g	IVPB	10:00 A.M. & 10:00 P.M.
Procrit (epoetin alfa)	3,000 units	subcutaneously	three times a week at 10:00 A.M.
digoxin	0.125 mg	PO	10:00 A.M.

1. Coumadin 10 mg; Lotensin 10 mg; Lasix 20 mg; Maxipime 1g, Procrit 3,000 units, digoxin 0.125 mg, Dilaudid 2 mg.
2. Dilaudid IV on 11/23 at 10:00 A.M.
3. Marie Colon, RN
4. subcutaneous
5. 9

Technology in the Medication Administration Process

Many healthcare agencies have computerized the medication process. Those who prescribe or administer medications must use security codes and passwords to access the computer system. Prescribers input orders and all other essential patient information directly into a computer terminal. This system may be referred to as **Computerized Physician Order Entry (CPOE)**. The order is received in the pharmacy, where a patient's drug profile (list of drugs) is maintained. The nurse verifies the order in the computer and inputs his or her digital ID after the medication is administered. A computer printout replaces the handwritten MAR.

One advantage of a computerized system is that handwritten orders do not need to be deciphered or transcribed. The computer program can also identify possible interactions among the patient's medications and automatically alert the pharmacist and persons administering the drugs.

Some institutions use *Automated Dispensing Cabinets (ADCs)* to dispense medications. See • **Figure 2.17.** The healthcare provider must still be vigilant when using such technology, and must be sure to follow the "Six Rights of Medication Administration"; refer to the ISMP guidelines for the safe use of ADCs.

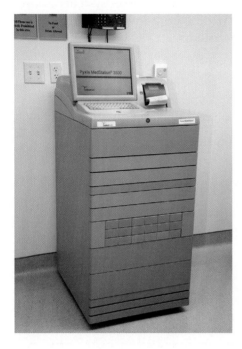

• **Figure 2.17**
Automated Dispensing Cabinet (ADC).

• **Figure 2.18** is a portion of a *computerized MAR* for a 24-hour period stated in military time. This MAR divides the day into three shifts. Note that

SCHEDULED	12/06/13–12/07/13 2301–0700	12/07/13 0701–1500	12/07/13 1501–2300
℞ Cefepime (Maxipime)		0840 2 g IVPB MAB	2015
℞ Emoxaparin Na (Lovenox)		1026 40 mg subcutaneous MAB	
℞ Furosemide (Lasix)	0611 20 mg IVP DJS		
℞ Hetastarch (he SPAN)		0920 250 mL IVPB MAB	
℞ KCl (Potassium chloride)		1026 20 mEq ER tab PO MAB	
℞ Metoprolol XL (Toprol XL)		1000 CANCEL MAB	2200
℞ Metronidazole (Flagyl)	0611 500 mg IVPB DJS	1324 500 mg IVPB MAB	2200
℞ NTG (Nitroglycerin)	0110 15 mg oint topical DJS 0611 15 mg oint topical DJS	1231 15 mg oint topical MAB	1800
℞ Pantoprazole (Protonix) 40 mg IVPB		1026 40 mg IVPB MAB	
PRN	**12/06/13–12/07/13 2301–0700**	**12/07/13 0701–1500**	**12/07/13 1501–2300**
℞ Saline flush	0110 2 mL IV flush DJS	0829 2 mL IV flush MAB	1600
℞ Morphine	0115 4 mg IVP DJS 0439 4 mg IVP DJS	1306 2 mg IVP MAB	
IV	**12/06/13–12/07/13 2301–0700**	**12/07/13 0701–1500**	**12/07/13 1501–2300**
℞ NS (NaCl, 0.9%, 1 L)		0810	2130

PRN ORDERS	
Hydrocodone 5 mg and Acetaminophen 500 mg	x 1–2 tab PO q4h prn process if pain
Saline flush	2 mL IV flush q8 at 0000/0800/1600 and prn
Insulin, human regular sliding scale {Novolin R SS}	See scale prn if BS 200–249 mg/dL give 4 Units of Reg insulin subcut

• **Figure 2.18**
A portion of a computerized MAR.

no medications have yet been recorded for the 3:01 P.M.–11:00 P.M. shift (1501h–2300h).

Scheduled (routine), IV, and PRN orders are shown. For each order administered, the MAR indicates the time, order, and the nurse's digital identification. Currently there is a variety of computerized medication systems in use. The healthcare provider has a responsibility to be both knowledgeable of the facility's policies and proficient in using its system.

EXAMPLE 2.5

Use the MAR in Figure 2.18 to answer the following questions:

1. Which drug was ordered in milliequivalents?

   _____

2. What drugs were administered at 6:11 A.M. on 12/06/2013?

   _____

3. Identify the dosage, route, and time that Flagyl was administered after noon on 12/07/2013.

   _____

4. Identify the name, dosage, route, and time of administration of the PRN drugs administered after noon on 12/07/2013.

   _____

5. What is the form and route of administration for nitroglycerin on 12/07/2013?

   _____

This is what you should have found:

1. KCl (Potassium chloride)
2. Furosemide (Lasix), Metronidazole (Flagyl), and NTG (Nitroglycerin)
3. 500 mg, IVPB at 1324h (1:24 P.M.)
4. Morphine 2 mg IVP was given at 1306h (1:06 P.M.)
5. Ointment, topical

Drug Labels

You will need to understand the information found on drug labels in order to calculate drug dosages. The important features of a drug label are identified in • Figure 2.19.

1. **Name of drug:** Mycobutin is the trade name. In this case, the name begins with an uppercase letter, is in large type, and is boldly visible on the label. The generic name is rifabutin, written in lowercase letters.

2. **Form of drug:** The drug is in the form of a capsule.

3. **National Drug Code (NDC) number:** 0013-5301-17.

4. **Bar code:** Has the NDC number encoded in it.

5. **Dosage strength:** 150 mg of the drug are contained in one capsule.

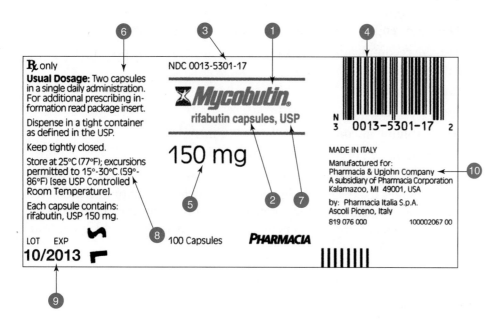

Always read the expiration date! After the expiration date, the drug may lose its potency or act differently in a patient's body. Follow the healthcare facility's policy regarding disposal of expired drugs. Never give expired drugs to patients!

• **Figure 2.19**
Drug label for Mycobutin.
(Reg. Trademark of Pfizer Inc. Reproduced with permission.)

6. **Dosage recommendations:** 2 capsules in a single daily administration. **Note that the manufacturer informs you to read the package insert.**

7. **USP:** This drug meets the standards of the United States Pharmacopeia.

8. **Storage directions:** Some drugs have to be stored under controlled conditions if they are to retain their effectiveness. This drug should be stored at 25°C (77°F).

9. **Expiration date:** The expiration date specifies when the drug should be discarded. After 10/2013 (October 31, 2013), the drug cannot be dispensed and should be discarded. For the sake of simplicity, not every drug label in this textbook will have an expiration date.

10. **Manufacturer:** Pharmacia & Upjohn.

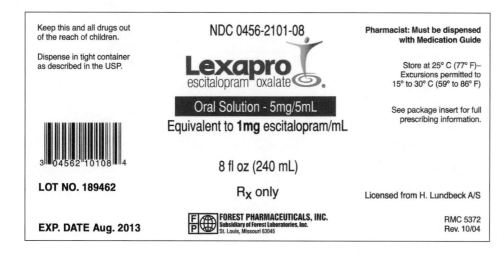

• **Figure 2.20**
Drug label for Lexapro.

The label in • **Figure 2.20** indicates the following information:

1. **Trade name:** Lexapro

2. **Generic name:** escitalopram oxalate

3. **Form:** oral solution

4. **Dosage strength:** 5 mg/5 mL, equivalent to 1 mg of escitalopram per mL

5. **Dosage recommendations:** See package insert for full prescribing information

6. **NDC number:** 0456-2101-08

7. **Expiration date:** August 2013

8. **Total volume in container:** 8 fl oz (240 mL)

9. **Manufacturer:** Forest Pharmaceuticals, Inc.

10. **Lot number** or **control number:** The lot number of this drug is 189462. This number identifies where and when a drug was manufactured. When there is a problem with particular batches of a drug and these batches must be recalled, lot numbers are useful for identifying which items are to be taken off the market.

EXAMPLE 2.6

Read the label in •Figure 2.21 and find the following:

1. Trade name: _____

2. Generic name: _____

3. Form: _____

4. Dosage strength: _____

5. NDC number: _____

6. Dosage and use: _____

7. Instructions for dispensing: _____

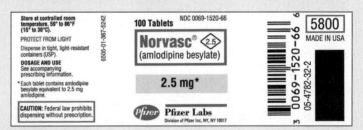

•**Figure 2.21**
Drug label for Norvasc.
(Reg - Trademark of Pfizer Inc. Reproduced with permission.)

The label for the antihypertensive drug Norvasc in Figure 2.21 indicates the following:

1. **Trade name:** Norvasc

2. **Generic name:** amlodipine besylate

3. **Form:** Tablets

4. **Dosage strength:** 2.5 mg per tablet

5. **NDC number:** 0069152066

6. **Dosage and use:** See accompanying information

7. **Instructions for dispensing:** Dispense in tight, light-resistant container

EXAMPLE 2.7

Examine the label shown in • Figure 2.22 and record the following information:

1. Trade name: _____
2. Generic name: _____
3. Form: _____
4. Dosage strength: _____
5. Amount of drug in container: _____
6. Storage temperature: _____
7. Special instructions: _____

This is what you should have found:

1. **Trade name:** Norvir
2. **Generic name:** ritonavir
3. **Form:** Oral solution
4. **Dosage strength:** 80 mg per mL
5. **Amount of drug in container:** 240 mL
6. **Storage temperature:** Do not refrigerate
7. **Special instructions:** ALERT: Find out about medicines that should NOT be taken with Norvir.

NDC 0074-1940-63

Norvir®
Ritonavir
Oral Solution

80 mg per mL

240 mL

Do Not Refrigerate

ALERT: Find out about medicines that should NOT be taken with NORVIR.

Note to Pharmacist: Do not cover ALERT box with pharmacy label.

04-A347-2/R5

Rx only   **Abbott**

• **Figure 2.22**
Drug label for Norvir.

EXAMPLE 2.8

Examine the label shown in • Figure 2.23 and record the following information:

1. Trade name: _____
2. Generic name: _____
3. Form: _____
4. Dosage strength: _____
5. Usual adult dosage: _____

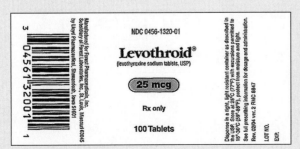

• **Figure 2.23**
Drug label for Levothroid.

This is what you should have found:

1. **Trade name:** Levothroid
2. **Generic name:** levothyroxine sodium
3. **Form:** tablets
4. **Dosage strength:** 25 mcg per tablet
5. **Usual adult dosage:** See full prescribing information

Combination Drugs

Combination drugs contain two or more generic drugs in one form. Both names and strengths of each drug are on the label. Two such medication labels follow.

Examine the label shown in • **Figure 2.24**. The label for this antidiabetic combination drug indicates that each tablet contains 50 milligrams of sitagliptin and 500 milligrams of metformin HCl.

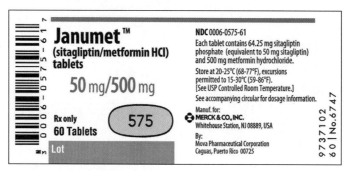

• **Figure 2.24**
Drug label for Janumet.

EXAMPLE 2.9

Examine the label shown in • Figure 2.25 and answer the following questions:

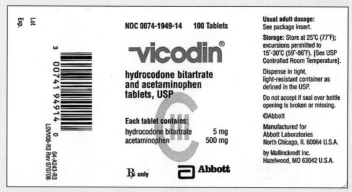

• **Figure 2.25**
Drug Label for Vicodin.

1. What is the trade name and dosage strength of the drug?

_____

2. What is the dosage strength of acetaminophen?

_____

3. What is the route of administration?

_____

4. What is the amount of drug in the container?

_____

5. What is the usual dosage?

_____

This is what you should have found:

1. Vicodin is the trade name, and the dosage strength is 5 mg/500 mg per tablet
2. 500 mg of acetaminophen per tablet
3. By mouth
4. 100 tablets
5. See package insert

Controlled Substances

Certain drugs which can lead to abuse or dependence are classified by law as **controlled substances.** These drugs are divided into five categories, called schedules. Schedule I drugs are those with the highest potential for abuse (e.g., heroin, marijuana). Schedule V drugs are those with the lowest potential for abuse (e.g., cough medications containing codeine). _Controlled substances_ must be stored, handled, disposed of, and administered according to regulations established by the _U.S. Drug Enforcement Agency (DEA)._ Hospitals and pharmacies must register with the _DEA_ and use their assigned numbers to purchase scheduled drugs. Those who prescribe medications must have a _DEA_ number to prescribe _controlled substances._

The _controlled substance_ OxyContin (oxycodone hydrochloride) is a Schedule II drug, as indicated by the CII on the label. (See the arrow in • **Figure 2.26.**)

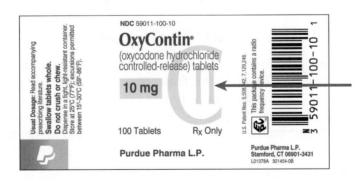

• **Figure 2.26**
Drug label for OxyContin.

Drug Information

In an effort to manage the risks of medications and reduce medical errors and adverse drug events, the U.S. Food and Drug Administration (FDA) mandates the format in which information about drugs is provided.

Drug information can be obtained online. Prescription drug information is also found on the package insert, whereas information on over-the-counter (OTC) drugs is found on the packaging itself.

Prescription Drug Package Inserts

The FDA has mandated that a new format for package inserts be phased in by 2016. The new categories for the format are:

- **Highlights of Prescribing Information:** provides immediate access to the most important facts.
- **Proprietary name, dosage form, route of administration, and initial U.S. approval (year):** gives the date of initial product approvals, thereby making it easier to determine how long a product has been on the market.
- **Boxed Warning:** identifies the dangers of the medication.
- **Recent Major Changes:** notes the changes made within the past year to ensure the most up-to-date information.
- **Indications and Usage:** includes conditions for which the product is effective.
- **Dosage and Administration:** describes the recommended dose and routes of administration.
- **Dosage Forms and Strengths:** indicates how the product is supplied and its strength (e.g., 10 mg/tab).
- **Contraindications:** gives reasons for which it is inadvisable to use the product.
- **Warnings and Precautions:** provides notice of things that may cause harm.
- **Adverse Reactions:** The following statement must be included in this section: "To report SUSPECTED ADVERSE REACTIONS, contact (manufacturer) at (phone # and Web address) or FDA at 1-800-FDA-1088 or www.fda.gov/medwatch.
- **Drug Interactions:** lists other drugs that, when taken in combination, may cause concern.
- **Use in Specific Populations:** indicates target populations, (e.g., pregnancy, nursing mothers, pediatric, and geriatric patients).

Over-the-Counter (OTC) Labels

Over-the-counter (OTC) medicines are drugs that can be obtained without a prescription. In the United States, the FDA decides which drugs are safe enough to sell over the counter. Taking OTC drugs still has risks. Some interact with other drugs, supplements, foods, or drinks, whereas others may cause problems for people with certain medical conditions. The FDA format for OTC drug labels is much simpler than that for prescription drugs. The categories are as follows:

- **Drug Facts:** includes the name of the drug and its purpose.
- **Uses:** indicates the conditions for which the drug is effective.
- **Warnings:** indicates the effects of the medication of which to be aware.
- **Directions:** specifies the quantity of the drug to take and how often to take it. For example, 2 tablets every 8 hours with water.
- **Other Information:** provides miscellaneous information, for example, expiration date and storage directions.

> **NOTE**
>
> Prescription drug information is accessible on "Daily Med," an interagency online health information clearing house created cooperatively by the FDA and the National Library of Medicine (NLM) at http://dailymed.nlm.nih.gov.

- **Inactive ingredients:** lists other substances in the drug that are not active ingredients.
- **Questions or comments:** provides a contact number for consumer questions.

• **Figure 2.27** shows an excerpt from the prescribing information for the drug ZyPREXA (olanzapine).

HIGHLIGHTS OF PRESCRIBING INFORMATION

These highlights do not include all the information needed to use ZYPREXA safely and effectively. See full prescribing information for ZYPREXA.

ZYPREXA (olanzapine) Tablet for Oral use
ZYPREXA ZYDIS (olanzapine) Tablet, Orally Disintegrating for Oral use
ZYPREXA IntraMuscular (olanzapine) Injection, Powder, For Solution for Intramuscular use

Initial U.S. Approval: 1996

WARNING: INCREASED MORTALITY IN ELDERLY PATIENTS WITH DEMENTIA-RELATED PSYCHOSIS

See full prescribing information for complete boxed warning.
- Elderly patients with dementia-related psychosis treated with antipsychotic drugs are at an increased risk of death. ZYPREXA is not approved for the treatment of patients with dementia-related psychosis. (5.1, 5.14, 17.2)
  When using ZYPREXA and fluoxetine in combination, also refer to the Boxed Warning section of the package insert for Symbyax.

-------------------------- **RECENT MAJOR CHANGES** -------------------------

Indications and Usage:

Schizophrenia (1.1)	12/2009
Bipolar I Disorder (Manic or Mixed Episodes) (1.2)	12/2009
Special Considerations in Treating Pediatric Schizophrenia and Bipolar I Disorder (1.3)	12/2009
ZYPREXA IntraMuscular: Agitation Associated with Schizophrenia and Bipolar I Mania (1.4)	12/2009

Dosage and Administration:

Schizophrenia (2.1)	12/2009
Bipolar I Disorder (Manic or Mixed Episodes) (2.2)	12/2009

Warnings and Precautions:

Orthostatic Hypotension (5.8)	05/2010
Leukopenia, Neutropenia, and Agranulocytosis (5.9)	08/2009
Hyperprolactinemia (5.15)	01/2010

--------------------------- **INDICATIONS AND USAGE** --------------------------

ZYPREXA® (olanzapine) is an atypical antipsychotic indicated:

As oral formulation for the:
- Treatment of schizophrenia. (1.1)
  - Adults: Efficacy was established in three clinical trials in patients with schizophrenia: two 6-week trials and one maintenance trial. (14.1)
  - Adolescents (ages 13-17): Efficacy was established in one 6-week trial in patients with schizophrenia (14.1). The increased potential (in adolescents compared with adults) for weight gain and hyperlipidemia may lead clinicians to consider prescribing other drugs first in adolescents. (1.1)
- Acute treatment of manic or mixed episodes associated with bipolar I disorder and maintenance treatment of bipolar I disorder. (1.2)
  - Adults: Efficacy was established in three clinical trials in patients with manic or mixed episodes of bipolar I disorder: two 3- to 4-week trials and one maintenance trial. (14.2)
  - Adolescents (ages 13-17): Efficacy was established in one 3-week trial in patients with manic or mixed episodes associated with bipolar I disorder (14.2). The increased potential (in adolescents compared with adults) for weight gain and hyperlipidemia may lead clinicians to consider prescribing other drugs first in adolescents. (1.2)
- Medication therapy for pediatric patients with schizophrenia or bipolar I disorder should be undertaken only after a thorough diagnostic evaluation and with careful consideration of the potential risks. (1.3)
- Adjunct to valproate or lithium in the treatment of manic or mixed episodes associated with bipolar I disorder. (1.2)
  - Efficacy was established in two 6-week clinical trials in adults (14.2). Maintenance efficacy has not been systematically evaluated.

As ZYPREXA IntraMuscular for the:
- Treatment of acute agitation associated with schizophrenia and bipolar I mania. (1.4)

- Efficacy was established in three 1-day trials in adults. (14.3)

As ZYPREXA and Fluoxetine in Combination for the:
- Treatment of depressive episodes associated with bipolar I disorder. (1.5)
  - Efficacy was established with Symbyax (olanzapine and fluoxetine in combination) in adults; refer to the product label for Symbyax.
- Treatment of treatment resistant depression (major depressive disorder in patients who do not respond to 2 separate trials of different antidepressants of adequate dose and duration in the current episode). (1.6)
  - Efficacy was established with Symbyax (olanzapine and fluoxetine in combination) in adults; refer to the product label for Symbyax.

---------------------- **DOSAGE AND ADMINISTRATION** ---------------------

Schizophrenia in adults (2.1)	Oral: Start at 5-10 mg once daily; Target: 10 mg/day within several days
Schizophrenia in adolescents (2.1)	Oral: Start at 2.5-5 mg once daily; Target: 10 mg/day
Bipolar I Disorder (manic or mixed episodes) in adults (2.2)	Oral: Start at 10 or 15 mg once daily
Bipolar I Disorder (manic or mixed episodes) in adolescents (2.2)	Oral: Start at 2.5-5 mg once daily; Target: 10 mg/day
Bipolar I Disorder (manic or mixed episodes) with lithium or valproate in adults (2.2)	Oral: Start at 10 mg once daily
Agitation associated with Schizophrenia and Bipolar I Mania in adults (2.4)	IM: 10 mg (5 mg or 7.5 mg when clinically warranted) Assess for orthostatic hypotension prior to subsequent dosing (max. 3 doses 2-4 hrs apart)
Depressive Episodes associated with Bipolar I Disorder in adults (2.5)	Oral in combination with fluoxetine: Start at 5 mg of oral olanzapine and 20 mg of fluoxetine once daily
Treatment Resistant Depression in adults (2.6)	Oral in combination with fluoxetine: Start at 5 mg of oral olanzapine and 20 mg of fluoxetine once daily

- Lower starting dose recommended in debilitated or pharmacodynamically sensitive patients or patients with predisposition to hypotensive reactions, or with potential for slowed metabolism. (2.1)
- Olanzapine may be given without regard to meals. (2.1)

ZYPREXA and Fluoxetine in Combination:
- Dosage adjustments, if indicated, should be made with the individual components according to efficacy and tolerability. (2.5, 2.6)
- Olanzapine monotherapy is not indicated for the treatment of depressive episodes associated with bipolar I disorder or treatment resistant depression. (2.5, 2.6)
- Safety of co-administration of doses above 18 mg olanzapine with 75 mg fluoxetine has not been evaluated. (2.5, 2.6)

--------------------- **DOSAGE FORMS AND STRENGTHS** --------------------
- Tablets (not scored): 2.5, 5, 7.5, 10, 15, 20 mg (3)
- Orally Disintegrating Tablets (not scored): 5, 10, 15, 20 mg (3)
- Intramuscular Injection: 10 mg vial (3)

---------------------------- **CONTRAINDICATIONS** --------------------------
- None with ZYPREXA monotherapy.
- When using ZYPREXA and fluoxetine in combination, also refer to the Contraindications section of the package insert for Symbyax®. (4)
- When using ZYPREXA in combination with lithium or valproate, refer to the Contraindications section of the package inserts for those products. (4)

---------------------- **WARNINGS AND PRECAUTIONS** ----------------------
- *Elderly Patients with Dementia-Related Psychosis:* Increased risk of death and increased incidence of cerebrovascular adverse events (e.g., stroke, transient ischemic attack). (5.1)
- *Suicide:* The possibility of a suicide attempt is inherent in schizophrenia and in bipolar I disorder, and close supervision of high-risk patients should accompany drug therapy; when using in combination with fluoxetine, also refer to the Boxed Warning and Warnings and Precautions sections of the package insert for Symbyax. (5.2)
- *Neuroleptic Malignant Syndrome:* Manage with immediate discontinuation and close monitoring. (5.3)

• **Figure 2.27**
Excerpts of package insert for ZyPREXA.

- *Hyperglycemia:* In some cases extreme and associated with ketoacidosis or hyperosmolar coma or death, has been reported in patients taking olanzapine. Patients taking olanzapine should be monitored for symptoms of hyperglycemia and undergo fasting blood glucose testing at the beginning of, and periodically during, treatment. (5.4)
- *Hyperlipidemia:* Undesirable alterations in lipids have been observed. Appropriate clinical monitoring is recommended, including fasting blood lipid testing at the beginning of, and periodically during, treatment. (5.5)
- *Weight Gain:* Potential consequences of weight gain should be considered. Patients should receive regular monitoring of weight. (5.6)
- *Tardive Dyskinesia:* Discontinue if clinically appropriate. (5.7)
- *Orthostatic Hypotension:* Orthostatic hypotension associated with dizziness, tachycardia, bradycardia and, in some patients, syncope, may occur especially during initial dose titration. Use caution in patients with cardiovascular disease, cerebrovascular disease, and those conditions that could affect hemodynamic responses. (5.8)
- *Leukopenia, Neutropenia, and Agranulocytosis:* Has been reported with antipsychotics, including ZYPREXA. Patients with a history of a clinically significant low white blood cell count (WBC) or drug induced leukopenia/neutropenia should have their complete blood count (CBC) monitored frequently during the first few months of therapy and discontinuation of ZYPREXA should be considered at the first sign of a clinically significant decline in WBC in the absence of other causative factors. (5.9)
- *Seizures:* Use cautiously in patients with a history of seizures or with conditions that potentially lower the seizure threshold. (5.11)
- *Potential for Cognitive and Motor Impairment:* Has potential to impair judgment, thinking, and motor skills. Use caution when operating machinery. (5.12)
- *Hyperprolactinemia:* May elevate prolactin levels. (5.15)
- *Use in Combination with Fluoxetine, Lithium or Valproate:* Also refer to the package inserts for Symbyax, lithium, or valproate. (5.16)
- *Laboratory Tests:* Monitor fasting blood glucose and lipid profiles at the beginning of, and periodically during, treatment. (5.17)

-------------------------------- ADVERSE REACTIONS --------------------------------

Most common adverse reactions (≥5% and at least twice that for placebo) associated with:

Oral Olanzapine Monotherapy:
- Schizophrenia (Adults) – postural hypotension, constipation, weight gain, dizziness, personality disorder, akathisia (6.1)
- Schizophrenia (Adolescents) – sedation, weight increased, headache, increased appetite, dizziness, abdominal pain, pain in extremity, fatigue, dry mouth (6.1)
- Manic or Mixed Episodes, Bipolar I Disorder (Adults) – asthenia, dry mouth, constipation, increased appetite, somnolence, dizziness, tremor (6.1)

- Manic or Mixed Episodes, Bipolar I Disorder (Adolescents) – sedation, weight increased, increased appetite, headache, fatigue, dizziness, dry mouth, abdominal pain, pain in extremity (6.1)

Combination of ZYPREXA and Lithium or Valproate:
- Manic or Mixed Episodes, Bipolar I Disorder (Adults) – dry mouth, weight gain, increased appetite, dizziness, back pain, constipation, speech disorder, increased salivation, amnesia, paresthesia (6.1)

ZYPREXA and Fluoxetine in Combination: Also refer to the Adverse Reactions section of the package insert for Symbyax. (6)

ZYPREXA IntraMuscular for Injection:
- Agitation with Schizophrenia and Bipolar I Mania (Adults) – somnolence (6.1)

To report SUSPECTED ADVERSE REACTIONS, contact Eli Lilly and Company at 1-800-LillyRx (1-800-545-5979) or FDA at 1-800-FDA-1088 or www.fda.gov/medwatch

-------------------------------- DRUG INTERACTIONS --------------------------------
- *Diazepam:* May potentiate orthostatic hypotension. (7.1, 7.2)
- *Alcohol:* May potentiate orthostatic hypotension. (7.1)
- *Carbamazepine:* Increased clearance of olanzapine. (7.1)
- *Fluvoxamine:* May increase olanzapine levels. (7.1)
- *ZYPREXA and Fluoxetine in Combination:* Also refer to the Drug Interactions section of the package insert for Symbyax. (7.1)
- *CNS Acting Drugs:* Caution should be used when taken in combination with other centrally acting drugs and alcohol. (7.2)
- *Antihypertensive Agents:* Enhanced antihypertensive effect. (7.2)
- *Levodopa and Dopamine Agonists:* May antagonize levodopa/dopamine agonists. (7.2)
- *Lorazepam (IM):* Increased somnolence with IM olanzapine. (7.2)
- *Other Concomitant Drug Therapy:* When using olanzapine in combination with lithium or valproate, refer to the Drug Interactions sections of the package insert for those products. (7.2)

----------------------- USE IN SPECIFIC POPULATIONS -----------------------
- *Pregnancy:* ZYPREXA should be used during pregnancy only if the potential benefit justifies the potential risk to the fetus. (8.1)
- *Nursing Mothers:* Breast-feeding is not recommended. (8.3)
- *Pediatric Use:* Safety and effectiveness of ZYPREXA in children <13 years of age have not been established. (8.4)

See 17 for PATIENT COUNSELING INFORMATION and FDA-approved Medication Guide

Revised: 05/2010

● **Figure 2.27**
(*Continued*)

EXAMPLE 2.10

Read the excerpts of the package insert in Figure 2.27 and fill in the requested information.

1. What is the generic name of the drug?

_____

2. For what condition is the intramuscular form of ZyPREXA used?

_____

3. What may occur if the drug is taken with diazepam?

_____

4. What is the recommended beginning oral dose for adults with schizophrenia?

_____

5. Should women who are breastfeeding use this drug?

_____

This is what you should have found:

1. olanzapine.
2. Acute agitation associated with Schizophrenia and Bipolar I mania in adults.
3. Orthostatic hypotension.
4. 5–10 mg once daily.
5. No.

EXAMPLE 2.11

Read the drug information in •Figures 2.28 and 2.29 and answer the following questions.

1. What is the trade name of the drug?

   _____

2. What is the active ingredient in this drug?

   _____

3. Can this drug be taken by mouth?

   _____

4. What danger may occur with prolonged exposure to this solution?

   _____

5. What should you do if you have questions about this drug?

   _____

Drug Facts

Active ingredient	Purpose
Povidone-iodine, 7.5% (0.75% available iodine)	Antiseptic

Uses
- for preparation of the skin prior to surgery
- helps to reduce bacteria that potentially can cause skin infection
- for handwashing to reduce bacteria on the skin
- significantly reduces the number of microorganisms on the hands and forearms prior to surgery or patient care

Warnings
For external use only

Do not use this product ■ in the eyes

Stop use and ask a doctor
- if irritation and redness develop
- in rare instances of local irritation or sensitivity

When using this product
- prolonged exposure to wet solution may cause irritation or, rarely, severe skin reactions
- in pre-operative prepping, avoid "pooling" beneath the patient

Keep out of reach of children. If swallowed, get medical help or contact a Poison Control Center right away.

Directions
A. Surgical hand scrub:
- wet hands with water
- spread about 5 cc (1 teaspoonful) of Scrub over both hands and forearms
- without adding more water, scrub thoroughly for 2 ½ to 3 minutes
- use a sponge if desired. Clean thoroughly under fingernails.
- add a little water and develop copious suds. Rinse thoroughly under running water.
- repeat the entire procedure using another 5 cc of Scrub

B. Antiseptic hand wash:
- wet hands with water and pour about 5 cc of Scrub on hands
- rub hands vigorously together for at least 15 seconds, covering all surfaces
- rinse and dry with a disposable towel

C. Patient pre-operative skin preparation:
- wet skin with water
- apply Scrub (1 cc is sufficient to cover an area of 20-30 square inches), develop lather and scrub thoroughly for about 5 minutes
- rinse off using sterile gauze saturated with water
- the area may then be painted with BETADINE Solution and allowed to dry

Other information
- store at 25°C (77°F); excursions permitted between 15°-30°C (59°-86°F)
- store in original container

Inactive ingredients ammonium nonoxynol-4 sulfate, nonoxynol-9, purified water, sodium hydroxide

Questions? 1-888-726-7535 (8am-5pm, EST, Mon.-Fri.)

•**Figure 2.28**
Information found on Betadine packaging.

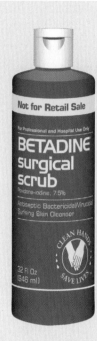

• **Figure 2.29**
Container of Betadine Surgical Scrub.

This is what you should have found:

1. Betadine surgical scrub.
2. Povidone-iodine 7.5%
3. No, the drug is for external use only.
4. May cause irritation or, rarely, severe skin reactions.
5. Call 1-888-726-7535.

Summary

In this chapter, the Medication Administration Process was discussed, including those who may administer drugs; the "six rights" and "three checks" of medication administration; and how to interpret prescriptions, medication orders, medication administration records, drug labels, and drug package inserts.

- The six rights of medication administration serve as a guide for *safe* administration of medications to patients.
- Failure to achieve any of the six rights constitutes a medication error.
- A person administering medications has a legal and ethical responsibility to report medication errors.
- Medication errors can occur at any point in the medication process.
- A drug should be prescribed using its generic name.
- Understanding drug orders requires the interpretation of common abbreviations.
- Never use any abbreviations on the Joint Commission "Official Do Not Use" list.
- Read drug labels carefully; many drugs have look-alike/sound-alike names.
- Carefully read the label to determine dosage strength and check calculations, paying special attention to decimal points.
- Medications must be administered in the form and via the route specified by the prescriber.
- The form of a drug affects its speed of onset, intensity of action, and route of administration.
- The *oral (PO)* route is the one most commonly used.
- *Buccal* and *sublingual* medications must be kept in the mouth until they are completely dissolved.
- *Topical* medications may have local and systemic effects. *Transdermal patches* are applied for their systemic effect.
- *Inhalation* medications may be administered with various devices, such as *nebulizers, dry powder,* and *metered dose inhalers.*

- *Parenteral* medications are injected into the body. To prevent infection, sterile technique must be used for their administration.
- Before administering any medication, it is essential to identify the patient.
- Medications should be documented immediately after, but never before, they are administered.
- No medication should be given without a legal order.
- If persons administering medications have difficulty understanding or interpreting the order, they must clarify the order with the prescriber.

- Medication administration process is rapidly becoming computerized.
- Drug package inserts contain detailed information about the drug indications and usage; dosage and administration; forms and strengths; contraindications; warnings and precautions; adverse reactions; drug interactions; use in special populations; and contact information to report suspected adverse reactions.
- Information for prescription drugs is found in package inserts, whereas information for OTC drugs is found on the packaging itself.

Practice Sets

The answers to *Try These for Practice* and *Exercises* are found in Appendix A. Ask your instructor for the answers to the *Additional Exercises*.

Try These for Practice

Test your comprehension after reading the chapter.
Study the labels in • **Figures 2.30** to **2.34** and answer the following five questions.

1. What is the trade name for losartan potassium?

   _____

2. What is the route of administration for Bystolic?

   _____

3. What is the generic name for Humira?

   _____

4. Which drug is a combination drug?

   _____

5. What is the dosage strength of paricalcitol?

   _____

Workspace

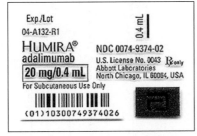

• **Figure 2.30**
Drug label for Humira.

Workspace

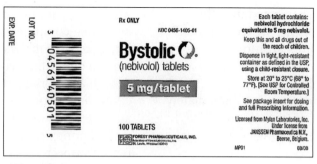

• **Figure 2.31**
Drug label for Bystolic.

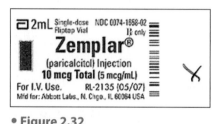

• **Figure 2.32**
Drug label for Zemplar.

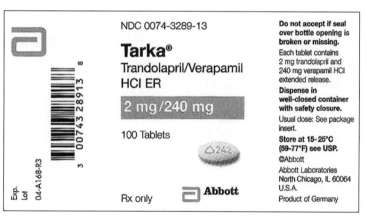

• **Figure 2.33**
Drug label for Tarka.

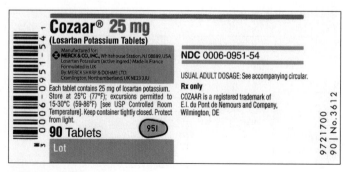

• **Figure 2.34**
Drug label for Cozaar.

Exercises

Reinforce your understanding in class or at home.

Use the information from drug labels in Figures 2.30 to 2.34 to complete Exercises 1 to 5.

1. What is the route of administration for paricalcitol?

_____

2. Write the trade name for the drug whose NDC number is 0074-3289-13.

_____

3. How many milliliters are contained in the container for the drug whose NDC number is 0074-9374-02?

_____

4. What is the dosage strength of adalimumab?

_____

5. How many milligrams of verapamil are contained in one tablet of Tarka?

_____

6. Study the portions of a MAR in • **Figures 2.35a, 2.35b,** and **2.35c** to answer the following questions.

Order Date	Exp Date	Medication Dosage Frequency & Route	Time	12/7	12/8	12/9	12/10	12/11	12/12
12/7	12/13	Neurontin (gabapentin) 100 mg PO t.i.d.	10 AM 2 PM 6 PM	MC MC JY	MC MC JY	MC MC JY	MC MC JY		
12/7	12/16	Vantin (cefpodoxime) 200 mg PO q12h for 10 days	8 AM 8 PM	SG JY	SG JY	SG JY	SG JY		
12/7	12/13	digoxin 0.125 mg PO daily	10 AM	MC	MC	MC	MC		
12/7	12/13	Levemir 7 units subcut at bedtime	10 PM	JY	JY	JY	JY		
12/7	12/13	Norvasc (amlodipine) 5 mg PO daily	10 AM	MC	MC	MC	MC		

• **Figure 2.35a**
Portion of a MAR.

Workspace

Workspace

PRN Medication		Medication Dosage Route & Time	Doses Given						
Order Date	Expiration Date		Date	12/10					
12/10	12/13	Darvocet N 100 tab 1 PO q4h prn mild-moderate pain	Time	10 PM					
			Init	JY					

• **Figure 2.35b**
Portion of a MAR.

Initial	Nurse's Signature	Initial	Nurse's Signature
SG	Sara Gordon RN		
MC	Marie Colon RN		
JY	Jim Young LPN		

• **Figure 2.35c**
Portion of a MAR.

(a) Which drug(s) were administered at 10 P.M. on 12/10/2013?

_____

(b) Using military time, designate the time(s) of day the patient received cefpodoxime.

_____

(c) How many doses of gabapentin were administered to the patient by nurse Colon?

_____

(d) What is the route of administration for Levemir?

_____

(e) Which drugs were administered by nurse Young on 12/8/2013?

_____

7. Study the portion of a physician's order sheet in • **Figure 2.36** to answer the following questions.

(a) Which drug(s) is/are given four times a day?

_____

(b) Which drug(s) is/are given daily?

_____

(c) How many times a day should the patient receive ciprofloxacin?

_____

(d) What is the route of administration for morphine?

_____

(e) How many times a day can the patient receive morphine?

_____

PHYSICIAN'S ORDERS

Order Date	Date Disc	
4/20/2013	4/30/2013	Cipro (ciprofloxacin HCl) 500 mg PO q12h
4/20/2013	4/27/2013	digoxin 0.125 mg PO daily
4/20/2013	4/27/2013	Crestor (rosuvastatin) 20 mg PO daily
4/20/2013	4/27/2013	Emex (metoclopramide HCl) 10 mg PO q.i.d. ac and hs. Give 30 minutes before meals and at bedtime.
4/20/2013	4/23/2013	morphine sulfate 5 mg IVP q4h prn moderate-severe pain
4/20/2013	4/27/2013	Lasix (furosemide) 40 mg PO daily

• **Figure 2.36**
Portion of a physician's order sheet.

8. Use the package insert shown in • **Figure 2.37** to answer the following questions.

(a) What is the generic name and form of the drug?

_____

(b) What condition is the drug used to treat?

_____

(c) What is the initial dose on the first day?

_____

(d) Can the drug be used for children?

_____

(e) What is the maximum daily dose?

_____

Workspace

Workspace

HIGHLIGHTS OF PRESCRIBING INFORMATION
These highlights do not include all the information needed to use Savella safely and effectively. See full prescribing information for Savella.
Savella® (milnacipran HCl) Tablets
Initial U.S. Approval: 2009

WARNING: SUICIDALITY AND ANTIDEPRESSANT DRUGS
See full prescribing information for complete boxed warning.
- **Increased risk of suicidal ideation, thinking, and behavior in children, adolescents, and young adults taking antidepressants for major depressive disorder (MDD) and other psychiatric disorders. Savella is not approved for use in pediatric patients (5.1)**

-------------- RECENT MAJOR CHANGES--------------------
Warnings and Precautions, Serotonin Syndrome or Neuroleptic Malignant Syndrome (NMS)-like Reactions (5.2) 06/2009

-------------------INDICATIONS AND USAGE------------------
Savella® is a selective serotonin and norepinephrine reuptake inhibitor (SNRI) indicated for the management of fibromyalgia (1)
Savella is not approved for use in pediatric patients (5.1)

-------------DOSAGE AND ADMINISTRATION-------------
- Administer Savella in two divided doses per day (2.1)
- Based on efficacy and tolerability, dosing may be titrated according to the following schedule (2.1):
  Day 1: 12.5 mg once
  Days 2-3: 25 mg/day (12.5 mg twice daily)
  Days 4-7: 50 mg/day (25 mg twice daily)
  After Day 7: 100 mg/day (50 mg twice daily)
- Recommended dose is 100 mg/day (2.1)
- May be increased to 200 mg/day based on individual patient response (2.1)
- Dose should be adjusted in patients with severe renal impairment (2.2)

------------DOSAGE FORMS AND STRENGTHS------------
- Tablets: 12.5 mg, 25 mg, 50 mg, 100 mg (3)

--------------------CONTRAINDICATIONS--------------------
- Use of monoamine oxidase inhibitors concomitantly or in close temporal proximity (4.1)
- Use in patients with uncontrolled narrow-angle glaucoma (4.2)

-------------WARNINGS AND PRECAUTIONS-------------
- Suicidality: Monitor for worsening of depressive symptoms and suicide risk (5.1)
- Serotonin Syndrome or Neuroleptic Malignant Syndrome (NMS)-like Reactions: Serotonin syndrome or NMS-like reactions have been reported with SNRIs and SSRIs. Discontinue Savella and initiate supportive treatment (5.2, 7)

- Elevated blood pressure and heart rate: Cases have been reported with Savella. Monitor blood pressure and heart rate prior to initiating treatment with Savella and periodically throughout treatment (5.3, 5.4)
- Seizures: Cases have been reported with Savella therapy. Prescribe Savella with care in patients with a history of seizure disorder (5.5)
- Hepatotoxicity: More patients treated with Savella than with placebo experienced mild elevations of ALT and AST. Rarely, fulminant hepatitis has been reported in patients treated with Savella. Avoid concomitant use of Savella in patients with substantial alcohol use or chronic liver disease (5.6)
- Discontinuation: Withdrawal symptoms have been reported in patients when discontinuing treatment with Savella. A gradual dose reduction is recommended (5.7)
- Abnormal Bleeding: Savella may increase the risk of bleeding events. Caution patients about the risk of bleeding associated with the concomitant use of Savella and NSAIDs, aspirin, or other drugs that affect coagulation (5.9)
- Male patients with a history of obstructive uropathies may experience higher rates of genitourinary adverse events (5.11)

--------------------ADVERSE REACTIONS--------------------
The most frequently occurring adverse reactions (≥ 5% and greater than placebo) were nausea, headache, constipation, dizziness, insomnia, hot flush, hyperhidrosis, vomiting, palpitations, heart rate increased, dry mouth, and hypertension (6.3)

To report SUSPECTED ADVERSE REACTIONS, contact Forest Pharmaceuticals, Inc., at (800) 678-1605 or FDA at 1-800-FDA-1088 or www.fda.gov/medwatch.

--------------------DRUG INTERACTIONS--------------------
- Savella is unlikely to be involved in clinically significant pharmacokinetic drug interactions (7)
- Pharmacodynamic interactions of Savella with other drugs can occur (7)

-------------USE IN SPECIFIC POPULATIONS--------------
- Pregnancy and nursing mothers: Use only if the potential benefit justifies the potential risk to the fetus or child (8.1, 8.3)
- To enroll in the Savella Pregnancy Registry call 1-877-643-3010 (toll free) or download data forms from the registry website: www.savellapregnancyregistry.com (8.1)

See 17 for PATIENT COUNSELING INFORMATION and Medication Guide.
Revised: May 2010

• Figure 2.37
Excerpt from package insert for Savella.

9. Fill in the following table with the equivalent times.

Standard Time	Military Time
7:30 A.M.	_____
_____	1743h
_____	2400h
8:20 P.M.	_____
_____	1257h
10:30 P.M.	_____
_____	1532h
4:15 A.M.	_____
_____	0004h
9:12 A.M.	_____

10. Interpret the following drug orders:
    (a) Norvasc (amlodipine) 10 mg PO daily, hold for SBP below 100
    (b) morphine sulfate 5 mg subcut q4h prn moderate-severe pain
    (c) Methergine (methylergonovine maleate) 0.2 mg IM stat, then 0.2 mg PO q6h for six doses
    (d) Ceftin (cefuroxime axetil) 1.5 g IVPB 30 minutes before surgery, then 750 milligrams IVPB q8h for 24h
    (e) heparin 5,000 units subcut q12h

11. Determine which part is missing for each of the following drug orders:
    (a) *cephalexin 500 mg q12h*
    (b) *Ziagen (abacavir sulfate) 300 mg PO*
    (c) *Vasotec (enalapril) via PEG hold for HR less than 60 and SBP less than 100*
    (d) *hydrocortisone sodium succinate 140 mg IVPB*
    (e) *acetaminophen PO*

Additional Exercises

Now, test yourself!

Use the information from drug labels in • **Figures 2.38** to **2.42** to complete Exercises 1 to 5.

1. Write the generic name for Kaletra.

   _____

2. Write the trade name for the drug whose NDC number is 0006-0117-54.

   _____

3. What is the total amount of solution in the bottle of Kaletra?

   _____

4. What is the dosage strength of Biaxin?

   _____

5. What is the dosage strength of the drug whose NDC number is 0006-0749-54?

   _____

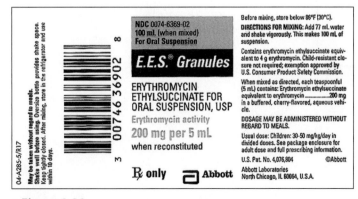

• **Figure 2.38**
Drug label for E.E.S. granules.

Workspace

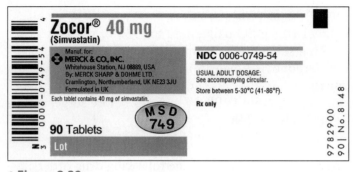

• Figure 2.39
Drug label for Zocor.

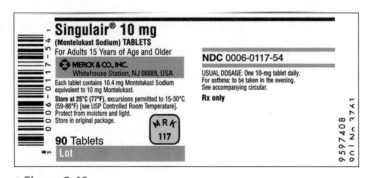

• Figure 2.40
Drug label for Singulair.

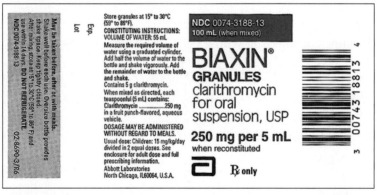

• Figure 2.41
Drug label for Biaxin.

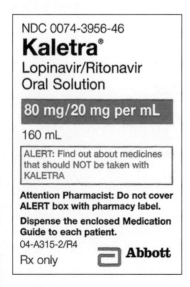

• Figure 2.42
Drug label for Kaletra.

6. Study the MAR in • **Figures 2.43a** and **2.43b** and answer the questions.

(a) Which drugs were administered at 10 p.m. on 12/10/2013?

_____

(b) Designate the time of the day the patient received ibandronate sodium.

_____

(c) How many doses of Dilantin were administered to the patient by nurse Young?

_____

(d) What drugs must be taken before breakfast?

_____

(e) What is the last date on which the patient will receive Bactrim?

_____

UNIVERSITY HOSPITAL

324689
Jane Ambery
2336 17th Avenue
Brooklyn, NY 10001

12/7/2013
5/01/47
Protestant
HIP

DAILY MEDICATION ADMINISTRATION RECORD

Dr. Mae Ling

PATIENT NAME _Jane Ambery_

ROOM # _112_

IF ANOTHER RECORDS IS IN USE ☐

ALLERGIC TO (RECORD IN RED): _sulfa, fish_

DATES GIVEN ⬇ MONTH/DAY   YEAR: _2013_

RED CHECK INITIAL	ORDER DATE	INITIAL	EXP DATE	MEDICATION, DOSAGE, FREQUENCY AND ROUTE	TIME	12/7	12/8	12/9	12/10	12/11	12/12	12/13
	12/7	MC	12/13	Dilantin (phenytoin) 100 mg	10AM	MC	MC	MC	MC			
				PO t.i.d.	2PM	MC	MC	MC	MC			
					6PM	JY	JY	JY	JY			
	12/7	SG	12/16	Bactrim DS 2tabs PO q12h	8AM	SG	SG	SG	SG			
				for 10 days	8PM	JY	JY	JY	JY			
	12/7	SG	12/13	Bonivar (ibandronate sodium)	6AM	SG	SG	SG	SG			
				2.5 mg PO daily. Take 60 minutes								
				before first food or drink of day								
				(except plain water)								
	12/7	SG	12/13	Humulin N insulin 15 units subcut	7:30AM	SG	SG	SG	SG			
				every morning								
				30 minutes before breakfast								
	12/7	SG	12/13	Humulin R insulin 8 units subcut	7:30AM	SG	SG	SG	SG			
				every morning								
				30 minutes before breakfast								

INT.	NURSES' FULL SIGNATURE AND TITLE	INT.	NURSES' FULL SIGNATURE AND TITLE
SG	Sara Gordon, RN		
MC	Marie Colon, RN		
JY	Jim Young, RN		

• **Figure 2.43a**
Medication Administration Record for Jane Ambery.

Workspace

Figure 2.43b
Medication Administration Record for Jane Ambery.

7. Study the physician's order sheet in • **Figure 2.44** and then answer the following questions.

   (a) Which drugs are ordered to be given once daily?

   _____

   (b) Which drug should be given four times a day?

   _____

   (c) What is the dose and route of administration of metoclopramide?

   _____

   (d) What is the route of administration for Duragesic?

   _____

   (e) Which drug is given every 12 hours?

   _____

8. Use the package insert shown in • **Figure 2.45** to answer the following questions.

   (a) What is an appropriate dose for use as a single-agent in non–small cell lung cancer?

   _____

   (b) What are the most common adverse reactions with single-agent use?

   _____

(c) Should the patient be instructed to take folic acid before Alimta is administered?

_____

(d) What is the route of administration of this drug?

_____

PHYSICIAN'S ORDERS

ORDER DATE	DATE DISC			
4/20/13	4/30/13	Omnicef (cefdinir) 300 mg PO q12h for 10 days		
4/20/13	4/27/13	digoxin 0.125 mg PO daily		
4/20/13	4/27/13	Glucophage (metformin HCl) 850 mg PO b.i.d. with breakfast and dinner		
4/20/13	4/27/13	Reglan (metoclopramide) 10 mg PO 30 minutes before meals and at bedtime		
4/20/13	4/23/13	Duragesic transdermal film ER 25 mg per hour. Remove in 72 hours.		
4/20/13	4/27/13	Lasix 40 mg PO daily		

PLEASE INDICATE BEEPER # →   222

2/28/52 Episcopal Aetna   *4/20/2013*

Jane Myers 23 College Ave Salt Lake City Utah 46022   *Dr. Juan Rodriguez #212332*

• **Figure 2.44**
Physician's order sheet for patient Jane Myers.

HIGHLIGHTS OF PRESCRIBING INFORMATION

These highlights do not include all the information needed to use ALIMTA safely and effectively. See full prescribing information for ALIMTA.

ALIMTA (pemetrexed disodium) Injection, Powder, Lyophilized, For Solution for Intravenous Use

Initial U.S. Approval: 2004

------------------------- INDICATIONS AND USAGE -------------------------

ALIMTA® is a folate analog metabolic inhibitor indicated for:
- Locally Advanced or Metastatic Nonsquamous Non-Small Cell Lung Cancer:
  - Initial treatment in combination with cisplatin. (1.1)
  - Maintenance treatment of patients whose disease has not progressed after four cycles of platinum-based first-line chemotherapy. (1.2)
  - After prior chemotherapy as a single-agent. (1.3)
- Mesothelioma: in combination with cisplatin. (1.4)

Limitations of Use:
- ALIMTA is not indicated for the treatment of patients with squamous cell non-small cell lung cancer. (1.5)

--------------------- DOSAGE AND ADMINISTRATION ---------------------
- Combination use in Non-Small Cell Lung Cancer and Mesothelioma: Recommended dose of ALIMTA is 500 mg/m^2 i.v. on Day 1 of each 21-day cycle in combination with cisplatin 75 mg/m^2 i.v. beginning 30 minutes after ALIMTA administration. (2.1)
- Single-Agent use in Non-Small Cell Lung Cancer: Recommended dose of ALIMTA is 500 mg/m^2 i.v. on Day 1 of each 21-day cycle. (2.2)
- Dose Reductions: Dose reductions or discontinuation may be needed based on toxicities from the preceding cycle of therapy. (2.4)

--------------------- DOSAGE FORMS AND STRENGTHS ---------------------
- 100 mg vial for injection (3)
- 500 mg vial for injection (3)

--------------------------- CONTRAINDICATIONS ---------------------------
History of severe hypersensitivity reaction to pemetrexed. (4)

----------------------- WARNINGS AND PRECAUTIONS -----------------------
- Premedication regimen: Instruct patients to take folic acid and vitamin B$_{12}$. Pretreatment with dexamethasone or equivalent reduces cutaneous reaction. (5.1)
- Bone marrow suppression: Reduce doses for subsequent cycles based on hematologic and nonhematologic toxicities. (5.2)
- Renal function: Do not administer when CrCl <45 mL/min. (2.4, 5.3)
- NSAIDs with renal insufficiency: Use caution in patients with mild to moderate renal insufficiency (CrCl 45-79 mL/min). (5.4)
- Lab monitoring: Do not begin next cycle unless ANC ≥1500 cells/mm^3, platelets ≥100,000 cells/mm^3, and CrCl ≥45 mL/min. (5.5)
- Pregnancy: Fetal harm can occur when administered to a pregnant woman. Women should be advised to use effective contraception measures to prevent pregnancy during treatment with ALIMTA. (5.6)

----------------------------- ADVERSE REACTIONS -----------------------------

The most common adverse reactions (incidence ≥20%) with single-agent use are fatigue, nausea, and anorexia. Additional common adverse reactions when used in combination with cisplatin include vomiting, neutropenia, leukopenia, anemia, stomatitis/pharyngitis, thrombocytopenia, and constipation. (6.1)

To report SUSPECTED ADVERSE REACTIONS, contact Eli Lilly and Company at 1-800-LillyRx (1-800-545-5979) or FDA at 1-800-FDA-1088 or www.fda.gov/medwatch.

----------------------------- DRUG INTERACTIONS -----------------------------
- NSAIDs: Use caution with ibuprofen or other NSAIDs. (7.1)
- Nephrotoxic drugs: Concomitant use of these drugs and/or substances which are tubularly secreted may result in delayed clearance. (7.2)

See 17 for PATIENT COUNSELING INFORMATION and FDA-approved patient labeling

Revised: 08/2010

• **Figure 2.45**
Excerpt of package insert for Alimta.

9. Fill in the following table with the equivalent times.

Standard Time	Military Time
9 A.M.	_____
_____	1500h
_____	1200h
6 P.M.	_____
_____	2015h
2:30 A.M.	_____
_____	1645h
6 A.M.	_____
_____	0000h

10. Interpret the following drug orders:
    (a) *digoxin 0.25 mg PO daily, hold if heart rate less then 60*
    (b) *Toradol (ketorolac) 15 mg IVP q6h × 4 doses*
    (c) *Milk of Magnesia 30 mL PO daily prn constipation*
    (d) *ibuprofen 800 mg PO t.i.d.*
    (e) *Novolin R insulin 5 units subcut stat*

11. Determine which part is missing for each of the following drug orders:
    (a) *Amoxicillin 500 mg q.i.d.*
    (b) *enalapril 10 mg via NGT daily*
    (c) *metoprolol 25 mg via PEG hold for HR less than 60 and SBP less than 100*
    (d) *Solu-Medrol 60 mg IVPB*
    (e) *aspirin po daily*

Dimensional Analysis and Ratio & Proportion

Learning Outcomes

$$\frac{2\,h}{1} \times \frac{60\ \text{min}}{1\,h}$$

After completing this chapter, you will be able to

1. Solve simple problems by using both Dimensional Analysis and Ratio & Proportion.
2. Identify some common units of measurement and their abbreviations.
3. Construct unit fractions and ratios from equivalences.
4. Convert a quantity expressed with a single unit of measurement to an equivalent quantity with another single unit of measurement.
5. Convert a quantity expressed as a rate to another rate.
6. Solve complex problems using both Dimensional Analysis and Ratio & Proportion.

I n this chapter, you will learn to use both *Dimensional Analysis* and *Ratio & Proportion* methods. Both methods are standard approaches to drug calculations that largely free you from the need to memorize formulas. Once these techniques are mastered, you will be able to calculate drug dosages quickly and safely. A third method, the Formula method, will be presented in Chapter 6. Students will chose the method with which they are most comfortable.

Dimensional Analysis

Introduction to Dimensional Analysis

In courses such as chemistry and physics, students learn to routinely change a quantity in one unit of measurement to an equivalent quantity in a different unit of measurement by cancelling matching units of measurement. The name Dimensional Analysis was chosen because the units of measure (e.g., feet and inches) are called *dimensions*, and these dimensions have to be *analyzed* to see how to do the problems.

The Mathematical Foundation for Dimensional Analysis

Dimensional Analysis relies on two simple mathematical concepts.

Concept 1   When a nonzero quantity is divided by the same amount, the result is 1.

For example: $7 \div 7 = 1$

Because you can also write a division problem in fractional form, you get

$$\frac{7}{7} = 1$$

Because $\frac{7}{7}$ is a fraction equal to 1, and the word "unit" means one, the fraction $\frac{7}{7}$ is called a **unit fraction**.

In the preceding unit fraction, you may *cancel* the 7s on the top and bottom. That is, you can divide both numerator and denominator by 7.

$$\frac{\cancel{7}}{\cancel{7}} = \frac{1}{1} = 1$$

Units of measurement are the "labels," such as *inches, feet, minutes,* and *hours*, which are sometimes written after a number. They are also referred to as **dimensions**, or simply **units**. For example, in the quantity 7 *days, days* is the unit of measurement.

The equivalent quantities you divide may contain **units of measurement.** For example: 7 days ÷ 7 days = 1

Or in fractional form: $\dfrac{7 \text{ days}}{7 \text{ days}} = 1$

In the preceding unit fraction, you may cancel the number 7 and the unit of measurement *days* on the top and bottom and obtain the following:

$$\frac{\cancel{7 \text{ days}}}{\cancel{7 \text{ days}}} = \frac{1}{1} = 1$$

Going one step further, now consider this *equivalence:* **7 days = 1 week**.

Because 7 *days* is the same quantity of time as 1 *week*, when you divide these quantities, you must get 1.

So, both 7 days ÷ 1 week = 1 **and** 1 week ÷ 7 days = 1

Or in unit fractional form: $\dfrac{7 \text{ days}}{1 \text{ week}} = 1$ **and** $\dfrac{1 \text{ week}}{7 \text{ days}} = 1$

Other unit fractions can be obtained from the equivalences found in Table 3.1.

Table 3.1 Equivalents for Common Units

12 inches (in)	=	1 foot (ft)
2 pints (pt)	=	1 quart (qt)
16 ounces (oz)	=	1 pound (lb)
60 seconds (sec)	=	1 minute (min)
60 minutes (min)	=	1 hour (h or hr)
24 hours (h or hr)	=	1 day (d)
7 days (d)	=	1 week (wk)
12 months (mon)	=	1 year (yr)

Concept 2   When a quantity is multiplied by 1, the quantity is unchanged.

In the following examples, the quantity 2 *weeks* will be multiplied by the number 1 and also by the unit fractions $\dfrac{7}{7}$, $\dfrac{7\text{ days}}{7\text{ days}}$, and $\dfrac{7\text{ days}}{1\text{ week}}$

$$2 \text{ weeks} \times 1 = \qquad\qquad 2 \text{ weeks}$$

$$2 \text{ weeks} \times \frac{7}{7} = 2 \text{ weeks} \times 1 = 2 \text{ weeks}$$

$$2 \text{ weeks} \times \frac{7 \text{ days}}{7 \text{ days}} = 2 \text{ weeks} \times 1 = 2 \text{ weeks}$$

$$2 \text{ weeks} \times \frac{7 \text{ days}}{1 \text{ week}} = 2 \text{ weeks} \times 1 = 2 \text{ weeks}$$

Consider the previous line again. This time you cancel the *week(s)!*

$$2 \text{ weeks} = 2 \text{ weeks} \times \frac{7 \text{ days}}{1 \text{ week}} = (2 \times 7) \text{ days} = 14 \text{ days}$$

So, 2 weeks = 14 days.

This shows how to convert a quantity measured in weeks (2 *weeks*) to an equivalent quantity measured in days (14 *days*). With the Dimensional Analysis method, you will be multiplying quantities by unit fractions to convert the units of measure. This procedure demonstrates the basic technique of Dimensional Analysis.

Many of the problems in dosage calculation require changing a quantity with a *single unit of measurement* into an equivalent quantity with a different *single unit of measurement*; for example, changing 2 *weeks* to 14 *days* as was shown.

Changing a Single Unit of Measurement to Another Single Unit of Measurement

Simple (One-Step) Problems with Single Units of Measurement Using Dimensional Analysis

Suppose you want to express 18 *months* in *years*. That is, you want to convert 18 *months* to an equivalent amount of time in *years*.

This is a **simple** problem. Simple problems have only three elements. The elements in this problem are

The given quantity:	18 months
The quantity you want to find:	? years
An equivalence between them:	1 year = 12 months

To begin the Dimensional Analysis process in a logical way, write the quantity you are given (18 *months*) on the left of an equal sign and the unit you want to change it to (*years*) on the right side, as follows:

$$18 \text{ months} = ? \text{ years}$$

It may help to write 18 *months* as the fraction $\dfrac{18 \text{ months}}{1}$

Thus, you now have

$$\frac{18 \text{ months}}{1} = ? \text{ years}$$

Formulate the Appropriate Unit Fraction To change *months* to *years*, you need an equivalence between *months* and *years*. That equivalence is

$$12 \text{ months} = 1 \text{ year}$$

From this equivalence, you can get two possible unit fractions:

$$\frac{12 \text{ months}}{1 \text{ year}} \quad \text{and} \quad \frac{1 \text{ year}}{12 \text{ months}}$$

But which of these fractions shall you choose? If you multiply $\dfrac{18 \text{ months}}{1}$ by the first of these fractions, you get

$$\frac{18 \text{ months}}{1} \times \frac{12 \text{ months}}{1 \text{ year}}$$

Notice that both the *months* units are in the numerators of the fractions.

Because no cancellation of the units is possible in this case, do not select this unit fraction.

If instead you multiply by the second of the unit fractions, you get the following:

$$\frac{18 \text{ months}}{1} \times \frac{1 \text{ year}}{12 \text{ months}} = ? \text{ years}$$

Notice that now *one of the months is in the numerator (top), and the other months is in the denominator (bottom) of a fraction.* Because cancellation of the *months* is now possible, this is the appropriate unit fraction to choose.

Cancel the Units of Measurement $\dfrac{18 \text{ months}}{1} \times \dfrac{1 \text{ year}}{12 \text{ months}} = ?$ years

After you cancel the *months*, notice that *year* (the unit of measurement that you want to find) is the only remaining unit on the left side.

$$\frac{18 \text{ months}}{1} \times \frac{1 \text{ year}}{12 \text{ months}} = ? \text{ years}$$

Cancel the Numbers and Finish the Multiplication After you are sure that you have *only the unit of measurement that you want (years) remaining on the left side and that it is on the top of a fraction,* you can complete the cancellation and multiplication of the numbers as follows:

$$\frac{\overset{3}{18 \text{ months}}}{1} \times \frac{1 \text{ year}}{\underset{2}{12 \text{ months}}} = \frac{3 \text{ years}}{2} \quad \text{or} \quad 1\frac{1}{2} \text{ years}$$

So, 18 *months* is equivalent to $1\frac{1}{2}$ *years.*

Ratio & Proportion

Ratios

A **ratio** compares two quantities. Ratios can be expressed in a variety of ways, including fractional form. For this reason, fractions are sometimes referred to as *rati*onal numbers.

Suppose a recipe indicates that 1 cup of sugar and 2 cups of flour are needed to make a certain type of cake. The relative amounts of sugar and flour in the cake are crucial to its quality. To compare the amount of sugar to the amount of flour in this recipe, any of the following equivalent *sugar-flour ratios* could be used:

> 1 cup of sugar *for every* 2 cups of flour
> 1 cup of sugar *per* 2 cups of flour
> 1 cup of sugar *to* 2 cups of flour
> 1 cup *to* 2 cups
> 1 to 2
> 1:2
> $\frac{1}{2}$

On the other hand, to compare the amount of flour to the amount of sugar in this recipe, the following equivalent *flour-sugar ratios* could be used:

> 2 cups of flour *for every* 1 cup of sugar
> 2 cups of flour *per* 1 cup of sugar
> 2 cups of flour *to* 1 cup of sugar
> 2 cups *to* 1 cup
> 2 to 1
> 2:1
> $\frac{2}{1}$

As you can see, the order of the numbers in the flour-sugar ratio is the reverse of the order in the sugar-flour ratio.

Now, if twice the amount of this cake were needed, the baker would need to double the amount of each of the ingredients in the recipe.

Therefore, instead of

1 cup of sugar and 2 cups of flour,
2 cups of sugar and 4 cups of flour

would be required, and the *sugar-flour ratio* would now be 2 to 4. Although the quantities of sugar and flour have each been increased, the ratio of sugar to flour has not changed; the ratio 1:2 is equivalent to the ratio 2:4. It is easy to see this equivalency when both the ratios are written in fractional form because $\frac{1}{2} = \frac{2}{4}$.

Recall that in Chapter 1 both *building and reducing* fractions were discussed, and $\frac{1}{2}$ could be "*built*" into $\frac{2}{4}$ by multiplying both numerator and denominator by 2, as follows:

$$\frac{1}{2} = \frac{1 \times 2}{2 \times 2} = \frac{2}{4}$$

Similarly, $\frac{2}{4}$ could be "*reduced*" to $\frac{1}{2}$ by dividing both numerator and denominator by 2 as follows:

$$\frac{2}{4} = \frac{2 \div 2}{4 \div 2} = \frac{1}{2}$$

So, $\frac{1}{2}$ and $\frac{2}{4}$ are equivalent ratios.

Next, suppose that three times the amount of the cake were needed. The baker would need to multiply the amount of each ingredient in the recipe by three.

Therefore, instead of using

1 cup of sugar and 2 cups of flour,
3 cups of sugar and 6 cups of flour

would be required.

Continuing this process, a table could be constructed showing the amount of sugar and the corresponding amount of flour needed in order to make various amounts of this cake. See Table 3.2.

Table 3.2 **Some Corresponding Amounts of Sugar and Flour for a 1 to 2 Sugar-Flour Ratio**	
Cups of Sugar	**Cups of Flour**
1	2
2	4
3	6
4	8
5	10
6	12

EXAMPLE 3.1

Suppose a recipe indicates that 1 cup of sugar and 2 cups of flour are needed to make a certain type of cake. If the baker wants to make some of this cake and decides to use 10 cups of flour, how much sugar would be needed?

Cups of Sugar	Cups of Flour
1	2
2	4
3	6
4	8
⑤ ←	⑩
6	12

The baker could look at Table 3.2 and see that for 10 cups of flour, 5 cups of sugar are needed.

Another way to solve the problem is to realize that the amount of flour (10 cups) is 5 times the amount of flour (2 cups) in the recipe. Whenever the amount of flour in the recipe is multiplied by 5, the amount of sugar in the recipe must also be multiplied by 5. So, the terms in the ratio of

1 cup of sugar to 2 cups of flour

are each multiplied by 5 to yield

5 cups of sugar to 10 cups of flour

and 5 cups of sugar would be needed.

EXAMPLE 3.2

Mary prepares her morning coffee by combining 5 parts black coffee with 2 parts milk.

(a)   What is the black coffee-milk ratio expressed in colon [:] form and in fractional form?

(b)   Mary wants to make some of her morning coffee and take it along in a thermos bottle. If she used 8 ounces of milk, how much black coffee must be added to the bottle?

(a)   The drink has 5 parts black coffee to 2 parts milk. This is a ratio of *5 parts to 2 parts* or a ratio of *5 to 2*. This ratio can also be written in colon form as *5:2* or in fractional form as $\frac{5}{2}$.

(b)   A table could be constructed showing the amount of black coffee and the corresponding amount of milk needed to make various amounts of this drink. See Table 3.3.

Table 3.3	**Some Corresponding Amounts of Black Coffee and Milk in a 5 to 2 Ratio**

Ounces of Black Coffee	**Ounces of Milk**
5	2
10	4
15	6
20	8
25	10
30	12

Mary could look at Table 3.3 and see that for 8 ounces of milk, 20 ounces of black coffee are needed.

Ounces of Black Coffee	**Ounces of Milk**
5	2
10	4
15	6
(20) ←	(8)
25	10
30	12

Rates

Rates are like ratios except that they compare two quantities with *different units of measurement.*

For example, a car might be traveling on a highway at a constant rate of speed of *50 miles per hour.* This rate has two different units of measurement, *miles* and *hours.* To compare the number of *miles* traveled to the number of *hours* driven, any of the following equivalent *rates of speed* could be used:

> 50 miles for every 1 hour driven
> 50 miles per each hour driven
> 50 miles per hour
> 50 miles : 1 hour
> 50 miles/1 hour
> 50 miles/hour

Notice that if the car drove twice the number of hours (2 hours), then the car would travel twice the distance (100 miles). However, the rate of speed would be the same.

Now, consider a worker's rate of pay. Suppose the pay rate is $60 for every 2 hours worked. To compare the amount of *dollars* paid to the number of *hours* worked, any of the following equivalent *rates of pay* could be used:

$60 for every 2 hours worked

$60 per 2 hours

$60:2 hours

$60/2 hours

$30 for every 1 hour worked

$30 per hour

$30:1 hour

$30/hour

Notice that if a person worked 2 hours for $60, or if the person worked 1 hour for $30, the rate of pay would be the same.

EXAMPLE 3.3

Each can of cola contains 12 ounces.

(a) How many ounces are contained in 6 cans?

(b) How many cans would contain 18 ounces?

Cans of Cola	Ounces of Cola
1	12
2	24
3	36
4	48
5	60
6 →	72

(a) A table could be constructed showing the number of 12-ounce cans and the corresponding number of ounces. The last line of the table indicates that 6 cans contain 72 ounces.

Another way to do the problem is to realize that the rate is 12 ounces per 1 can. In this case the number of cans is multiplied by 6, so the number of ounces must also be multiplied by 6.

So, the terms in the rate of

12 ounces per 1 can

are each multiplied by 6 to yield

72 ounces per 6 cans

(b) If the number of cans in the rate is multiplied by $\frac{1}{2}$, the number of ounces must also be multiplied by $\frac{1}{2}$.

So, the terms in the rate of

12 ounces per 1 can

are each multiplied by $\frac{1}{2}$ to yield

6 ounces per $\frac{1}{2}$ can

Put these two rates into a table as follows:

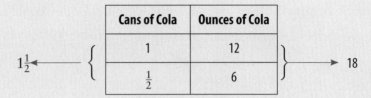

Cans of Cola	Ounces of Cola
1	12
$\frac{1}{2}$	6

By adding the two rows of the preceding table, it can be concluded that 18 ounces of cola are contained in $1\frac{1}{2}$ cans.

EXAMPLE 3.4

(a) An object is moving at a rate of 72 inches in 2 hours. Express this rate in terms of inches/hour.

(b) An object is moving at a rate of 240 inches per hour. Express this rate in terms of inches/min.

(c) An object is moving at a rate of 2 feet per minute. Express this rate in terms of feet/hour.

You can do this problem in many different ways.

(a) The rate *72 inches in 2 hours*, in fractional form, is $\frac{72\ in}{2\ h}$.

It is already in the form of inches/hour, so merely reduce the fraction as follows:

$$\frac{72\ in}{2\ h} = \frac{72}{2}\ \frac{in}{h} = 36\ in/h$$

(b) To change *240 inches/hour* to *inches/minute*, substitute 60 minutes for 1 hour as follows:

$$\frac{240\ in}{1\ h} = \frac{240\ in}{60\ min} = \frac{240}{60}\ \frac{in}{min} = 4\ in/min$$

(c) To change *2 feet/minute* to *feet/hour*, multiply both numerator and denominator by 60 because 60 min = 1h.

$$\frac{2\ ft \times 60}{1\ min \times 60} = \frac{120\ ft}{60\ min} = \frac{120\ ft}{1\ h} = 120\ ft/h$$

Proportions

A **proportion** is a statement or equation indicating that two ratios or two rates are equal. For example,

$$\frac{2}{4} = \frac{5}{10}\ \text{is a proportion.}$$

True proportions have an interesting property. If the true proportion is written in fractional form, when you cross multiply, the products obtained are equal.

Cross multiply:

$$\frac{2}{4} = \frac{5}{10}$$

$$(5)(4) = (2)(10)$$

$$20 = 20$$

The products each equal 20.

The proportion $\frac{2}{4} = \frac{5}{10}$ may also be written using the colon form as follows:

$$2 : 4 = 5 : 10$$

In this form, the equivalent to cross multiplication is to multiply the means and the extremes (inside numbers and outside numbers) as follows:

$$2 \times 10 = 20$$

$$2 : 4 = 5 : 10$$

$$4 \times 5 = 20$$

Again, these products are both equal to 20.

EXAMPLE 3.5

Verify that $\frac{30}{1,000} = \frac{6}{200}$ is a true proportion.

To verify that this proportion is true, cross multiply. If the products obtained are equal, then the proportion is true.

Cross multiply

$$\frac{30}{1,000} = \frac{6}{200}$$

$$(6)(1000) = (30)(200)$$

$$6,000 = 6,000$$

Because the products are equal, it is a true proportion.

EXAMPLE 3.6

Is $\frac{30}{120} = \frac{6}{18}$ a true portion?

To determine if this proportion is true, cross multiply. If the products obtained are equal, then the proportion is true.

Cross multiply

$$\frac{30}{120} = \frac{6}{18}$$

$$(6)(120) = (30)(18)$$

$$720 \neq 540$$

Because the products are not equal, $\frac{30}{120} = \frac{6}{18}$ is not a true proportion.

The Mathematics Needed to Solve Proportions

Your first step toward understanding how to solve proportions is a review of a few basic arithmetic and algebraic concepts.

Using Parentheses to Indicate Multiplication

In algebra, letters are used to stand for numbers. The letter x is the symbol most commonly used to represent an unknown number, but the times sign $\times$ is also a symbol for multiplication. To avoid confusion between the two meanings of the same symbol, *the times sign $\times$ will generally be avoided* throughout the remainder of the textbook. Instead of using $\times$ to represent multiplication, a pair of parentheses will be used.

So, $3 \times 4 = 12$ will often be written as $(3)(4) = 12$.

Multiplying by 1

The rules of algebra are generalizations of the rules of arithmetic. In arithmetic, when 1 is multiplied by 7, the result is 7. When 1 is multiplied by 52, the result is 52. In general, *when 1 is multiplied by any number, the result is that same number*. In algebraic terms, 1 multiplied by x equals x. This can be summarized as:

$$(1)(x) = x$$

Dividing by 1

In arithmetic, when 9 is divided by 1 the result is 9, and when 23 is divided by 1 the result is 23. In general, *when any number is divided by 1 the result is that same number*. In algebraic terms, x divided by 1 equals x. This can be summarized as:

$$\frac{x}{1} = x$$

Shorthand for Multiplication

When a known number is multiplied by an unknown number, 7 times x, for example, this product could be represented as $(7)(x)$. The product of the two numbers (7) and (x) is usually written in the shorthand $7x$. This can be summarized as:

$$(7)(x) = 7x$$

EXAMPLE 3.7

Simplify the expression: $(45)(x)$

When a known number (45) is multiplied by an unknown number (x), the product may be written in the simplified shorthand form of $45x$.

Commutative Property

In arithmetic, when you multiply numbers, the order of the factors does not matter. You may **commute** the factors (*switch their positions*) without changing the product. For example,

$$3 \times 4 = 12 \quad \text{and} \quad 4 \times 3 = 12,$$

therefore,

$$3 \times 4 = 4 \times 3$$

You may want to use this commutative property when you have to multiply an unknown number by a known number. To multiply an unknown number by 12, you could write $(x)(12)$. But reversing the order of the factors gives $(12)(x)$, and the shorthand for this is $12x$.

Similarly,

$$(x)(37) = (37)(x) = 37x$$

EXAMPLE 3.8

Simplify the expression: $(x)(13)$

Because the order does not matter when you multiply two numbers, you may write

$$(x)(13) \text{ as } (13)(x)$$

The shorthand for $(13)(x)$ is $13x$.

Cancelling

In arithmetic a fraction can be reduced by cancelling. For example, the fraction $\frac{21}{28}$ could be reduced as follows. Write the numerator and denominator in factored form.

$$\frac{21}{28} = \frac{(7)(3)}{(7)(4)}$$

Now cancel the (7)s.

$$\frac{21}{28} = \frac{(\cancel{7})(3)}{(\cancel{7})(4)} = \frac{3}{4}$$

So, $\frac{21}{28} = \frac{3}{4}$

This cancelling technique will be used in solving simple equations.

Solving Simple Equations

In the process of solving proportions, you will frequently encounter simple equations like:

$$3x = 6$$

This equation states that 3 times a number equals 6. To solve this equation means to find a value of x that will make the equation true. Because 3 times 2 equals 6, the solution is 2.

Not every simple equation can easily be solved mentally. So, the technique for solving such equations is to manipulate them so that x is alone on one side of the equal sign. This can be accomplished by dividing both sides of the equation by the **coefficient of x** (the number multiplying the x).

$$\textcircled{3}x = 6$$

coefficient of x

In the term $3x$, the coefficient of x is 3, so you should divide both sides of the equation by 3.

$$\frac{3x}{3} = \frac{6}{3}$$

Now cancel the 3s

$$\frac{\cancel{3}x}{\cancel{3}} = \frac{6}{3}$$

This gives

$$x = \frac{6}{3}$$

Simplify $\frac{6}{3}$

$$x = 2$$

EXAMPLE 3.9

Solve the equation $5x = 35$

To solve this equation means to find the value of x that will make the equation true. The technique is to manipulate the equation so that x is alone on one side of the equation. This can be accomplished by dividing both sides of the equation by the coefficient of x, which is 5 in this case.

$$\textcircled{5}x = 35$$

coefficient of x

Divide by 5

$$\frac{5x}{5} = \frac{35}{5}$$

Now cancel

$$\frac{\cancel{5}x}{\cancel{5}} = \frac{35}{5}$$

This gives

$$x = 7$$

Solving Proportions

Throughout the textbook you will encounter **proportions** in which one of the four numbers in the proportion is unknown. For example,

$$\frac{2}{?} = \frac{5}{10}.$$

In this proportion, the denominator of the first fraction is not known. Unknown numbers are often represented by letters of the alphabet, x in particular. So this equation might also be written as

$$\frac{2}{x} = \frac{5}{10}$$

Finding this unknown number x that makes the proportion true is called "*solving the proportion.*" In general, solving a proportion involves two steps:

1. *Cross multiply* to obtain a simple equation
2. To solve the simple equation, *divide both sides of the equation by the coefficient of x*

Because the proportion is written in fractional form, when you cross multiply, the products obtained are equal.

$$\frac{2}{x} = \frac{5}{10}$$
$$(5)(x) = (2)(10)$$

Simplifying, you get the simple equation

$$5x = 20$$

Divide by 5, the coefficient of x

$$\frac{5x}{5} = \frac{20}{5}$$

Cancel

$$\frac{5x}{5} = \frac{20}{5}$$

This gives

$$x = 4$$

So, 4 is the solution of the equation.

You may *check your answer* by substituting 4 for x in the original proportion as follows:

$$\frac{2}{4} = \frac{5}{10}$$

Now cross multiply

$$\frac{2}{4} = \frac{5}{10}$$
$$(5)(4) = (2)(10)$$
$$20 = 20$$

Because the products are equal, the solution 4 is correct.

NOTE

You should always check your answers to proportion problems by substituting the answer into the proportion, cross multiplying, and seeing if the products are equal.

EXAMPLE 3.10

Solve the proportion $\frac{5}{12} = \frac{x}{6}$

The first step in solving the proportion is to cross multiply

$$\frac{5}{12} = \frac{x}{6}$$

$$(12)(x) = (5)(6)$$

Simplify

$$12x = 30$$

Divide both sides by 12, the coefficient of x

$$\frac{12x}{12} = \frac{30}{12}$$

Cancel

$$\frac{\cancel{12}x}{\cancel{12}} = \frac{30}{12}$$

This gives

$$x = \frac{30}{12}$$

Simplify

$$x = 2.5$$

EXAMPLE 3.11

Solve: $\frac{x}{26} = \frac{10.1}{13}$

Cross multiply

$$\frac{x}{26} = \frac{10.1}{13}$$

$$(10.1)(26) = 13x$$

At this point, there are two different approaches that may be used to finish the problem.

Method 1: Multiply 10.1 by 26 to obtain 262.6

$$262.6 = 13x$$

Divide both sides by 13, which is the coefficient of x

$$\frac{262.6}{13} = \frac{13x}{13}$$

Cancel

$$\frac{262.6}{13} = \frac{\cancel{13}x}{\cancel{13}}$$

Simplify

$$20.2 = x$$

Method 2: Do not multiply 10.1 by 26 to obtain 262.6, but leave the left side of the equation in factored form as follows:

$$(10.1)(26) = 13x$$

Divide both sides by 13 which is the coefficient of x

$$\frac{(10.1)(26)}{13} = \frac{13x}{13}$$

Cancel

$$\frac{(10.1)(\overset{2}{\cancel{26}})}{\underset{1}{\cancel{13}}} = \frac{\cancel{13}\,x}{\cancel{13}}$$

$$(10.1)(2) = x$$

Multiply

$$20.2 = x$$

The advantage of *Method 2* in this case is that it avoids the creation of the large number 262.6 and its subsequent division by 13.

Table 3.1 contains equivalents for several common units of measurement including the equivalence 7 *days* = 1 *week*.

This equivalence can be used to determine the solution to the problem of finding the number of weeks in 21 days. In this problem there are two quantities: *weeks* and *days*. You know that 1 week is equivalent to 7 days, and you need to find the unknown number of weeks which would contain 21 days.

Think of the problem this way:

$$7 \text{ days} = 1 \text{ week}$$

$$21 \text{ days} = ? \text{ weeks}$$

To determine if a proportion exists between *days* and *weeks*, ask yourself the question "if the number of *weeks* is doubled, is the number of *days* doubled?" If the answer were no, then days and weeks would not be proportional and a proportion would not be used to solve the problem.

But the answer is yes because for a given period of time, whenever the number of weeks is doubled, the number of days would be doubled. So the number of days and the number of weeks are proportional, and a proportion could be used to solve the problem.

The proportion could be set up in either of the following two ways:

$$\frac{weeks}{days} = \frac{weeks'}{days'}$$

or

$$\frac{days}{weeks} = \frac{days'}{weeks'}$$

The same answer will be obtained regardless of which of the two forms is used.

In mathematics the **prime notation** (') is commonly used to link together two quantities. The primed quantities are linked together, and the unprimed quantities are linked. In this case *days* and *weeks* are associated together, whereas *days'* (read, *days prime*) is associated with *weeks'*.

Because you know that 1 week equals 7 days, you can substitute those numbers, *1* and *7, for weeks* and *days*, respectively. Because you need to find the number of weeks (*x*) containing 21 days, you can substitute those quantities, *x and 21, for weeks'* and *days'*, respectively.

Substituting into the second form $\dfrac{days}{weeks} = \dfrac{days'}{weeks'}$

you obtain

$$\frac{7\ days}{1\ week} = \frac{21\ days}{x\ weeks}$$

Eliminate the units of measurement

$$\frac{7}{1} = \frac{21}{x}$$

cross multiply

$$\frac{7}{1} \diagup\!\!\!\!= \diagdown\!\!\! \frac{21}{x}$$

$$(21)(1) = (7)(x)$$

Simplify

$$21 = 7x$$

Divide both sides by 7, the coefficient of *x*

$$\frac{21}{7} = \frac{7x}{7}$$

Cancel

$$\frac{21}{7} = \frac{\cancel{7}x}{\cancel{7}}$$

Simplify

$$3 = x$$

You have just used the ratio and proportion method to convert a given amount of time measured in one unit of measurement (21 days) to an equivalent amount of time measured in another unit of measurement (3 weeks).

Simple (One-Step) Problems with Single Units of Measurement Using Ratio & Proportion

Suppose that you want to express 18 months as an equivalent amount of time measured in years. That is,

$$18\ months = ?\ years$$

Both *18 months* and *? years* are quantities that have single units of measurement. This problem can be solved by using a proportion. The steps to follow in solving a proportion problem are:

1. *Identify the two units of measurement in the problem.*
   In this problem there are two quantities: *months* and *years*.

2. *Write a known equivalence between the units of measurement.*
   You need to know that 12 months is equivalent to 1 year.

3. *Let x stand for the amount you are trying to find and write an equivalence involving x.*
   You have to find the unknown number of years (x) that would contain 18 months.

   So, think of the problem this way:

   $$12 \text{ months} = 1 \text{ year}$$

   $$18 \text{ months} = x \text{ years}$$

4. *Write a proportion using the two units of measurement.*
   Because the number of months and the number of years are proportional, a proportion could be used to solve the problem. The proportion could be set up in either of the following two ways:

   $$\frac{yr}{mon} = \frac{yr'}{mon'}$$

   or

   $$\frac{mon}{yr} = \frac{mon'}{yr'}$$

   You will get the same answer regardless of which of the two forms you use.

5. *Substitute into the proportion.*
   Because you know that 1 year equals 12 months, you can substitute those numbers, *1* and *12, for years* and *months*, respectively. And because you need to find the number of years (x) containing 18 months, you can substitute those quantities *(x and 18) for years'* and *months'*, respectively.

   Substituting into the second form $\dfrac{mon}{yr} = \dfrac{mon'}{yr'}$

   you obtain

   $$\frac{12 \text{ } mon}{1 \text{ } yr} = \frac{18 \text{ } mon}{x \text{ } yr}$$

6. *Eliminate the units of measurement*

   $$\frac{12}{1} = \frac{18}{x}$$

7. *Cross multiply*

   $$\frac{12}{1} \diagdown \frac{18}{x}$$

   $$(18)(1) = (12)(x)$$

   Simplify

   $$18 = 12x$$

8. *Divide both sides of the equation by 12, the coefficient of x.*

$$\frac{18}{12} = \frac{12x}{12}$$

9. *Cancel*

$$\frac{18}{12} = \frac{\cancel{12}x}{\cancel{12}}$$

Simplify

$$1\tfrac{1}{2} = x$$

So, 18 months is equivalent to $1\tfrac{1}{2}$ years.

10. *Check your answer.*

In the proportion, replace x by $1\tfrac{1}{2}$, cross multiply, and see if the cross products are equal.

$$\frac{12}{1} = \frac{18}{1\tfrac{1}{2}}$$

Cross multiply

$$(18)(1) = (12)(1\tfrac{1}{2})$$

Simplify

$$18 = 18$$

Because the products are equal, the answer is verified.

In summary the steps in solving a proportion are:

1. Identify the two units of measurement in the problem.
2. Write a known equivalence between the units of measure.
3. Let x stand for the amount you are trying to find and write an equivalence involving x.
4. Write a proportion using the two units of measurement.
5. Substitute into the proportion.
6. Eliminate the units.
7. Cross multiply.
8. Divide both sides of the equation by the coefficient of x (unless it is 1).
9. Cancel and simplify.
10. Check your answer by substituting and cross multiplying.

For each of the following examples, Dimensional Analysis and Ratio & Proportion methods will be shown side by side for comparison purposes.

Simple (One-Step) Problems with Single Units of Measurement

EXAMPLE 3.12

Change $2\frac{1}{4}$ *hours* to an equivalent amount of time in *minutes*.

DIMENSIONAL ANALYSIS

The elements in this problem are

The given quantity: $2\frac{1}{4}$ hours

The quantity you
want to find: ? minutes

An equivalence
between them: 1 hour = 60 minutes

$$2\frac{1}{4}\text{hours} = \text{? minutes}$$

NOTE

When a unit of measure follows a numeric fraction, write the unit of measure in the numerator (top) of the fraction. For example, write $\frac{1}{2}$ hour as $\dfrac{1 \text{ hour}}{2}$.

Avoid doing multiplication with mixed numbers; change them to improper fractions or decimal numbers. In this case, you can write $2\frac{1}{4}$ *hours* as the improper fraction $\frac{9}{4}$ *hours*. It is better to write the quantity $\frac{9}{4}$ *hours* as $\dfrac{9 \text{ hours}}{4}$ to make it clear that the unit of measurement (*hours*) is in the numerator of the fraction, not in the denominator.

So, the problem becomes $\dfrac{9 \text{ hours}}{4} = \text{? minutes}$.

Formulate the Appropriate Unit Fraction. You want to change *hours* to *minutes*, so you need an equivalence between *hours* and *minutes*. That equivalence is

1 hour = 60 minutes

RATIO & PROPORTION

In this problem there are two quantities: *minutes* and *hours*. You need to know that 60 minutes is equivalent to 1 hour, and you have to find the unknown number of minutes that would contain $2\frac{1}{4}$ hours.

So, think of the problem this way:

$$60 \text{ minutes} = 1 \text{ hour}$$
$$\text{? minutes} = 2\frac{1}{4} \text{ hours}$$

Because the number of minutes and the number of hours are proportional, a proportion could be used to solve the problem. The proportion could be set up as

$$\frac{\text{min}}{hr} = \frac{\text{min}'}{hr'}$$

Because 60 minutes equals 1 hour, you can substitute the numbers *60* and *1* for *minutes* and *hours*, respectively. And because you need to find the number of minutes (x) equal to $2\frac{1}{4}$ hours, you can substitute those quantities (x and $2\frac{1}{4}$) for *minutes'* and *hours'*, respectively.

Substituting, you get

$$\frac{60 \text{ } min}{1 \text{ } hr} = \frac{x \text{ } min}{2\frac{1}{4} \text{ } hr}$$

Eliminate the units of measurement

$$\frac{60}{1} = \frac{x}{2\frac{1}{4}}$$

Cross multiply

$$\frac{60}{1} \diagdown \frac{x}{2\frac{1}{4}}$$

$$(x)(1) = (60)(2\tfrac{1}{4})$$

Simplify

$$x = 135$$

From this equivalence, you get two possible fractions, which are both equal to 1:

$$\frac{1 \text{ hour}}{60 \text{ minutes}} \quad \text{and} \quad \frac{60 \text{ minutes}}{1 \text{ hour}}$$

But which of these fractions will lead to cancellation? Because you want to eliminate (cancel) the *hours*, and because *hours* are on the top, as follows:

$$\frac{9 \text{ hours}}{4} = ? \text{ minutes}$$

you need to multiply by the unit fraction with *hour* on the bottom, as follows:

$$\frac{9 \text{ hours}}{4} \times \frac{60 \text{ minutes}}{1 \text{ hour}} = ? \text{ minutes}$$

This is what you want because cancellation of the *hour(s)* is now possible.

Cancel the Units

$$\frac{9 \text{ hours}}{4} \times \frac{60 \text{ minutes}}{1 \text{ hour}} = ? \text{ minutes}$$

NOTE

To eliminate a particular unit of measurement in the numerator, use a unit fraction with that same unit of measurement in the denominator.

After you cancel the *hour(s)*, make sure that *minutes* (the unit you want) is the only remaining unit of measurement and that it is in a numerator (top) of a fraction.

$$\frac{9 \text{ hours}}{4} \times \frac{60 \text{ minutes}}{1 \text{ hour}} = ? \text{ minutes}$$

Cancel the Numbers and Finish the Multiplication

$$\frac{9 \text{ hours}}{\underset{1}{4}} \times \frac{\overset{15}{60} \text{ minutes}}{1 \text{ hour}} = 135 \text{ minutes}$$

So, $2\frac{1}{4}$ hours is equivalent to 135 minutes.

EXAMPLE 3.13

Change 4.5 *feet* to an equivalent length measured in *inches*.

DIMENSIONAL ANALYSIS

Given quantity: 4.5 *feet*

Quantity you want to find: ? *inches*

Equivalence between the
two quantities: $1\,foot = 12\,inches$

$$4.5\,feet = ?\,inches$$

You want to cancel the *feet* and get the answer in *inches*, so choose a fraction with *feet* (or *foot*) on the bottom and *inches* on top. You need a fraction in the form of $\dfrac{?\,inches}{?\,feet}$.

Because 1 *foot* = 12 *inches*, the fraction you need is $\dfrac{12\,inches}{1\,foot}$

$$\frac{4.5\;\cancel{feet}}{1} \times \frac{12\;inches}{1\;\cancel{foot}} = 54\;inches$$

RATIO & PROPORTION

In this problem there are two quantities: *inches* and *feet*. You need to know that 12 inches is equivalent to 1 foot, and you have to find the unknown number of inches that would be equivalent to 4.5 feet.

So, think of the problem this way:

$$12 \text{ inches} = 1 \text{ feet}$$
$$x \text{ inches} = 4.5 \text{ feet}$$

Because the number of inches and the number of feet are proportional, a proportion could be used to solve the problem. The proportion could be set up as

$$\frac{in}{ft} = \frac{in'}{ft'}$$

Because 12 inches equals 1 foot, you can substitute those numbers, *12* and *1*, for *feet* and *inches*, respectively. And because you need to find the number of inches (*x*) containing 4.5 feet, you can substitute those quantities, *x* and 4.5, for *inches'* and *feet'*, respectively.

Substituting you get

$$\frac{12\ in}{1\ ft} = \frac{x\ in}{4.5\ ft}$$

Eliminate the units of measurement

$$\frac{12}{1} = \frac{x}{4.5}$$

Cross multiply

$$\frac{12}{1} = \frac{x}{4.5}$$

$$(x)(1) = (12)(4.5)$$

Simplify

$$x = 54$$

So, 4.5 feet is equivalent to 54 inches.

EXAMPLE 3.14

An infant weighs 6 pounds 5 ounces. What is the weight of the infant in ounces?

DIMENSIONAL ANALYSIS

6 *pounds 5 ounces* means 6 pounds + 5 ounces

First, convert 6 *pounds* to *ounces*.

The given quantity: 6 pounds

The quantity you
want to find: ? ounces

An equivalence
between them: 1 pound = 16 ounces

$$6 \text{ pounds} = ? \text{ ounces}$$

$$\frac{6 \text{ pounds}}{1} = ? \text{ ounces}$$

You want to cancel *pounds* and get the answer in *ounces*. So, choose a fraction with *pounds* on the bottom and *ounces* on top; that is, a fraction that looks like $\frac{? \text{ ounces}}{? \text{ pounds}}$

Since 1 pound = 16 ounces, the fraction is $\frac{16 \text{ ounces}}{1 \text{ pounds}}$

$$\frac{6 \text{ pounds}}{1} \times \frac{16 \text{ ounces}}{1 \text{ pound}} = 96 \text{ ounces}$$

RATIO & PROPORTION

Because 6 *pounds 5 ounces* means 6 *pounds* + 5 *ounces*, you need to first convert 6 pounds to ounces.

There are two quantities: *ounces* and *pounds*. You need to know that 16 ounces is equivalent to 1 pound, and you have to find the unknown number of ounces that would be equivalent to 6 pounds.

So, think of the problem this way:

$$16 \text{ ounces} = 1 \text{ pound}$$
$$x \text{ ounces} = 6 \text{ pounds}$$

Because the number of ounces and the number of pounds are proportional, a proportion could be set up as

$$\frac{oz}{lb} = \frac{oz'}{lb'}$$

Because 16 ounces equals 1 pound, you can substitute those numbers, *16* and *1*, for *ounces* and *pound*, respectively. And because you need to find the number of ounces (*x*) containing 6 pounds, you can substitute those quantities, *x* and *6*, for *ounces'* and *pound'*, respectively.

Substituting, you get

$$\frac{16 \text{ } oz}{1 \text{ } lb} = \frac{x \text{ } oz}{6 \text{ } lb}$$

Eliminate the units of measurement and cross multiply

$$\frac{16}{1} = \frac{x}{6}$$

$$(x)(1) = (16)(6)$$

Simplify

$$x = 96$$

Because 6 pounds equals 96 ounces, the infant weighs 96 ounces + 5 ounces, or 101 ounces.

As part of Example 3.14, the number of ounces that is equivalent to 6 pounds was found. The proportion used was in the form:

(1)
$$\frac{oz}{lb} = \frac{oz'}{lb'}$$

Other proportions which students may choose to use to solve the problem are:

(2)
$$\frac{lb}{oz} = \frac{lb'}{oz'}$$

(3)
$$\frac{oz}{oz'} = \frac{lb}{lb'}$$

(4)
$$\frac{lb}{lb'} = \frac{oz}{oz'}$$

Any of these forms will give the correct answer. However, for simplicity, this textbook uses only types 1 and 2.

Both Dimensional Analysis and Ratio & Proportion can be applied to a wide variety of problems, as illustrated in the next example.

EXAMPLE 3.15

Suppose that the currency exchange rate in Mexico is 0.076 *U.S. dollar* for 1 *Mexican peso*. At this rate how many *Mexican pesos* would be exchanged for 190 *U.S. dollars*?

DIMENSIONAL ANALYSIS

Given quantity: 190 *dollars*

Quantity you want
to find: ? *pesos*

Equivalence
between them: 0.076 *dollar* = 1 *peso*

$$190 \ dollars = ? \ pesos$$

You want to cancel the *dollars* and get the answer in *pesos*, so choose a fraction with *dollars* on the bottom and *pesos* on top. You need a unit fraction in the form of $\dfrac{? \ pesos}{? \ dollars}$

Because 0.076 *dollar* = 1 *peso*, the fraction you need is $\dfrac{1 \ peso}{0.076 \ dollar}$

$$\frac{190 \ \cancel{dollars}}{1} \times \frac{1 \ peso}{0.076 \ \cancel{dollar}}$$

$$= \frac{190}{0.076} \ pesos \ \text{ or } 2{,}500 \ pesos$$

RATIO & PROPORTION

In this problem there are two quantities: *pesos* and *dollars*. You know that 1 peso is equivalent to 0.076 dollar, and you have to find the unknown number of pesos that would be equivalent to 190 dollars.

So think of the problem this way:

$$1 \ peso = 0.076 \ dollar$$
$$? \ pesos = 190 \ dollars$$

Because the number of pesos and the number of dollars are proportional, a proportion could be set up as

$$\frac{pesos}{dollars} = \frac{pesos'}{dollars'}$$

Because you know that 1 peso equals 0.076 dollar, you can substitute those numbers, *1* and *0.076*, for *pesos* and *dollars*, respectively. And because you need to find the number of pesos (*x*) containing 190 dollars, you can substitute those quantities, *x* and 190, for *pesos'* and *dollars'*, respectively.

Substituting, you obtain

$$\frac{1 \ peso}{\$0.076} = \frac{x \ pesos}{\$190}$$

Eliminate the units of measurement and cross multiply

$$\frac{1}{0.076} \diagdown \frac{x}{190}$$

$$(x)(0.076) = (1)(190)$$

Simplify

$$x = \frac{190}{0.076} \quad or \quad 2{,}500$$

So, $190 will be exchanged for 2,500 pesos.

Complex (Multi-Step) Problems with Single Units of Measurement

Sometimes you will encounter problems that will require the procedures used previously to be repeated one or more times. We call such problems **complex**. In a complex problem, multiplication by more than one unit fraction is required. The method is very similar to that used with simple problems.

EXAMPLE 3.16

Convert 4 *hours* to an equivalent time in *seconds*.

DIMENSIONAL ANALYSIS

The given quantity: 4 hours

The quantity you want to find: ? seconds

An equivalence between them: ?

Most people do not know the direct equivalence between hours and seconds. But you do know the following two equivalences related to the units of measurement in this problem: 1 hour = 60 minutes and 1 minute = 60 seconds.

So the problem is

$$4 \text{ hours} = \text{? seconds}$$

First, you want to cancel *hours*. To do this, you must use an equivalence containing *hours* and a unit fraction with *hours* on the bottom. Because 1 hour = 60 minutes, this fraction will be $\dfrac{60 \text{ minutes}}{1 \text{ hour}}$

$$\frac{4 \, \cancel{\text{hours}}}{1} \times \frac{60 \text{ minutes}}{1 \, \cancel{\text{hour}}} = \text{? seconds}$$

After the *hours* are cancelled, as shown previously, only *minutes* remain on the left side. So, what you have done at this point is changed 4 *hours* to (4 × 60 = 240) *minutes*, but you want to obtain the answer in *seconds*.

RATIO & PROPORTION

In this problem there are two quantities: *seconds* and *hours*. Most people have not memorized the direct equivalence between seconds and hours. But they do know equivalences between *hours* and *minutes* and between *minutes* and *seconds*, namely,

$$1 \text{ hour} = 60 \text{ minutes}$$

and

$$1 \text{ minute} = 60 \text{ seconds}$$

This problem will be done in two steps; first change the 4 *hours* to *minutes*, and then change the resulting *minutes* to *seconds*.

Think of *Step 1* this way:

$$1 \text{ hour} = 60 \text{ minutes}$$
$$4 \text{ hours} = x \text{ minutes}$$

The first proportion could be

$$\frac{min}{h} = \frac{min'}{h'}$$

Substitute 60 and 1 for *min* and *h*, and *x* and 4 for *min'* and *h'*, respectively

$$\frac{60 \, min}{1 \, h} = \frac{x \, min}{4 \, h}$$

Therefore, the *minutes* must now be cancelled. Because *minutes* is in the numerator, a fraction with *minutes* in the denominator is required.

Because 1 *minute* = 60 *seconds*, the fraction is $\dfrac{60 \text{ seconds}}{1 \text{ minute}}$

Now multiplying by this unit fraction, you get

$$\frac{4 \text{ hours}}{1} \times \frac{60 \text{ minutes}}{1 \text{ hour}} \times \frac{60 \text{ seconds}}{1 \text{ minute}} = ? \text{ seconds}$$

Cancel the *minutes* and notice that the only unit of measurement remaining on the left side is *seconds*, the unit that you want to find!

$$\frac{4 \text{ hours}}{1} \times \frac{60 \text{ minutes}}{1 \text{ hour}} \times \frac{60 \text{ seconds}}{1 \text{ minute}} = ? \text{ seconds}$$

Now that you have the unit of measurement that you want (seconds) on the left side, cancel the numbers (not possible in this example) and finish the multiplication:

$$\frac{4 \text{ hours}}{1} \times \frac{60 \text{ minutes}}{1 \text{ hour}} \times \frac{60 \text{ seconds}}{1 \text{ minute}} = 14{,}400 \text{ seconds}$$

Eliminate the units of measurement and cross multiply

$$\frac{60}{1} = \frac{x}{4}$$

$$(x)(1) = (60)(4)$$
$$x = 240$$

So, 4 hours is equivalent to 240 minutes.

In *Step 2*, change *240 minutes to seconds*.

Think of *Step 2* this way:

$$1 \text{ minute} = 60 \text{ seconds}$$
$$240 \text{ minutes} = x \text{ seconds}$$

The second proportion could be

$$\frac{\text{min}}{\text{sec}} = \frac{\text{min}'}{\text{sec}'}$$

Substitute 1 and 60 for *min* and *sec*, and *240* and *x* for *min'* and *sec'*, respectively

$$\frac{1 \text{ min}}{60 \text{ sec}} = \frac{240 \text{ min}}{x \text{ sec}}$$

Eliminate the units of measurement and cross multiply

$$\frac{1}{60} = \frac{240}{x}$$

$$(240)(60) = (1)(x)$$
$$14{,}400 = x$$

So, 4 hours is equivalent to 14,400 seconds.

EXAMPLE 3.17

Convert 50,400 *minutes* to an equivalent time in *days*.

DIMENSIONAL ANALYSIS

The given quantity: 50,400 minutes

The quantity you want to find: ? days

Equivalences between them: ?

You might not know the direct equivalence between minutes and days. But you do know the following two equivalences related to the

RATIO & PROPORTION

In this problem, there are two quantities: *minutes* and *days*. Most people have not memorized the direct equivalence between minutes and days. But they do know that

60 minutes is equivalent to 1 hour

and

24 hours is equivalent to 1 day

units in this problem: 60 minutes = 1 hour and 24 hours = 1 day.

$$50{,}400 \text{ minutes} = ? \text{ days}$$

You want to cancel *minutes*. To do this, you must use an equivalence containing *minutes* and make a unit fraction with *minutes* on the bottom. Because 60 minutes = 1 hour, this fraction will be $\dfrac{1 \text{ hour}}{60 \text{ minutes}}$.

$$50{,}400 \text{ minutes} \times \frac{1 \text{ hour}}{60 \text{ minutes}} = ? \text{ days}$$

After the *minutes* are cancelled as shown, only *hour* remains on the left side, but you want to obtain the answer in *days*. Therefore, the *hour* must now be cancelled. This will require a unit fraction with *hours* in the denominator. Because 1 day = 24 hours, this fraction is $\dfrac{1 \text{ day}}{24 \text{ hours}}$.

After cancelling the *hours*, you now have

$$50{,}400 \text{ minutes} \times \frac{1 \text{ hour}}{60 \text{ minutes}} \times \frac{1 \text{ day}}{24 \text{ hours}} = ? \text{ days}$$

Because only *day* (in the numerator) is on the left side, the numbers can be cancelled.

$$\overset{840}{50{,}400} \text{ minutes} \times \frac{1 \text{ hour}}{\underset{1}{60} \text{ minutes}} \times \frac{1 \text{ day}}{24 \text{ hours}}$$

$$= \frac{840}{24} \text{ days} = 35 \text{ days}$$

This problem will be done in two steps; first change the *50,400 minutes to hours*, and then change the resulting *hours to days*.

Think of *Step 1* this way:

$$60 \text{ minutes} = 1 \text{ hour}$$
$$50{,}400 \text{ minutes} = x \text{ hours}$$

The first proportion could be

$$\frac{min}{h} = \frac{min'}{h'}$$

You can substitute those numbers *1* and *60* for *h* and *min*, and *x* and *50,400* for *h'* and *min'*, respectively

$$\frac{60 \; min}{1 \; h} = \frac{50{,}400 \; min}{x \; h}$$

Eliminate the units of measurement and cross multiply

$$\frac{60}{1} = \frac{50{,}400}{x}$$

$$(50{,}400)(1) = (60)(x)$$
$$50{,}400 = 60x$$

Divide by 60 and cancel

$$\frac{50{,}400}{60} = \frac{60 \, x}{60}$$

$$840 = x$$

So 50,400 minutes is equivalent to 840 hours.

In *Step 2* you change the *840 hours* to *days*

Think of *Step 2* this way:

$$24 \text{ hours} = 1 \text{ day}$$
$$840 \text{ hours} = x \text{ days}$$

The second proportion could be

$$\frac{d}{h} = \frac{d'}{h'}$$

Substitute those numbers *1* and *24* for *d* and *h*, and you can substitute *x* and *840* for *d'* and *h'*, respectively

$$\frac{1 \; d}{24 \; h} = \frac{x \; d}{840 \; h}$$

Eliminate the units of measurement and cross multiply

$$\frac{1}{24} = \frac{x}{840}$$

$$(x)(24) = (1)(840)$$
$$24x = 840$$

Divide by 24 and cancel.

$$\frac{24x}{24} = \frac{840}{24}$$
$$x = 35$$

So, 50,400 minutes is equivalent to 35 days.

EXAMPLE 3.18

Kim is having a party for 24 people and is serving hot dogs. Each person will eat 2 hot dogs. How much will the hot dogs for the party cost if a package of 8 hot dogs costs $2.50?

DIMENSIONAL ANALYSIS

The given single unit
of measurement: 24 people or 24 persons

The single unit of
measurement
you want to find: ? Cost ($)

You might not know the direct equivalence between people and cost. But you do know the following equivalences supplied in this problem:

2 hot dogs per person
2 hot dogs = 1 person
1 package of hot dogs is $2.50
1 package = $2.50
1 package has 8 hot dogs
1 package = 8 hot dogs

But where do you start?

In this problem, there are two single units of measurement—one that is given (persons) and one you have to find (cost). Cost involves a single unit of measurement, namely dollars ($). *Because you are looking for a quantity measured in a single unit of measurement ($), you should start with the given single unit of measurement* (persons).

24 persons = ? $

RATIO & PROPORTION

In this problem, there are three important quantities: *people*, *hot dogs*, and *dollars*. Here are the relationships given in the problem:

24 people will require *? dollars*
1 person eats *2 hot dogs*
8 hot dogs cost *$2.50*

This problem will be done in two steps; first determine the number of hot dogs 24 people will eat, and then determine the cost of those hot dogs.

Think of *Step 1* this way:

1 person = 2 hot dogs
24 persons = x hot dogs

The first proportion could be

$$\frac{person}{hot\ dogs} = \frac{person'}{hot\ dogs'}$$

Substituting, you get

$$\frac{1\ person}{2\ hot\ dogs} = \frac{24\ persons}{x\ hot\ dogs}$$

You want to cancel *persons*. To do this, you must use an equivalence containing *person(s)* to make a fraction with *person(s)* on the bottom. From the preceding equivalence, 2 hot dogs = 1 person, this fraction will be $\dfrac{2 \text{ hot dogs}}{\text{person}}$.

$$24 \,\overline{\text{persons}} \times \frac{2 \text{ hot dogs}}{\overline{\text{person}}} = ? \ \$$$

NOTE

Don't stop multiplying by unit fractions until the unit of measurement you are looking for is the only remaining unit on the left side. Remember that the unit you are looking for must be in the numerator of a fraction.

After the *person(s)* are cancelled, only *hot dogs* remains on the left side, and it indicates that 48 *hot dogs* are needed. But you want to obtain the answer in $. Therefore, the *hot dogs* must now be cancelled. This will require a fraction with *hot dogs* in the denominator. From the equivalence 1 package = 8 hot dogs, the unit fraction is $\dfrac{1 \text{ package}}{8 \text{ hot dogs}}$

Thus, you now have

$$24 \,\overline{\text{persons}} \times \frac{2 \,\overline{\text{hot dogs}}}{\overline{\text{person}}} \times \frac{1 \text{ package}}{8 \,\overline{\text{hot dogs}}} = ? \ \$$$

After the *hot dogs* are cancelled, only *package* remains on the left side, and (if you do the mathematics now) it indicates the number of *packages* (6) that are needed. But you want to obtain the answer in $. Therefore, the *package* must now be cancelled. This will require a fraction with *package* in the denominator. From the equivalence 1 package = $2.50, the unit fraction is $\dfrac{\$2.50}{1 \text{ package}}$.

Eliminate the units of measurement and cross multiply

$$\frac{1}{2} \diagup\!\!\!\!= \frac{24}{x}$$

$$48 = x$$

So, 48 hot dogs are needed.

In *Step 2*, you "change" 48 hot dogs to dollars.

Think of *Step 2* this way:

$$48 \text{ hot dogs} = x \text{ dollars}$$
$$8 \text{ hot dogs} = 2.50 \text{ dollars}$$

The second proportion could be set up as

$$\frac{hot\ dogs}{dollars} = \frac{hot\ dogs'}{dollars'}$$

Substituting you get

$$\frac{48\ hot\ dogs}{x\ dollars} = \frac{8\ hot\ dogs}{2.50\ dollars}$$

Eliminate the units of measurement and cross multiply

$$\frac{48}{x} \diagup\!\!\!\!= \frac{8}{2.50}$$

$$(8)(x) = (48)(2.50)$$
$$8x = 120$$

Divide by 8 and cancel

$$\frac{\cancel{8}\,x}{\cancel{8}} = \frac{120}{8}$$

$$x = 15$$

$$24 \text{ persons} \times \frac{2 \text{ hot dogs}}{\text{person}} \times \frac{1 \text{ package}}{8 \text{ hot dogs}}$$

$$\times \frac{\$2.50}{1 \text{ package}} = ? \$$$

Because you now have only $ (in the numerator) on the left side, the numbers can be cancelled and the multiplication finished.

$$\overset{3}{24} \text{ persons} \times \frac{2 \text{ hot dogs}}{\text{person}} \times \frac{1 \text{ package}}{\underset{1}{8} \text{ hot dogs}}$$

$$\times \frac{\$2.50}{1 \text{ package}} = \$15$$

So, the hot dogs for the party will cost $15.

Changing One Rate to Another Rate

A *rate* is a fraction with different units of measurement on top and bottom. For example, 50 *miles* per *hour* written as 50 miles/hour and 3 *pounds* per *week* written as 3 pounds/week are rates. In dosage calculation, the bottom unit of measurement is frequently time (e.g., *hours* or *minutes*). We sometimes want to change one rate into another rate. These problems are done in a manner similar to the method that was used to do the single-unit-to-single-unit problems.

Rate conversion will not be needed in this textbook until flow rates are encountered beginning in Chapter 10. Therefore, some students may prefer to study the rest of this chapter at that time.

Simple (One-Step) Problems with Rates

In dealing with rate conversions, students generally find it easier to use Dimensional Analysis or other techniques rather than Ratio & Proportion. However, in the following examples both methods will be shown along with some of the other techniques.

EXAMPLE 3.19

Convert *5 feet per hour* to an equivalent rate of speed in *inches per hour*.

DIMENSIONAL ANALYSIS

The given rate: 5 feet per hour
The rate you want to find: ? inches per hour

RATIO & PROPORTION

In this problem, there are two rates.

Think of the problem this way:

$$\frac{5 \text{ feet}}{hour} = \frac{? \text{ inches}}{hour}$$

Because you are looking for a rate, you start with the *given* rate:

$$5 \text{ feet per hour} = ? \text{ inches per hour}$$

Write these rates as fractions:

$$\frac{5 \text{ feet}}{\text{hour}} = \frac{? \text{ inches}}{\text{hour}}$$

Notice that you are given a rate with *hour* in the denominator, and the rate you are looking for also has *hour* in the denominator. Therefore, *the denominator does not have to be changed!*

But the given rate has *feet* in the numerator, and the rate you want has a different unit, *inches*, in the numerator. Therefore, *feet* must be changed.

To cancel *feet*, you must use an equivalence containing *feet*, namely, 12 *inches* = 1 *foot*. Because *feet* is in the numerator, you need a unit fraction with *feet* in the denominator. This unit fraction is $\dfrac{12 \text{ inches}}{1 \text{ foot}}$.

After the *feet* are cancelled, *inches* remain on top, and *hour* remains on the bottom, and those are the units you want. Finally, do the multiplication of the numbers.

$$\frac{5 \text{ feet}}{\text{hour}} \times \frac{12 \text{ inches}}{1 \text{ foot}} = \frac{60 \text{ inches}}{\text{hour}}$$

Notice that the given rate and the rate you are looking for both have the same denominator, *hour*. Therefore, the denominator does not have to be changed. But the given rate has *feet* in the numerator, and the rate you want has a different unit, *inches*, in the numerator. Therefore, the problem becomes

$$5 \text{ feet} = x \text{ inches}$$

The proportion could be set up as

$$\frac{ft}{in} = \frac{ft'}{in'}$$

Because you know that 1 foot equals 12 inches, you can substitute to obtain

$$\frac{1 \, ft}{12 \, in} = \frac{5 \, ft}{x \, in}$$

Eliminate the units of measurement and cross multiply

$$\frac{1}{12} = \frac{5}{x}$$

$$(5)(12) = (1)(x)$$

Simplify

$$60 = x$$

Therefore, *5 feet per hour* equals *60 inches per hour.*

EXAMPLE 3.20

Convert 90 *feet per hour* to an equivalent rate in *feet per minute.*

DIMENSIONAL ANALYSIS

The given rate: 90 ft/h

The rate you want to find: ? ft/min

Because you are looking for a rate, you start with the given rate,

$$90 \text{ ft per h} = ? \text{ ft/min}$$

$$\frac{90 \text{ ft}}{h} = \frac{? \text{ ft}}{min}$$

RATIO & PROPORTION

In this problem, there are two rates. Think of the problem this way:

$$\frac{90 \text{ feet}}{1 \text{ hour}} = ? \frac{ft}{min}$$

Notice that the given rate and the rate you are looking for both have the same numerator, *feet*. Therefore, the numerator does not have to

Notice that you are given a rate with *ft* in the numerator, and the answer you are looking for also has *ft* in the numerator. Therefore, the numerator does not have to be changed!

But the given rate has *h* in the denominator, and the rate you want has a different unit, *min*, in the denominator. Therefore, *h* must be eliminated. Since *h* is in the denominator, you need a fraction with *h* in the numerator.

Use the equivalence 1 h = 60 min. This unit fraction is $\dfrac{1\,h}{60\,min}$.

$$\frac{90\,(ft)}{h} \times \frac{1\,h}{60\,(min)} = \frac{?\,ft}{min}$$

After the *h* is cancelled, *ft* remains on top and *min* is on the bottom, and those are the units you want. Cancel the numbers and finish the multiplication.

$$\frac{\overset{3}{90}\,ft}{h} \times \frac{1\,h}{\underset{2}{60}\,min} = \frac{3\,ft}{2\,min} = \frac{1.5\,ft}{min}$$

be changed. But the given rate has *hour* in the denominator, and the rate you want has a different unit, *minute*, in the denominator.

This change can be accomplished by replacing 1 hour with 60 minutes in the rate $\frac{90\,ft}{1\,h}$ as follows:

$$\frac{90\,ft}{1\,h} = \frac{90\,ft}{60\,min} = \frac{90}{60}\,\frac{ft}{min}$$

Because $\frac{90}{60} = 1.5$

$$\frac{90}{60}\,\frac{ft}{min} = 1.5\frac{ft}{min}$$

So, *90 feet/hour* is equivalent to *1.5 feet per minute*.

EXAMPLE 3.21

Convert *3 ounces per day* to an equivalent rate measured in *ounces per week*.

DIMENSIONAL ANALYSIS

Given rate: 3 oz/d

Rate you want to find: ? oz/wk

You want to change one rate to another rate.

$$\frac{3\,oz}{d} = ?\,\frac{oz}{wk}$$

The numerators are both in *ounces*. The denominators do not match, therefore the *d must be changed to wk*. Because *d* is in the denominator, you must use an equivalent unit fraction with *d* in the numerator. This fraction will be $\dfrac{7\,d}{1\,wk}$

$$\frac{3\,oz}{d} \times \frac{7\,d}{1\,wk} = \frac{21\,oz}{wk}$$

MULTIPLYING NUMERATOR AND DENOMINATOR OF A RATE BY THE SAME NUMBER

You want to change one rate to another rate.

$$\frac{3\,oz}{d} = ?\,\frac{oz}{wk}$$

The numerators are both in *ounces*. The denominators do not match, therefore the *d must be changed to wk*. Because 7 day = 1 week, an easy way to do this example is to multiply the given rate by $\dfrac{7}{7}$.

$$\frac{3\,oz}{d} \times \frac{7}{7} = \frac{21\,oz}{7\,d} \;\text{ or }\; \frac{21\,oz}{wk}$$

So, *3 ounces per day* is equivalent to *21 ounces per week*.

EXAMPLE 3.22

Convert *4 pints per day* to an equivalent rate measured in *quarts per day*.

DIMENSIONAL ANALYSIS

You want to change one rate to another rate.

$$\frac{4\,pt}{d} = ?\,\frac{qt}{d}$$

The denominators are both in *days*. The numerators do not match, therefore the *pt must be changed to qt*. Because *pt* is in the numerator, you must use an equivalent unit fraction with *pt* in the denominator. This fraction will be $\frac{1\,qt}{2\,pt}$

$$\frac{4\,\cancel{pt}}{d} \times \frac{1\,qt}{2\,\cancel{pt}} = \frac{2\,qt}{d}$$

RATIO & PROPORTION

You want to change one rate to another rate.

$$\frac{4\,pt}{d} = ?\,\frac{qt}{d}$$

Because the denominators are the same, you need only change 4 *pints* to *quarts*.

Think of the problem as

$$4\,pt = x\,qt$$
$$2\,pt = 1\,qt$$

Use the proportion,

$$\frac{qt}{pt} = \frac{qt'}{pt'}$$

Substituting into a proportion you get

$$\frac{x\,qt}{4\,pt} = \frac{1\,qt}{2\,pt}$$

Eliminate the units of measurement and cross multiply

$$\frac{x}{4} = \frac{1}{2}$$

$$(1)(4) = (x)(2)$$
$$4 = 2x$$
$$2 = x$$

So, *4 pints per day* is equivalent to *2 quarts per day*.

Complex (Multi-Step) Problems with Rates

When using Dimensional Analysis these examples will involve more than one unit fraction, and when using Ratio & Proportion they will require more than one step.

EXAMPLE 3.23

Convert $10\frac{1}{2}$ *feet/hour* to an equivalent rate in *inches/minute*.

DIMENSIONAL ANALYSIS

The given rate: $10\frac{1}{2}$ feet/hour

The rate you want to find: ? inches/minute

Since you are looking for a rate, you should start with a rate.

$$10\frac{1}{2} \text{ feet/hour} = \text{? inches/minute}$$

Write $10\frac{1}{2}$ as the improper fraction $\frac{21}{2}$

$$\frac{21 \text{ ft}}{2 \text{ h}} = \frac{? \text{ in}}{\min}$$

You want to cancel *ft*. To do this, you must use an equivalence containing *ft* on the bottom. Because you want to convert to *inches*, use the equivalence 12 *inches* = 1 *foot*, and the unit fraction will be $\frac{12 \text{ in}}{1 \text{ ft}}$.

$$\frac{21 \text{ ft}}{2 \text{ h}} \times \frac{12 \text{ in}}{1 \text{ ft}} = \frac{? \text{ in}}{\min}$$

After the *ft* are cancelled, *in* is on top, which is what you want. But *h* is on the bottom and it must be cancelled. This will require a fraction with *h* in the numerator. From the equivalence 1 hour = 60 minutes, the unit fraction is $\frac{1 \text{ h}}{60 \text{ min}}$.

After cancelling the hours, you now have

$$\frac{21 \text{ ft}}{2 \text{ h}} \times \frac{12 \text{ in}}{1 \text{ ft}} \times \frac{1 \text{ h}}{60 \text{ min}} = \frac{? \text{ in}}{\min}$$

You now have *in* on top and *min* on the bottom, so do the cancelling and multiplications of the numbers.

$$\frac{21 \text{ ft}}{2 \text{ h}} \times \frac{\overset{1}{12} \text{ in}}{1 \text{ ft}} \times \frac{1 \text{ h}}{\underset{5}{60} \text{ min}} = \frac{21 \text{ in}}{10 \text{ min}} \text{ or } \frac{2.1 \text{ in}}{\min}$$

RATIO & PROPORTION

In this problem there are two rates.

$$\frac{10\frac{1}{2} \text{ feet}}{1 \text{ hour}} = \text{?} \frac{\text{inches}}{\text{minute}}$$

Notice that the given rate and the rate you are looking for both have different numerators and different denominators. Therefore, both must be changed. $10\frac{1}{2}$ feet must be changed to inches, and 1 hour must be changed to minutes.

First change $10\frac{1}{2}$ *feet* to *inches* using the proportion

$$\frac{\text{feet}}{\text{inches}} = \frac{\text{feet'}}{\text{inches'}}$$

Think of the problem as

$$10\frac{1}{2} \text{ feet} = x \text{ inches}$$
$$1 \text{ foot} = 12 \text{ inches}$$

Substituting into a proportion you get

$$\frac{1 \text{ foot}}{12 \text{ inches}} = \frac{10\frac{1}{2} \text{ feet}}{x \text{ inches}}$$

Eliminate the units of measurement and cross multiply

$$\frac{1}{12} = \frac{10\frac{1}{2}}{x}$$

$$(10\tfrac{1}{2})(12) = (1)(x)$$
$$126 = x$$

So, $10\frac{1}{2}$ feet equals 126 inches, and the problem becomes

$$\frac{126 \text{ inches}}{1 \text{ hour}} = \text{?} \frac{\text{inches}}{\text{minute}}$$

Now you need to change 1 hour to minutes. You replace 1 hour by 60 minutes

$$\frac{126 \text{ inches}}{1 \text{ hour}} = \frac{126 \text{ inches}}{60 \text{ minutes}} = \frac{126}{60} \frac{\text{inches}}{\text{minute}}$$

but $\frac{126}{60} = 2.1$

So, $10\frac{1}{2}$ *feet/hour* to an equivalent 2.1 *inches/minute*.

EXAMPLE 3.24

Write 3.2 *inches/second* in *feet/minute*.

DIMENSIONAL ANALYSIS

The given rate: 3.2 in/sec

The rate you want to find: ? ft/min

Since you are looking for a **rate**, you should start with a **rate**.

$$\frac{3.2 \text{ in}}{\text{sec}} = \frac{? \text{ ft}}{\text{min}}$$

You want to cancel *in*. To do this, you must use an equivalence containing *in* on the bottom. This fraction will be $\dfrac{1 \text{ ft}}{12 \text{ in}}$

$$\frac{3.2 \text{ in}}{\text{sec}} \times \frac{1 \text{ ft}}{12 \text{ in}} = \frac{? \text{ ft}}{\text{min}}$$

Now, *ft* is on top, which is what you want. But *sec* is on the bottom and it must be cancelled. This will require a fraction with *sec* in the numerator: $\dfrac{60 \text{ sec}}{1 \text{ min}}$.

Now cancel and multiply the numbers.

$$\frac{3.2 \text{ in}}{\text{sec}} \times \frac{1\,\text{ft}}{12\,\text{in}} \times \frac{\overset{5}{\cancel{60}}\,\text{sec}}{1\,\text{min}} = \frac{16 \text{ ft}}{\text{min}}$$

RATIO & PROPORTION

In this problem there are two rates. Think of the problem this way:

$$\frac{3.2 \text{ in}}{1 \text{ sec}} = \frac{? \text{ ft}}{\text{min}}$$

Notice that the given rate and the rate you want have different numerators and different denominators. Therefore, both must be changed. The inches must be changed to feet, and the seconds must be changed to minutes.

You can change the denominator (1 sec) to minutes by multiplying both numerator and denominator by 60 as follows:

$$\frac{3.2 \text{ in}}{1 \text{ sec}} \times \frac{60}{60} = \frac{192 \text{ in}}{60 \text{ sec}}$$

Replace 60 seconds with 1 minute

$$\frac{192 \text{ in}}{60 \text{ sec}} = \frac{192 \text{ in}}{1 \text{ min}}$$

Now the problem becomes

$$\frac{192 \text{ in}}{1 \text{ min}} = \frac{? \text{ feet}}{\text{min}}$$

Now, only the numerator must be changed. Change 192 inches to feet using the proportion

$$\frac{feet}{inches} = \frac{feet'}{inches'}$$

Think of the problem as

$$192 \text{ feet} = x \text{ inches}$$
$$1 \text{ foot} = 12 \text{ inches}$$

Substituting into a proportion you get

$$\frac{1 \text{ foot}}{12 \text{ inches}} = \frac{x \text{ feet}}{192 \text{ inches}}$$

Eliminate the units of measurement and cross multiply

$$\frac{1}{12} = \frac{x}{192}$$

$$(x)(12) = (1)(192)$$
$$12x = 192$$

Divide by 12 and cancel

$$\frac{\cancel{12}\,x}{\cancel{12}} = \frac{192}{12}$$

$$x = 16$$

Therefore, *3.2 inches/second* equals *16 feet/minute*.

EXAMPLE 3.25

A person drinks water at *2 qt per day*. Convert this to an equivalent rate measured in *pints per week*.

DIMENSIONAL ANALYSIS

Given rate: *2 qt/d*

Rate you want to find: *? pt/wk*

You want to change one rate to another rate.

$$\frac{2\,qt}{d} = ?\,\frac{pt}{wk}$$

Neither the units on the tops (*qt* and *pt*), nor those on the bottoms (*d* and *wk*) match, therefore both the *pt* and the *sec* must be changed (cancelled). Suppose you start with *qt*. Because *qt* is on the top, you must use an equivalent unit fraction with *qt* on the bottom. This fraction will be $\frac{2\,pt}{1\,qt}$

$$\frac{2\,qt}{d} \times \frac{2\,pt}{1\,qt} = ?\,\frac{pt}{wk}$$

Now, *pt* is on the top, which is what you want. But *d* is on the bottom and it must be cancelled. This will require a unit fraction with *d* in the numerator. This fraction will be $\frac{7\,d}{1\,wk}$

After you cancel all the units, multiply the numbers

$$\frac{2\,\cancel{qt}}{\cancel{d}} \times \frac{2\,pt}{1\,\cancel{qt}} \times \frac{7\,\cancel{d}}{wk} = 28\,\frac{pt}{wk}$$

RATIO & PROPORTION

We need to change one rate to another.

$$\frac{2\,qt}{d} = ?\,\frac{pt}{wk}$$

Notice that the given rate and the rate you are looking for both have the different numerators and different denominators. Therefore, both must be changed; 2 *quarts* must be changed to *pints*, and 1 *day* must be changed to *weeks*.

We know the equivalence: *7 days = 1 week*

If you multiply the given rate by the fraction $\frac{7}{7}$, you get

$$\frac{2\,qt}{d} \times \frac{7}{7} = \frac{14\,qt}{7\,d} \ or \ \frac{14\,qt}{wk}$$

So the problem becomes

$$\frac{14\,qt}{wk} = ?\,\frac{pt}{wk}$$

Now change *14 quarts* to *pints*.

Think of the problem as

14 quarts = x pints

1 quarts = 2 pints

Use the proportion

$$\frac{qt}{pt} = \frac{qt'}{pt'}$$

Substituting into a proportion you get

$$\frac{14\,qt}{x\,pt} = \frac{1\,qt}{2\,pt}$$

Eliminate the units of measurement and cross multiply

$$\frac{14}{x} = \frac{1}{2}$$

$$(1)(x) = (14)(2)$$
$$x = 28$$

So, *2 quarts per day* is equivalent to *28 pints per week*.

EXAMPLE 3.26

A person gains *96 ounces per year*. Convert this rate to *pounds per month*.

DIMENSIONAL ANALYSIS

Given rate: 96 oz/yr

Rate you want to find: ? *lb/mon*

You want to change one rate to another rate.

$$\frac{96\,oz}{yr} = ?\,\frac{lb}{mon}$$

Neither the units on the tops (*lb* and *oz*), nor those on the bottoms (*mon* and *yr*) match, therefore both the *oz* and the *yr* must be changed (cancelled). Suppose you start with *oz*. Because *oz* is on the top, you must use an equivalent unit fraction with *oz* on the bottom. This fraction will be $\frac{16\,oz}{1\,lb}$

$$\frac{96\,oz}{yr} \times \frac{1\,lb}{16\,oz} = ?\,\frac{lb}{mon}$$

Now, *lb* is on the top, which is what you want. But *yr* is on the bottom and it must be cancelled. This will require a unit fraction with *yr* in the numerator. This fraction will be $\frac{1\,yr}{12\,mon}$

After you cancel all the units, then cancel and multiply the numbers.

$$\frac{96\,oz}{yr} \times \frac{1\,lb}{16\,oz} \times \frac{1\,yr}{12\,mon} = 0.5\,\frac{lb}{mon}$$

RATIO & PROPORTION

We need to change one rate to another:

$$\frac{96\,oz}{1\,yr} = ?\,\frac{lb}{mon}$$

Notice that the given rate and the rate you are looking for both have the different numerators and different denominators. Therefore, both must be changed; 96 *ounces* must be changed to *pounds*, and 1 *year* must be changed to *months*.

We know the equivalence: 12 *months* = *1 year*

If you replace 1 year by 12 months in the given rate, the problem becomes

$$\frac{96\,oz}{12\,mon} = ?\,\frac{lb}{mon}$$

or

$$\frac{8\,oz}{1\,mon} = ?\,\frac{lb}{mon}$$

The denominators now match, so now change *8 ounces* to *pounds.*

Think of the problem as

$$8\,oz = x\,lb$$
$$16\,oz = 1\,lbs$$

Substituting into a proportion you get

$$\frac{8\,oz}{x\,lb} = \frac{16\,oz}{1\,lb}$$

Eliminate the units of measurement and cross multiply

$$\frac{8}{x} = \frac{16}{1}$$

$$(16)(x) = (8)(1)$$
$$x = 0.5$$

So, *96 ounces per year* is equivalent to *0.5 pounds per month*.

Summary

In this chapter the methods of Dimensional Analysis and Ratio & Proportion were introduced.

For Dimensional Analysis:

Mathematical concepts were reinforced:
- A nonzero number divided by itself equals 1.
- A fraction equal to 1 is called a unit fraction.
- When a quantity is multiplied (or divided) by 1, the quantity is unchanged.
- Cancellation always involves a quantity in a numerator and another quantity in a denominator.

Simple (one-step) single-unit-to-single-unit problems:
- Start with the **given** single unit of measure on the left side of the = sign.
- Write the single unit of measure you want to **find** on the right side of the = sign.
- Identify an **equivalence** containing the units of measure in the problem.
- Use the equivalence to make a unit fraction with the **given** unit of measure in the **denominator**.
- Multiply by the unit fraction.
- Cancel the units of measure. The only unit of measurement remaining on the left side (in a numerator) will match the unit of measure on the right side.
- Cancel the numbers and finish the multiplication.

Simple (one-step) rate-to-rate problems:
- Start with the given rate on the left side of the equal sign.
- Write the rate you want to **find** on the right side of the equal sign.

- Identify a unit of measure that must be cancelled.
- Find an **equivalence** containing the unwanted unit of measure you want to cancel.
- Choose a unit fraction that leads to cancellation of the unwanted unit of measurement.
- Cancel the units of measurement. The only units of measurement remaining on the left side (in a numerator) will match the units of measure on the right side.
- Cancel the numbers and finish the multiplication.
- In medical dosage calculations involving rates of flow, time (in minutes or hours) will always be in the denominator.

Complex (multi-step) problems:
- Repeat the preceding steps until the only unit of measurement(s) remaining on the left side is the same as the unit of measurement(s) on the right side.

For Ratio & Proportion:

- A ratio is a comparison of two numbers.
- A ratio can be written as a fraction.
- Ratios are equal if their fractional forms are equivalent fractions.
- Order matters: a ratio of *2 to 3* is not the same as a ratio of *3 to 2*.
- A rate compares two quantities that have different units of measurement.
- Rates often have a unit of time in the denominator.
- A proportion can be written as an equation with a ratio on each side of the equal sign.
- A proportion is true if the products of cross multiplication are equal.

- Two quantities are proportional if, whenever you double one of the quantities, you double the other.
- The steps in solving a proportion are:
  1. Identify the two units of measurement in the problem.
  2. Write a known equivalence between the units of measure.
  3. Let x stand for the unit you are trying to find and write an equivalence involving x.
  4. Write a proportion using the two units of measurement.
  5. Substitute into the proportion.
  6. Eliminate the units.
  7. Cross multiply.
  8. Divide both sides of the equation by the coefficient of x (unless the coefficient is 1).
  9. Cancel and simplify if possible.
  10. Check the answer by substituting and cross multiplying.

Workspace

Practice Sets

The answers to *Try These for Practice* and *Exercises* appear in Appendix A at the end of the book. Ask your instructor for the answers to the *Additional Exercises*.

Try These for Practice

Test your comprehension after reading the chapter.

1. How many seconds are in 3.5 minutes? _____

2. What is the weight in ounces of an infant who weighs 6 pounds 9 ounces? _____

3. How many hours are equivalent to 720 minutes? _____

4. A bucket is being filled with water at the rate of 1.5 quarts per minute. Find the equivalent flow rate in quarts per hour. _____

5. A ball is rolling at the speed of 2 feet per minute. Find this speed in inches per minute. _____

Exercises

Reinforce your understanding in class or at home.

1. 0.25 hours = _____ minutes

2. $5\frac{1}{4}$ years = _____ months

3. $2\frac{1}{3}$ days = _____ hours

4. 2.5 lb = _____ oz

5. $\frac{3}{4}$ h = _____ min

6. 18 mon = _____ yr

7. 36 in = _____ ft

8. 40 oz = _____ lb

9. An infant weighs 6 pounds 5 ounces at birth. What is the weight in ounces?
_____

10. There are 12 cans of soda in a case. Each can contains 16 ounces of soda. Every 24 ounces of soda contains 1 cup of sugar. How many cups of sugar are in 3 cases of soda? _____

11. What fraction of an hour is 1,350 seconds? _____

12. What is the height in inches of a person who is 6 feet 2 inches tall? _____

13. Write 604,800 seconds as an equivalent amount of time in weeks. _____

14. If a person measures 54 inches in height, what does the person measure in feet? _____

15. 4 pt/min = ? qt/min

16. 2 pt/min = ? pt/hr

17. 0.2 pt/min = ? qt/hr

18. 2 in/min = ? ft/hr

19. 2 oz/d = ? lb/wk

20. 0.02 inches per second is equivalent to how many feet per hour?

Additional Exercises

Now, test yourself!

1. 1.5 min = _____ sec

2. $5\frac{1}{2}$ years = _____ months

3. $4\frac{1}{4}$ days = _____ h

4. 40 ounces = _____ lb

5. $\dfrac{3}{4}$ hour = _____ min

6. 51 mon = _____ yr

7. 3 qt = _____ pt

8. 3 lb = _____ oz

9. $\dfrac{12 \text{ inches}}{\text{second}}$ = _____ $\dfrac{\text{feet}}{\text{second}}$

10. $\dfrac{30 \text{ pints}}{\text{minute}}$ = _____ $\dfrac{\text{pints}}{\text{sec}}$

11. An infant weighs 8 pounds 10 ounces at birth. What is the weight in ounces?
_____

12. What is the height in inches of a person who is 6 feet 4 inches tall? _____

13. If 3 feet = 1 yard, convert 4 yards to an equivalent distance in inches.
_____

Workspace

Workspace

14. If a person measures 42 inches in height, what does the person measure in feet? _____

15. What fraction of an hour is 2,700 seconds? _____

16. Change $6 \frac{\text{pints}}{\text{h}}$ to an equivalent rate in $\frac{\text{quarts}}{\text{day}}$. _____

17. Change $6 \frac{\text{quarts}}{\text{day}}$ to an equivalent rate in $\frac{\text{pints}}{\text{hour}}$. _____

18. Change 1,680 hours to weeks. _____

19. Write 1,209,600 seconds as an equivalent amount of time in weeks. _____

20. There are 24 cans of soda in a case. Each can contains 12 ounces of soda. Every 60 ounces of soda contains 1 cup of sugar. How many cups of sugar are in 5 cases of soda? _____

Unit

2

Systems of Measurement

CHAPTER 4

The Household and Metric Systems

CHAPTER 5

Converting from One System of Measurement to Another

Chapter 4

The Household and Metric Systems

Learning Outcomes

$$0.4\,g = 400\,mg$$

After completing this chapter, you will be able to

1. Identify the units of measurement in the household and metric systems.
2. Recognize the abbreviations for the units of measurement in the two systems.
3. State the equivalents for the units of volume.
4. State the equivalents for the units of weight.
5. State the equivalents for the units of length.
6. Convert from one unit to another within each of the two systems.

Historically, the United States has used three different systems to measure drugs: the apothecary, household, and metric systems.

The **apothecary** system is the oldest of the three systems, and it is difficult to use. Because its use led to many medication errors, the Joint Commission, FDA, and ISMP have suggested that it be discontinued. Package inserts and other drug references no longer use the apothecary system for recommended medication dosages. Therefore, the apothecary system is not included in this chapter. However, for those interested in the apothecary system, see Appendix G.

The **household** system is designed so that dosages can be measured at home using ordinary containers found in the kitchen, such as cups and teaspoons. The household system is sometimes referred to as the English system.

The **metric** system is the most logically organized and easiest to use of all the systems of measurement. It was first adopted by France a few years after the French revolution of 1789. It is also referred to as the *International System of Units*. It can be abbreviated as SI, which are the first two initials of its French name, *Système International d'Unités*. The metric system will eventually replace all other systems of measurement used in health care.

In this chapter you will be introduced to the household and metric systems.

The Household System

Liquid Volume in the Household System

Occasionally, household measurements are used when prescribing liquid medication. Table 4.1 lists equivalent values, with their abbreviations, for units of liquid measurement in the household system.

Table 4.1 Household Equivalents of Liquid Volume

1 quart (qt)	=	2 pints (pt)
1 pint (pt)	=	2 measuring cups
1 measuring cup	=	8 ounces (oz)
1 glass (usually)	=	8 ounces (oz)
1 ounce (oz)	=	2 tablespoons (T)
1 tablespoon (T)	=	3 teaspoons (t)

You can use dimensional analysis to convert from one unit of measurement to an equivalent unit of measurement within the household system the same way you converted units of measurement in Chapter 3. You multiply the given measurement by a unit fraction that is equal to 1; the unit fraction has the **given units of measurement on the bottom** (the denominator) and the **desired units of measurement on top** (the numerator), as the following examples show.

EXAMPLE 4.1

A patient drank 24 oz of the laxative agent COLYTE. How many glasses did this patient drink?

DIMENSIONAL ANALYSIS

$$24 \text{ oz} = ? \text{ glasses}$$

Cancel the ounces and obtain the equivalent amount in glasses.

$$24 \text{ oz} \times \frac{? \text{ glasses}}{? \text{ oz}} = ? \text{ glasses}$$

Because 1 glass = 8 ounces, the unit fraction is $\frac{1 \text{ glass}}{8 \text{ oz}}$

$$\overset{3}{\cancel{24 \text{ oz}}} \times \frac{1 \text{ glass}}{\underset{1}{\cancel{8 \text{ oz}}}} = 3 \text{ glasses}$$

RATIO & PROPORTION

Think of the problem this way:

$$8 \text{ ounces} = 1 \text{ glass} \quad [\text{known equivalent}]$$
$$24 \text{ ounces} = x \text{ glasses}$$

Because the number of ounces and the number of glasses are proportional, a proportion could be used to solve the problem. One way to set up the proportion is

$$\frac{oz}{glasses} = \frac{oz'}{glasses'}$$

Substituting, you obtain

$$\frac{8 \, oz}{1 \, glass} = \frac{24 \, oz}{x \, glasses}$$

Eliminate the units of measurement

$$\frac{8}{1} = \frac{24}{x}$$

Cross multiply

$$\frac{8}{1} \diagdown \frac{24}{x}$$

$$(24)(1) = (8)(x)$$

Simplify

$$24 = 8x$$

Divide both sides of the equation by 8, the coefficient of x

$$\frac{24}{8} = \frac{8x}{8}$$

Cancel

$$\frac{24}{8} = \frac{8x}{8}$$

Simplify

$$3 = x$$

24 oz is approximately the same as 3 glasses, so the patient drank 3 glasses of COLYTE.

EXAMPLE 4.2

NOTE

In the household system for quantities less than 1, either decimal numbers or fractions may be used. However, fractions are preferred. For example, $\frac{1}{2}$ qt is preferred over 0.5 qt.

A patient needs to drink $1\frac{1}{2}$ ounces of an elixir per day. How many teaspoons would be equivalent to this dosage?

DIMENSIONAL ANALYSIS

$$1\frac{1}{2} \; ounces = ? \; teaspoons$$

If you do not know a direct equivalence between *ounces* and *teaspoons*, then this will be a complex (multistep) problem, which

NOTE

Teaspoon is sometimes abbreviated as *tsp*, and tablespoon is sometimes abbreviated as *tbs*.

RATIO & PROPORTION

In this problem, there are two quantities: *ounces* and *teaspoons*.

Because you may not know the direct equivalence between ounces and teaspoons, you will first change 1½ ounces to an equivalent number of tablespoons, and then change the resulting tablespoons to teaspoons. This problem, then, requires two steps.

Step 1   *Change $1\frac{1}{2}$ ounces to tablespoons*

1 ounce = 2 tablespoons [known equivalence]

$1\frac{1}{2}$ ounces = x tablespoons

requires first changing *ounces* to *tablespoons* and then changing *tablespoons* to *teaspoons*.

$$1\tfrac{1}{2}\ ounces \rightarrow ?\ tablespoons \rightarrow ?\ teaspoons$$

Because calculating with mixed numbers is difficult, you should write $1\tfrac{1}{2}$ *ounces* as either $1.5\ ounces$ or $\dfrac{3\ ounces}{2}$

Now you want to cancel the *ounces* and get the answer in *tablespoons*, so choose a unit fraction with *ounces* on the bottom and *tablespoons* on top. That is, you need a unit fraction in the form of

$$\frac{?\ tablespoons}{?\ ounces}$$

Because 1 *ounce* = 2 *tablespoons*, the fraction you need is $\dfrac{2\ tablespoons}{1\ ounce}$

Cancel the *ounces*

$$\frac{3\ \cancel{ounces}}{2} \times \frac{2\ \boxed{tablespoons}}{1\ \cancel{ounce}} = ?\ teaspoons$$

After cancelling the *ounces* as shown, only *tablespoons* remain in the numerator on the left side. But you want the answer to be in *teaspoons*, so you must cancel the *tablespoons*. This requires a second unit fraction with *tablespoons* in the denominator. The fraction is $\dfrac{3\ teaspoons}{1\ tablespoon}$

$$\frac{3\ \cancel{ounces}}{2} \times \frac{2\ \cancel{tablespoons}}{1\ \cancel{ounce}} \times$$

$$\frac{3\ \boxed{teaspoons}}{1\ \cancel{tablespoon}} = ?\ teaspoons$$

After cancelling the *tablespoons* as shown, only *teaspoons* remain in the numerator on the left side. *Teaspoons* is the unit you want on the left side, so now focus on the numbers. Cancel the twos and multiply as shown below:

$$\frac{3\ oz}{2} \times \frac{2\ T}{1\ oz} \times \frac{3\ t}{1\ T} = 9t$$

So, $1\tfrac{1}{2}$ oz is equivalent to 9 teaspoons

One way to set up the proportion is

$$\frac{oz}{T} = \frac{oz'}{T'}$$

Substituting, you obtain

$$\frac{1\ oz}{2\ T} = \frac{1\tfrac{1}{2}\ oz}{x\ T}$$

Eliminate the units of measurement

$$\frac{1}{2} = \frac{1\tfrac{1}{2}}{x}$$

Cross multiply

$$\frac{1}{2} \underset{\searrow}{=} \frac{1\tfrac{1}{2}}{x}$$

$$\left(1\tfrac{1}{2}\right)(2) = (1)(x)$$

$$3 = x$$

So, $1\tfrac{1}{2}$ oz is equivalent to 3 tablespoons.

Step 2   *Change 3 tablespoons to teaspoons*

$$1\ tablespoon = 3\ teaspoons \quad [\text{known equivalence}]$$

$$3\ tablespoons = x\ teaspoons$$

One way to set up the proportion is

$$\frac{t}{T} = \frac{t'}{T'}$$

Substituting, you obtain

$$\frac{3t}{1\ T} = \frac{xt}{3\ T}$$

Eliminate the units of measurement

$$\frac{3}{1} = \frac{x}{3}$$

Cross multiply

$$\frac{3}{1} \underset{\searrow}{=} \frac{x}{3}$$

$$x = 9$$

Weight in the Household System

The only units of weight used in the household system of medication administration are ounces (oz) and pounds (lb), as shown in Table 4.2.

Table 4.2   Household Equivalents of Weight

1 pound (lb)	=	16 ounces (oz)

EXAMPLE 4.3

An infant weighs 5 lb 8 oz. What is the weight of the infant in ounces?

DIMENSIONAL ANALYSIS

First change the 5 lb to ounces

$$5 \text{ lb} = ? \text{ oz}$$

Cancel the pounds and obtain the equivalent amount in ounces

$$5 \text{ lb} \times \frac{? \text{ oz}}{? \text{ lb}} = ? \text{ oz}$$

Because 16 oz = 1 lb, the unit fraction is $\dfrac{16 \text{ oz}}{1 \text{ lb}}$

$$5 \text{ lb} \times \frac{16 \text{ oz}}{1 \text{ lb}} = 80 \text{ oz}$$

Now add the extra 8 ounces

$$80 \text{ oz} + 8 \text{ oz} = 88 \text{ oz}$$

RATIO & PROPORTION

First change the 5 lb to ounces. Think:

$$16 \text{ ounces} = 1 \text{ pound} \quad \text{[known equivalence]}$$
$$x \text{ ounces} = 5 \text{ pounds}$$

One way to set up the proportion is

$$\frac{oz}{lb} = \frac{oz'}{lb'}$$

Substituting, you obtain

$$\frac{16 \, oz}{1 \, lb} = \frac{x \, oz}{5 \, lb}$$

Eliminate the units of measurement and cross multiply

$$\frac{16}{1} \diagdown \frac{x}{5}$$
$$x = 80$$

Now, add the extra 8 ounces

$$80 \text{ oz} + 8 \text{ oz} = 88 \text{ oz}$$

So, the 5 lb 8 oz infant weighs 88 oz.

Length in the Household System

The only units of length used in the household system for medication administration are feet (ft) and inches (in), as shown in Table 4.3.

Table 4.3   Household Equivalents for Length

1 foot (ft)	=	12 inches (in)

EXAMPLE 4.4

A child is 3 ft 2 in tall. Find the child's height in inches.

DIMENSIONAL ANALYSIS

First, change the 3 feet to inches.

$$3\,feet = ?\,inches$$

You want to cancel the *feet* and get the answer in *inches*, so choose a fraction with *feet* on the bottom and *inches* on top. You need a unit fraction in the form of $\dfrac{?\,inches}{?\,feet}$

Because $1\,foot = 12\,inches$, the fraction you need is $\dfrac{12\,inches}{1\,foot}$

$$\frac{3\,\cancel{feet}}{1} \times \frac{12\,\cancel{inches}}{1\,\cancel{foot}} = 36\,inches$$

So, 3 *feet* is equivalent to 36 *inches*. Now add the extra 2 *inches*

$$36\,in + 2\,in = 38\,inches$$

RATIO & PROPORTION

First, change the 3 feet to inches.

Think of the problem this way:

$$1\,ft = 12\,in \quad [\text{known equivalent}]$$
$$3\,ft = x\,in$$

Because the number of feet and the number of inches are proportional, a proportion could be used to solve the problem. One way to set up the proportion is

$$\frac{ft}{in} = \frac{ft'}{in'}$$

Substituting, you obtain

$$\frac{1\,ft}{12\,in} = \frac{3\,ft}{x\,in}$$

Eliminate the units of measurement

$$\frac{1}{12} = \frac{3}{x}$$

Cross multiply

$$\frac{1}{12} \diagup\!\!\!= \frac{3}{x}$$

$$(12)(3) = (1)(x)$$

Simplify

$$36 = x$$

So, 3 feet equal 36 inches. Now, add the extra 2 inches

$$36\,in + 2\,in = 38\,in$$

The 3 *feet* 2 *inch* child is 38 *inches* tall.

Decimal-Based Systems

As seen in Chapter 1, our *place-value number system* is a *decimal* system, that is, it is based on the number 10. The *U.S. monetary system* and the *metric system* are also decimal systems.

The *U.S. monetary system* uses the dollar as its fundamental unit. All other denominations are decimal multiples or fractions of the dollar.

hundred-dollar bill	ten-dollar bill	dollar bill	dime	penny

An amount of money measured in one denomination can be easily converted to another denomination by merely moving the decimal point the appropriate number of places.

For example, to convert *60 dimes* to *pennies*, see in the chart that *dime* to *penny* is one jump to the *right*.

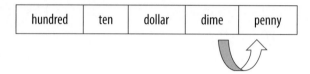

So, move the decimal point in 60 dimes one place to the *right* as follows:

60 dimes = 60.0 dimes = 6 0 0 . pennies, or 600 pennies

To convert *80 dollars* to *ten dollar bills*, see in the chart that *dollar* to *ten* is one jump to the *left*.

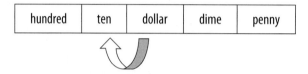

So, move the decimal point in 80 dollars one place to the *left*, as follows:

80 dollars = 80. dollars = 8 . 0 tens = 8 tens

To convert *4 hundred-dollar bills* to *dimes*, see in the chart that *hundred* to *dime* is a jump of *3 places to the right*.

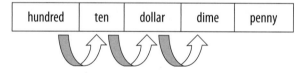

So, move the decimal point in 4 hundreds *3 places to the right*.

4 hundreds = 4.000 hundreds = 4 0 0 0 . dimes or 4,000 dimes.

The Metric System

The metric system is the most widely used general system of measurement in the world today, with the United States being the only exception among developed countries. However, in all countries, the metric system is the preferred system for prescribing medications.

Because the *metric system* is based on 10, converting quantities in this system can also be accomplished by merely shifting the decimal point. The simplicity of its decimal basis has encouraged the proliferation of the metric system.

At the heart of the *metric* system are the *fundamental* or *base units*. The **base units** needed for medical dosages are *gram (g)*, *liter (L)*, and *meter (m)*; these base units are used to measure weight, liquid volume, and length, respectively.

Decimal multiples of any of the base units are obtained by appending standard *metric prefixes* to the base unit. Table 4.4 shows both the base units and their **metric prefixes** with their abbreviations. Note that only the prefixes in blue are used in dosage calculation.

Table 4.4   Format of the Metric System

Name	kilo	hecto	deka	BASE UNIT	deci	centi	milli	*	*	micro
Abbreviation	k	h	da	g, L, m	d	c	m	*	*	mc
Multiple of the Base	1,000	100	10	1	0.1	0.01	0.001	*	*	0.000001

In the metric system, the prefixes indicate multiples of 10 times the base unit, or the base unit divided by multiples of 10. The meanings of the necessary prefixes are found in Table 4.5.

Table 4.5   Metric Prefixes Used in Health Care

Metric Prefixes			
kilo	means	one thousand	(1,000 times the base)
deci	means	one tenth	(0.1 times the base)
centi	means	one hundredth	(0.01 times the base)
milli	means	one thousandth	(0.001 times the base)
micro	means	one millionth	(0.000001 times the base)

The metric prefixes are appended to the base units. For example,

$$1 \underline{\text{kilo}}\text{gram} = 1{,}000 \text{ grams}$$

and

$$1 \underline{\text{centi}}\text{meter} = 0.01 \text{ meter}.$$

Fractions, such as $\frac{1}{2}$, are not formally used in the metric system. For example, $3\frac{1}{2}$ grams is written as 3.5 grams.

Liquid Volume in the Metric System

Drugs in liquid form are measured by volume. The volume of a liquid is the amount of space it occupies. In dosage calculations for liquid volumes only, *liters* and *milliliters* are used (see Table 4.6).

Table 4.6   Metric Equivalents of Liquid Volume

1 cubic centimeter (cc or cm^3)	=	1 milliliter (mL)
1,000 milliliters (mL)	=	1 liter (L)

Milliliters are used for smaller amounts of fluids. The prefix milli means $\frac{1}{1{,}000}$, so

$$1 \text{ liter (L)} = 1{,}000 \text{ milliliters (mL)}$$

NOTE

Deciliters (dL) may be encountered in lab reports. However, deciliters are not used in calculating medical dosages.

NOTE

In example 4.5 when converting 0.5 L to 500 mL, the unit of measurement got smaller, whereas the number got larger.

Milliliters are equivalent to *cubic centimeters* (cm³ or cc), so

$$1 \text{ mL} = 1 \text{ cm}^3 = 1 \text{ cc}$$

You must be able to convert from one unit of measurement to another within the metric system. With liquids in the metric system you need to make conversions only between *liters* and *milliliters*. Of course, you could make such conversions by using *dimensional analysis* or *ratio and proportion*. However, conversions involving metric-system units can be done by merely *moving the decimal point*. In Example 4.5, two of the three methods will be compared.

In the remaining examples of this chapter, the methods of solution shown will alternate between *Dimensional Analysis* and *Ratio & Proportion*. The method of *Moving the Decimal Point* will also shown for each example.

EXAMPLE 4.5

If the prescriber ordered 0.5 L of 5% dextrose in water, how many milliliters were ordered?

RATIO & PROPORTION

In this problem there are two quantities: *liters* and *milliliters*. Think of the problem like this:

$1 \text{ L} = 1,000 \text{ mL}$ [known equivalence]

$0.5 \text{ L} = x \text{ mL}$

One way to set up the proportion is

$$\frac{L}{mL} = \frac{L'}{mL'}$$

Substituting, you obtain

$$\frac{1 \text{ L}}{1,000 \text{ mL}} = \frac{0.5 \text{ L}}{x \text{ mL}}$$

Eliminate the units of measurement and cross multiply

$$\frac{1}{1,000} \diagdown \frac{0.5}{x}$$

$$500 = x$$

MOVING THE DECIMAL POINT

The metric system for liters has the following format, but only the units in blue are used in dosage calculations of liquid volume:

kilo	hecto	deka	Base Unit	deci	centi	milli	*	*	micro
kL	hL	daL	liter (L)	dL	cL	mL			mcL

Because for liquid volume the only units needed for medical dosage calculations are liter (L) and milliliter (mL), the jump will always be three places.

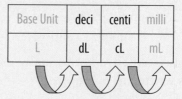

Base Unit	deci	centi	milli
L	dL	cL	mL

For this example, to convert *liters* to *milliliters* is a jump of *3 places to the right*, so, in the quantity 0.5 L, move the decimal point *3 places to the right*, as follows:

0.5 L = 0.500 L = 0 5 0 0. mL = 500. mL = 500 mL.

ALERT

Write 0.5 L instead of $\frac{5}{10}$ L or $\frac{1}{2}$ L because in the metric system, quantities are written as decimal numbers instead of fractions.

So, the prescriber ordered 500 milliliters of 5% dextrose in water.

EXAMPLE 4.6

The patient is to receive *1,750 milliliters of 0.9% NaCl IV q12h*. What is this volume in liters?

NOTE

When converting 1,750 mL to 1.75 L, the unit of measurement got larger, whereas the number got smaller.

DIMENSIONAL ANALYSIS

$$1{,}750 \text{ mL} = ? \text{ L}$$

Cancel the milliliters and obtain the equivalent amount in liters.

$$\frac{1{,}750 \text{ mL}}{1} \times \frac{? \text{ L}}{? \text{ mL}} = ? \text{ L}$$

Because 1,000 mL = 1 L, the unit fraction you want is $\dfrac{1 \text{ L}}{1{,}000 \text{ mL}}$

$$\frac{1{,}750 \text{ mL}}{1} \times \frac{1 \text{ L}}{1{,}000 \text{ mL}} = \frac{1{,}750 \text{ L}}{1{,}000} = 1.75 \text{ L}$$

MOVING THE DECIMAL POINT

For this example, to convert *1,750 milliliters* to *liters* is a jump of *3 places to the left,*

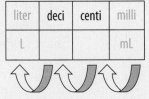

liter	deci	centi	milli
L			mL

So, in 1,750 mL move the decimal point *3 places to the left* as follows:

$$1{,}750 \text{ mL} = 1{,}750. \text{ mL} = 1\,.\,7\,5\,0 \text{ L} = 1.750 \text{ L} = 1.75 \text{ L}$$

So, 1,750 mL of 0.9% NaCl is the same amount as 1.75 L of 0.9% NaCl.

Weight in the Metric System

Drugs in dry form are generally measured by weight. In dosage calculations, *kilograms, grams, milligrams,* and *micrograms* (written in order of size) are used to measure weight. *Kilograms* are the largest of these units of measurement, and *micrograms* are the smallest (see Table 4.7).

ALERT

The abbreviation for microgram, mcg, is preferred over the abbreviation μg because μg may be mistaken for the abbreviation for milligram, mg. This error would result in a dose that would be 1,000 times greater than the prescribed dose.

Table 4.7 Metric Equivalents of Weight

1 kilogram (kg)	=	1,000 grams (g)
1 gram (g)	=	1,000 milligrams (mg)
1 milligram (mg)	=	1,000 micrograms (mcg)

Kilograms are used for the weight of patients. The prefix kilo means 1,000, so

$$1 \textbf{ kilo}\text{gram (kg)} = 1{,}000 \text{ grams (g)}$$

Milligrams are used for measuring the weight of drugs, and *micrograms* are used for very small weights of drugs.

The prefix milli means $\frac{1}{1{,}000}$, and micro means $\frac{1}{1{,}000{,}000}$, so

$$1 \text{ gram (g)} = 1{,}000 \textbf{ milli}\text{grams (mg)}$$

$$1 \text{ milligram (mg)} = 1{,}000 \textbf{ micro}\text{grams (mcg)}$$

The metric system for weight (grams) features the following format. Only the units in blue are needed for dosage calculations involving weight:

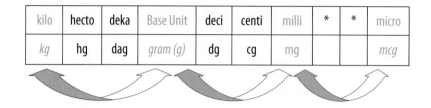

kilo	hecto	deka	Base Unit	deci	centi	milli	*	*	micro
kg	**hg**	**dag**	*gram (g)*	**dg**	**cg**	*mg*			*mcg*

For weight, the only units needed for medical dosage calculations are *kilogram (kg), gram (g), milligram (mg),* and *microgram (mcg).* Because these units are all 3 places apart, the jumps between them will always be three jumps. The following shortened version of the metric weight chart will be useful in the next few examples:

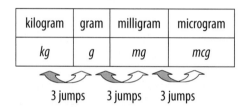

kilogram	gram	milligram	microgram
kg	*g*	*mg*	*mcg*

3 jumps   3 jumps   3 jumps

EXAMPLE 4.7

The order reads *125 mcg of Lanoxin (digoxin) PO daily.* How many milligrams of this cardiac medication would you administer to the patient?

RATIO & PROPORTION

In this problem there are two quantities: *micrograms* and *milligrams.* Think of the problem like this:

$$1{,}000 \text{ mcg} = 1 \text{ mg} \quad \text{[known equivalence]}$$
$$125 \text{ mcg} = x \text{ mg}$$

MOVING THE DECIMAL POINT

In this problem, you convert from mcg to mg. The movement from mcg to mg in the following chart is a movement of one column to the left.

Therefore, the conversion is accomplished by moving the decimal point three places to the left.

One way to set up the proportion is

$$\frac{mcg}{mg} = \frac{mcg'}{mg'}$$

Substituting you obtain

$$\frac{1,000\,mcg}{1\,mg} = \frac{125\,mcg}{x\,mg}$$

Eliminate the units of measurement and cross multiply

$$\frac{1,000}{1} = \frac{125}{x}$$

$$125 = 1,000x$$

Divide both sides by 1,000 $\dfrac{125}{1,000} = \dfrac{1,000x}{1,000}$

$$0.125 = x$$

Kilo-	Fundamental Unit	Milli-	Micro-
kilogram (kg)	gram (g)	milligram (mg)	microgram (mcg)

125 mcg = 125. mcg = . 1 2 5 mg

= .125 mg = 0.125 mg

So, 125 mcg is the same amount as 0.125 mg, and you would administer 0.125 mg of digoxin.

EXAMPLE 4.8

The order reads *Glucotrol (glipizide) 15 mg PO daily ac breakfast*. How many grams of this hypoglycemic agent would you administer?

DIMENSIONAL ANALYSIS

$$15 \text{ mg} = ? \text{ g}$$

Cancel the milligrams and obtain the equivalent amount in grams.

$$15 \text{ mg} \times \frac{?\text{ g}}{?\text{ mg}} = ? \text{ g}$$

$$15 \text{ mg} \times \frac{1 \text{ g}}{1,000 \text{ mg}} = \frac{15}{1,000} \text{ g} = 0.015 \text{ g}$$

MOVING THE DECIMAL POINT

In this problem, you convert from mg to g. The movement from mg to g in the following chart is a movement of one column to the left. Therefore, the conversion is accomplished by moving the decimal point three places to the left.

Kilo-	Fundamental Unit	Milli-	Micro-
kilogram (kg)	gram (g)	milligram (mg)	microgram (mcg)

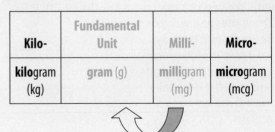

15 mg = 15. mg = . 0 1 5 g

= .015 g = 0.015 g

So, 15 mg is the same amount as 0.015 g, and you would administer 0.015 g of Glucotrol.

EXAMPLE 4.9

Convert 4.5 kilograms to an equivalent amount in grams.

RATIO & PROPORTION

In this problem there are two quantities: *kilograms* and *grams*. Think of the problem like this:

$$1 \, \text{kg} = 1,000 \, \text{g} \quad \text{[known equivalence]}$$
$$4.5 \, \text{kg} = x \, \text{g}$$

One way to set up the proportion is $\dfrac{\text{kg}}{\text{g}} = \dfrac{\text{kg}'}{\text{g}'}$

Substituting you obtain

$$\frac{1 \, kg}{1,000 \, g} = \frac{4.5 \, kg}{x \, g}$$

Eliminate the units of measurement and cross multiply

$$\frac{1}{1,000} = \frac{4.5}{x}$$

$$4,500 = x$$

MOVING THE DECIMAL POINT

To convert kg to g, jump *3 places to the right.*

kilogram	gram	milligram	microgram
kg	g	mg	mcg

Move the decimal point *3 places to the right.*

$$4.5 \text{ kg} = 4.500 \text{ kg} = 4\,5\,0\,0\,.\,g = 4,500 \text{ g}$$

So, 4.5 kilograms is equivalent to 4,500 grams.

Length in the Metric System

The metric system for meters has the following format, but only the units in blue are used in measuring lengths.

Centimeters (cm) and *millimeters (mm)* are the only metric units of length used in this textbook. A patient's height might be measured in *centimeters*, and the diameter of a tumor might be measured in *centimeters* or *millimeters*.

kilo	hecto	deka	Base Unit	deci	centi	milli
km	hm	dam	meter(m)	dm	cm	mm

1 jump

Because *centimeters* and *millimeters* are adjacent units, conversion between them will require a movement of one decimal place. See table 4.8.

NOTE

In metric conversions of liquid volumes and weights, the decimal point is always moved 3 places. However, in metric conversions of length (*cm* and *mm*) the decimal point is moved only one place.

Table 4.8 **Metric Equivalents of Length**
1 centimeter (cm) = 10 millimeters (mm)

EXAMPLE 4.10

A wound has a length of 0.7 centimeters. What is the length of this wound in millimeters?

DIMENSIONAL ANALYSIS

$$0.7 \text{ cm} = ? \text{ mm}$$

$$0.7 \text{ } centimeters = ? \text{ } millimeters$$

You want to cancel the *centimeters* and get the answer in *millimeters*, so choose a unit fraction with *centimeters* on the bottom and *millimeters* on top. You need a fraction in the form of $\dfrac{?\,mm}{?\,cm}$

Because 1 *centimeter* = 10 *millimeters*, the fraction you need is $\dfrac{10\,mm}{1\,cm}$

$$\frac{0.7 \text{ } \cancel{cm}}{1} \times \frac{10 \text{ } \widehat{mm}}{1 \text{ } \cancel{cm}} = 7 \text{ } mm$$

NOTE

The basic metric units of meter, liter, and gram have the following relationship: 1 cubic centi<u>meter</u> of water has a volume of 1 milli<u>liter</u> and weighs 1 <u>gram</u>.

MOVING THE DECIMAL POINT

To convert *centimeters* to *millimeters*, jump *1 place to the right.*

meter	decimeter	centimeter	millimeter
m	dm	cm	mm

So, in 0.7 cm move the decimal point *1 place to the right.*

$$0.7 \text{ cm} = 0\,7\!.\text{ mm} = 7.\text{ mm} = 7 \text{ mm}$$

So, the wound has a length of 7 millimeters.

Summary

In this chapter, the household and metric systems of measurement were introduced.

- The metric system is the dominant system used in health care.
- The apothecary system is being phased out.
- It is important to memorize the equivalences between the various units of measurement of the household and metric systems.
- It is important to memorize the abbreviations for the various units of measurement.
- To convert units of measure in the household system, use dimensional analysis or ratio & proportion.

- To convert units of measure in the metric system, use dimensional analysis, ratio & proportion, or the shortcut method of moving the decimal point. Always jump 3 places except for cm-mm conversions, which use a 1 place jump.
- Remember, each jump is 3 places in this chart:

kilogram	gram	milligram	microgram
kg	g, L	mg, mL	mcg

- Abbreviations for units of measurement are not followed by periods.
  Example: *40 mg and 5 t* (not 40 mg. and 5 t.).

- Abbreviations for units of measurement are not made plural by adding the letter s.
  Example: *70 mcg and 3 oz*
        (not 70 mcgs and 3 ozs).
- Insert a leading zero for decimal numbers less than 1.
  Example: *0.05 g and 0.34 mL*
        (not .05 g and .34 mL).
- Omit trailing zeros for decimal numbers.
  Example: *7.3 mL and 0.07 g*
        (not 7.30 mL and 0.070 g).

- Numbers greater than 999 need commas.
  Example: *2,500 mL and 20,000 mcg*
        (not 2500 mL and 20000 mcg).
- Leave space between the number and the unit of measurement.
  Example: *60 mL and 100 g*
        (not 60mL and 100g).
- Avoid the use of fractions with metric units of measurement.
  Example: *0.5 mL and 1.5 g*
        (not $\frac{1}{2}$ mL and $1\frac{1}{2}$ g).

Workspace

Practice Sets

The answers to *Try These for Practice*, *Exercises*, and *Cumulative Review Exercises* are found in Appendix A. Ask your instructor for the answers to the *Additional Exercises*.

Try These for Practice

Test your comprehension after reading the chapter.

1. You need to memorize all the metric and household equivalents. To test yourself, fill in the missing numbers in the following chart.

Metric System

(a) 1 L   = _____ mL

(b) 1 mL   = _____ cc

(c) 1 L   = _____ cm^3

(d) 1 kg   = _____ g

(e) 1 g   = _____ mg

(f) 1 mg   = _____ mcg

(g) 1 cm   = _____ mm

Household System

(a) 1 qt   = _____ pt

(b) 1 pt   = _____ cups

(c) 1 glass   = _____ oz

(d) 1 measuring cup = _____ oz

(e) 1 oz   = _____ T

(f) 1 T   = _____ t

(g) 1 ft   = _____ in

(h) 1 lb   = _____ oz

2. Use the label on the bottle in •**Figure 4.1** to determine the number of micrograms in one tablet of the drug.

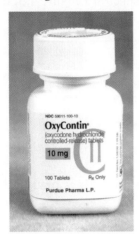

•**Figure 4.1**
Bottle of OxyContin.

3. The prescriber ordered *ProBanthine (propantheline bromide) 30 mg PO ac and hs*. How many grams of ProBanthine will the patient receive in one week?

4. The urinary output of a patient with an indwelling Foley catheter is 1,400 milliliters. How many liters of urine are in the bag?

5. How many tablespoons are equivalent to 3 ounces?

Exercises

Reinforce your understanding in class or at home.

1. 9.6 mg = _____ mcg

2. 0.06 g = _____ mg

3. 40 mg = _____ g

4. 6.25 L = _____ mL

5. 21 mm = _____ cm

6. $2\frac{1}{2}$ pt = _____ cups

7. 24 mL = _____ cc

8. 250,000 mcg = _____ mg

9. 3.5 qt = _____ pt

10. 4 T = _____ t

11. 2 cups = _____ oz

12. 0.35 kg = _____ g

13. Use the label in •**Figure 4.2** to determine the number of micrograms in one Biaxin tablet.

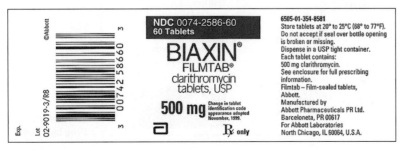

•**Figure 4.2**
Drug label for Biaxin.

14. Order: *doxycycline 100 mg po b.i.d.* What is this dose in grams?

15. According to the portion of the physician's order sheet in • **Figure 4.3,** how many grams of Avandia will the patient receive in 7 days?

Date	Time	Order
8/9/2013	1430 h	Avandia (rosiglitazone maleate) 2 mg po b.i.d.

• **Figure 4.3**
Portion of a Physician's Order Sheet.

16. Order: Amoxil (amoxicillin) *oral susp 1 tsp po q8h.* How many tablespoons of Amoxil will the patient receive in 3 full days?

17. Read the label in • **Figure 4.4** to determine the number of grams of Norvir contained in 1 mL of the Norvir solution.

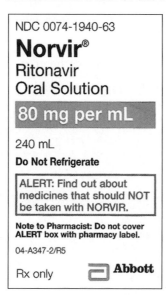

• **Figure 4.4**
Drug label for Norvir.

18. Read the label in • **Figure 4.5** and determine how many grams of Isentress are contained in one tablet.

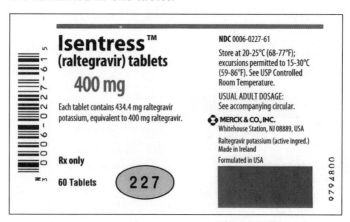

• **Figure 4.5**
Drug label for Isentress.

19. An infant weighs 3.1 kg. How much does the infant weigh in grams?

20. Read the portion of the package insert in •**Figure 4.6** and determine whether or not this order is a safe starting dose: *Dilaudid (hydromorphone HCl) 1.7 mg IM q6h prn for pain.*

DOSAGE AND ADMINISTRATION

DILAUDID INJECTION
   The usual starting dose is 1–2 mg subcutaneously or intramuscularly every 4 to 6 hours as necessary for pain control.

•**Figure 4.6**
Portion of the package insert for Dilaudid.

Additional Exercises

Now, test yourself!

1. 400 mg = _____ g

2. 0.003 g = _____ mg

3. 0.07 g = _____ mg

4. 3 L = _____ mL

5. 2,500 mL = _____ L

6. 600 mcg = _____ mg

7. 1.7 L = _____ mL

8. $4\frac{1}{2}$ qt = _____ pt

9. 2.5 kg = _____ g

10. 4 T = _____ t

11. 5 T = _____ oz

12. 32 oz = _____ pt

13. Using the label in •**Figure 4.7**, determine the number of grams in two tablets of Depakote ER.

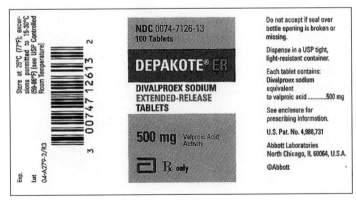

•**Figure 4.7**
Drug label for Depakote ER.

14. The physician ordered a loading dose of *digoxin 520 mcg PO stat*. How many milligrams are in this dose?

15. According to the package insert information in •**Figure 4.8,** would the following order be safe or not: *Uniphyl (theophylline, anhydrous) 400 mg po b.i.d.*

Workspace

> **UNIPHYL®**
> Tablets
> (theophylline, anhydrous)
> **400 mg and 600 mg**
>
> **DOSAGE AND ADMINISTRATION**
> Uniphyl® 400 or 600 mg Tablets can be taken once a day in the morning or evening.
>
> It is recommended that Uniphyl be taken with meals. Patients should be advised that if they choose to take Uniphyl with food it should be taken consistently with food and if they take it in a fasted condition it should routinely be taken fasted. It is important that the product whenever dosed be dosed consistently with or without food.

● **Figure 4.8**
Portion of the package insert for Uniphyl.

16. Read the label in ● **Figure 4.9** to determine the number of milligrams in 2 tablets of Levothroid.

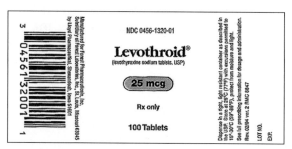

● **Figure 4.9**
Drug label for Lovothroid.

17. According to the physician's order sheet in ● **Figure 4.10,** what is the dose in grams of the chlorpromazine?

		PHYSICIAN'S ORDERS	CHART COPY

FORM 01 109
12065 - 0389

DATE	TIME		
7/3/2013	4 PM	chlorpromazine 50 mg	
		PO t.i.d.	

PLEASE INDICATE BEEPER # →

PATIENT CERTIFICATION

12/24/30 Buddhist Aetna
28945 Abdul Danuish 2 Otter St. Boulder, Co 43612
7/3/13
Mae Ling MD

● **Figure 4.10**
Portion of a physician's order sheet.

18. A patient is drinking $\frac{1}{2}$ pint of orange juice every two hours. At this rate, how many quarts of orange juice will the patient drink in eight hours?

19. An infant weighs 3,400 grams. How much does the infant weigh in kilograms?

20. 5 ft = _____ in

Cumulative Review Exercises

Reinforce your mastery of previous chapters.

1. 1.3 g = _____ mg

2. 24 oz = _____ cups

3. 4.2 L = _____ mL

4. 9 T = _____ t

5. 900 mL = _____ L

6. $1\frac{1}{2}$ pt = _____ cups

7. Convert 560 mg to grams.

8. How many ounces are contained in 12 teaspoons?

9. Order: *Motrin (ibuprofen) 200 mg po q4h prn back pain.* What is the maximum number of milligrams of Motrin that the patient could receive in any 6-hour period?

10. Order: *ampicillin 250 mg t.i.d.* What is missing from this order?

11. If a patient receives a drug *40 mg po b.i.d.*, how many mg would be administered in a 24-hour period?

12. If a patient receives a drug *40 mg po q12h*, how many mg would be administered in a 24-hour period?

13. If a patient receives a drug *40 mg po daily in two divided doses*, how many mg would be administered in a 24-hour period?

14. Write 9:30 P.M. in military time.

15. A patient must receive a drug *q6h*. If the patient gets one dose at 1900 h, at what time would the next dose be administered?

nursing.pearsonhighered.com
Prepare for success with animated examples, practice questions, challenge tests, and interactive assignments.

Chapter

5 Converting from One System of Measurement to Another

Learning Outcomes

1 kilogram (kg)
≈
2.2 pounds (lb)

After completing this chapter, you will be able to

1. State the equivalent units of weight between the metric and household systems.
2. State the equivalent units of volume between the metric and household systems.
3. State the equivalent units of length between the metric and household systems.
4. Convert a quantity measured in metric units to its equivalent measured in household units.
5. Convert a quantity measured in household units to its equivalent measured in metric units.

When calculating drug dosages, you will sometimes need to convert a quantity expressed in one system of measurement to an equivalent quantity expressed in a different system of measurement. For example, you might need to convert a quantity measured in ounces to the same quantity measured in milliliters. This chapter will show you how to accomplish such conversions.

Equivalents of Common Units of Measurement

To get started, you will need to learn some basic equivalent values of the various units in the different systems. Table 5.1 lists some common equivalent values for weight, volume, and length in the metric and household systems of measurement. Although these equivalents are considered standards, all of them are approximations.

A useful summary of the relationships that you should know among all the equivalents of liquid volume is provided in Table 5.2.

Table 5.1	**Approximate Equivalents between Metric and Household Units of Volume, Weight, and Length**		
	Metric		**Household**
Volume	5 milliliters (mL)	≈	1 teaspoon (t)
	15 milliliters (mL)	≈	1 tablespoon (T)
	30 milliliters (mL)	≈	1 ounce (oz)
	240 milliliters (mL)	≈	1 cup
	500 milliliters (mL)	≈	1 pint (pt)
	1,000 milliliters (mL)	≈	1 quart (qt)
Weight	1 kilogram (kg)	≈	2.2 pounds (lb)
Length	2.5 centimeters (cm)	≈	1 inch (in)

Table 5.2	**Summary Table of Equivalents within and Approximate Equivalents between Metric and Household Units of Volume**	
	1 teaspoon	≈ 5 mL
	1 tablespoon = 3 teaspoons	≈ 15 mL
	1 ounce = 2 tablespoons = 6 teaspoons	≈ 30 mL
	1 cup = 8 ounces = 16 tablespoons	≈ 240 mL
	1 pint = 2 cups = 16 ounces	≈ 500 mL
	1 quart = 2 pints = 4 cups = 32 ounces	≈ 1,000 mL = 1L

NOTE

Some books use these approximations:

$$250 \, \text{mL} \approx 1 \text{ cup}$$
$$480 \text{ mL} \approx 1 \text{ pt}$$

NOTE

Unlike all the approximations in Tables 5.1 and 5.2, an inch is defined to be exactly 2.54 cm.

You can use dimensional analysis to convert from one system to another in exactly the same way you converted from one unit to another within the same system. •**Figure 5.1** depicts medication cups with units of measurement from various systems.

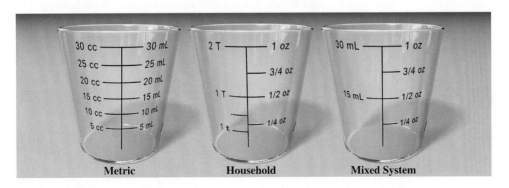

• **Figure 5.1**
Medication cups showing equivalent units.

The surface, called the meniscus, of a liquid in a medication cup is not flat (•**Figure 5.2**). It is curved. Read the amount of liquid at the level of the bottom of the meniscus.

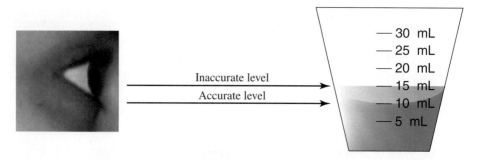

• **Figure 5.2**
Medication cup filled to 10 mL.

Metric-Household Conversions

Volume Conversions

EXAMPLE 5.1

Convert 8 teaspoons to an equivalent volume measured in milliliters.

DIMENSIONAL ANALYSIS

$$8\,t = ?\,mL$$

You want to cancel the teaspoons and obtain the equivalent in milliliters.

$$8\,t \times \frac{?\,mL}{?\,t} = ?\,mL$$

You use the equivalence $5\,mL = 1\,t$.

So, the unit fraction is $\dfrac{5\,mL}{1t}$

$$8\,t \times \frac{5\,mL}{1\,t} = 40\,mL$$

RATIO & PROPORTION

$$8\,t = ?\,mL$$

In this problem, there are two quantities: *teaspoons* and *milliliters*.

Think of the problem this way:

$$8\,t = x\,mL$$
$$1\,t = 5\,mL \quad \text{[known equivalent]}$$

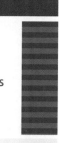

NOTE

Although 1 t is approximately equal to 5 mL, in Example 5.1, for simplicity, the equal sign is used. This practice will be followed throughout the textbook.

Because the number of teaspoons and the number of milliliters are proportional, a proportion could be used to solve the problem. One way to set up the proportion is

$$\frac{t}{mL} = \frac{t'}{mL'}$$

Substituting, you obtain

$$\frac{8t}{x\,mL} = \frac{1\,t}{5\,mL}$$

Eliminate the units of measurement

$$\frac{8}{x} = \frac{1}{5}$$

Cross multiply and simplify

$$\frac{8}{x} = \frac{1}{5}$$

$$(x)(1) = (8)(5)$$
$$x = 40$$

So, 8 teaspoons is equivalent to 40 milliliters.

EXAMPLE 5.2

Change $1\frac{1}{2}$ pints to milliliters.

DIMENSIONAL ANALYSIS

$$1\frac{1}{2} \text{ pt} = ? \text{ mL}$$

You want to cancel the pints and obtain the equivalent amount in milliliters.

$$\frac{3 \text{ pt}}{2} \times \frac{? \text{ mL}}{? \text{ pt}} = ? \text{ mL}$$

Because $500 \text{ mL} = 1 \text{ pt}$, the unit fraction is $\dfrac{500 \text{ mL}}{1 \text{ pt}}$

$$\frac{3 \text{ pt}}{\underset{1}{2}} \times \frac{\overset{250}{500} \text{ mL}}{1 \text{ pt}} = 750 \text{ mL}$$

RATIO & PROPORTION

$$1\frac{1}{2} \text{ pt} = ? \text{ mL}$$

Think of the problem this way:

$$1\frac{1}{2} \text{ pt} = x \text{ mL}$$

$$1 \text{ pt} = 500 \text{ mL} \quad \text{[known equivalent]}$$

One way to set up the proportion is

$$\frac{pt}{mL} = \frac{pt'}{mL'}$$

Substituting, you obtain

$$\frac{1\frac{1}{2} \, pt}{x \, mL} = \frac{1 \, pt}{500 \, mL}$$

Eliminate the units of measurement

$$\frac{1\frac{1}{2}}{x} = \frac{1}{500}$$

Cross multiply and simplify

$$\frac{1\frac{1}{2}}{x} = \frac{1}{500}$$

$$(x)(1) = \left(1\frac{1}{2}\right)(500)$$

$$x = 750$$

So, $1\frac{1}{2}$ pints is equivalent to 750 milliliters.

EXAMPLE 5.3

A patient is to receive 60 milliliters of a medication. How many ounces will the patient receive?

DIMENSIONAL ANALYSIS

$$60\,milliliters\ =\ ?\,ounces$$

You want to cancel the *milliliters* and get the answer in *ounces,* so choose a fraction with *milliliters* on the bottom and *ounces* on top.

You need a fraction in the form of $\dfrac{?\,oz}{?\,mL}$

Because $1\,oz = 30\,mL$, the unit fraction you need is $\dfrac{1\,oz}{30\,mL}$

$$\dfrac{\overset{2}{\cancel{60}}\,\cancel{mL}}{1} \times \dfrac{1\,oz}{\underset{1}{\cancel{30}\,\cancel{mL}}} = 2\,oz$$

NOTE

Example 5.3 could be done mentally by understanding that, because 1 ounce = 30 milliliters, then twice as many ounces (2 oz) will equal twice as many milliliters (60 mL). That is, 2 oz = 60 mL.

RATIO & PROPORTION

Think of the problem this way:

$$60\,mL = x\,oz$$
$$30\,mL = 1\,oz \quad \text{[known equivalent]}$$

One way to set up the proportion is

$$\frac{mL}{oz} = \frac{mL'}{oz'}$$

Substituting, you obtain

$$\frac{60\,mL}{x\,oz} = \frac{30\,mL}{1\,oz}$$

Eliminate the units of measurement

$$\frac{60}{x} = \frac{30}{1}$$

Cross multiply and simplify

$$\frac{60}{x} \diagdown \frac{30}{1}$$

$$(x)(30) = (1)(60)$$
$$30x = 60$$

Divide by 30 and cancel

$$\frac{\cancel{30}x}{\cancel{30}} = \frac{60}{30}$$
$$x = 2$$

So, the patient will receive 2 ounces of the medication.

EXAMPLE 5.4

A medication cup contains 22.5 milliliters of a solution. How many tablespoons are in the medication cup?

DIMENSIONAL ANALYSIS

$$22.5\,milliliters = ?\,tablespoons$$

You want to cancel the *milliliters* and get the answer in *tablespoons*, so choose a fraction with *milliliters* on the bottom and *tablespoons* on top. You need a fraction in the form of $\dfrac{?\,T}{?\,mL}$

Because $15\,milliliters = 1\,tablespoon$, the unit fraction you need is $\dfrac{1\,T}{15\,mL}$

$$\frac{22.5\,\cancel{mL}}{1} \times \frac{1\,T}{15\,\cancel{mL}} = 1.5\,T$$

RATIO & PROPORTION

Think of the problem this way:

$$22.5\,mL = x\,T$$
$$15\,mL = 1\,T \quad \text{[known equivalent]}$$

One way to set up the proportion is

$$\frac{mL}{T} = \frac{mL'}{T'}$$

Substituting, you obtain

$$\frac{22.5\,mL}{x\,T} = \frac{15\,mL}{1\,T}$$

Eliminate the units of measurement, cross multiply, and simplify

$$\frac{22.5}{x} = \frac{15}{1}$$

$$(x)(15) = (1)(22.5)$$
$$15x = 22.5$$

Divide by 15 and cancel

$$\frac{\cancel{15}x}{\cancel{15}} = \frac{22.5}{15}$$

$$x = 1.5$$

So, the medication cup contains $1\frac{1}{2}$ *tablespoons*.

Weight Conversions

EXAMPLE 5.5

A patient weighs 150 pounds. What is the patient's weight measured in kilograms?

DIMENSIONAL ANALYSIS

$$150\,pounds = ?\,kilograms$$

You want to cancel the *pounds* and get the answer in *kilograms*, so choose a fraction with *pounds* on the bottom and *kilograms* on top.

You need a fraction in the form of $\dfrac{?\,kg}{?\,lb}$

RATIO & PROPORTION

Think of the problem this way:

$$1.50\,lb = x\,kg$$
$$2.2\,lb = 1\,kg \quad \text{[known equivalent]}$$

One way to set up the proportion is

$$\frac{lb}{kg} = \frac{lb'}{kg'}$$

Because 2.2 *pounds* = 1 *kilogram*, the unit fraction you need is $\dfrac{1\,kg}{2.2\,lb}$

$$\frac{150\ \cancel{lb}}{1} \times \frac{1\,kg}{2.2\ \cancel{lb}} \approx 68.1818\,kg$$

Substituting, you obtain

$$\frac{150\,lb}{x\,kg} = \frac{2.2\,lb'}{1\,kg'}$$

Eliminate the units of measurement, cross multiply, and simplify

$$\frac{150}{x} = \frac{2.2}{1}$$

$$(x)(2.2) = (1)(150)$$
$$2.2x = 150$$

Divide by 2.2 and cancel

$$\frac{\cancel{2.2}\,x}{\cancel{2.2}} = \frac{150}{2.2}$$
$$x = 68.18$$

So, the patient weighs 68 kilograms.

EXAMPLE 5.6

Jennifer weighs 115 pounds 8 ounces. What is her weight in kilograms?

DIMENSIONAL ANALYSIS

115 lb 8 oz   means   115 lb + 8 oz

First determine Jennifer's weight in pounds. To do this, convert 8 ounces to pounds.

$$8\text{ oz} = ?\text{ lb}$$

You want to cancel ounces and obtain the equivalent amount in pounds.

$$8\text{ oz} \times \frac{?\text{ lb}}{?\text{ oz}} = ?\text{ lb}$$

Because 1 lb = 16 oz, the unit fraction is $\dfrac{1\text{ lb}}{16\text{ oz}}$

$$\overset{1}{\cancel{8}}\ \cancel{oz} \times \frac{1\text{ lb}}{\underset{2}{\cancel{16}}\ \cancel{oz}} = \frac{1}{2}\text{ lb}$$

So, Jennifer weighs 115 lb + $\frac{1}{2}$ lb or 115.5 pounds.

RATIO & PROPORTION

115 lb 8 oz   means   115 lb + 8 oz

First, determine Jennifer's weight in pounds. To do this, convert 8 ounces to pounds.

Think of the problem this way:

$$8\text{ oz} = x\text{ lb}$$
$$16\text{ oz} = 1\text{ lb}\quad\text{[known equivalent]}$$

One way to set up the proportion is

$$\frac{8\text{ oz}}{x\text{ lb}} = \frac{16\text{ oz}}{1\text{ lb}}$$

Eliminate the units of measurement, cross multiply, and simplify

$$\frac{8\text{ oz}}{x\text{ lb}} = \frac{16\text{ oz}}{1\text{ lb}}$$

$$(16)(x) = (8)(1)$$
$$16x = 8$$

Now, convert 115.5 pounds to kilograms

$$115.5 \text{ lb} = ? \text{ kg}$$

You want to cancel pounds and obtain the equivalent amount in kilograms

$$115.5 \text{ lb} \times \frac{? \text{ kg}}{? \text{ lb}} = ? \text{ kg}$$

Because $1 \text{ kg} = 2.2 \text{ lb}$, the unit fraction is $\dfrac{1 \text{ kg}}{2.2 \text{ lb}}$

$$115.5 \text{ lb} \times \frac{1 \text{ kg}}{2.2 \text{ lb}} = 52.5 \text{ kg}$$

NOTE

In Example 5.6, the 8 ounces could have been changed to $\frac{1}{2}$ pound mentally by understanding that because 16 ounces = 1 pound, then one-half as many ounces (8 oz) will equal one-half as many pounds ($\frac{1}{2}$ lb). That is, $8 \text{ oz} = \frac{1}{2} \text{ lb}$.

Divide by the coefficient of x, cancel, and simplify

$$\frac{16x}{16} = \frac{8}{16}$$

$$x = \frac{1}{2}$$

Jennifer weighs $115\frac{1}{2}$ pounds.
Now, change 115.5 pounds to kilograms.
To change 115.5 pounds to kilograms, think of the problem as

$$115.5 \text{ lb} = x \text{ kg}$$
$$2.2 \text{ lb} = 1 \text{ kg} \quad \text{[known equivalent]}$$

One way to set up the proportion is

$$\frac{115.5 \, lb}{x \, kg} = \frac{2.2 \, lb}{1 \, kg}$$

Eliminate the units of measurement, cross multiply, and simplify

$$\frac{115.5 \, lb}{x \, kg} = \frac{2.2 \, lb}{1 \, kg}$$

$$(2.2)(x) = (115.5)(1)$$
$$2.2x = 115.5$$

Divide by the coefficient of x, cancel, and simplify

$$\frac{2.2x}{2.2} = \frac{115.5}{2.2}$$

$$x = 52.5$$

So, Jennifer weighs 52.5 kilograms.

EXAMPLE 5.7

An infant weighs 4 kilograms. What is the infant's weight measured in pounds and ounces?

DIMENSIONAL ANALYSIS

$$4 \, kilograms = ? \, pounds$$

You want to cancel the *kilograms* and get the answer in *pounds*, so choose a fraction with *kilograms* on the bottom and *pounds* on top. You need a fraction in the form of $\dfrac{? \, lb}{? \, kg}$

Because 1 *kilogram* = 2.2 *pounds*, the unit fraction you need is $\dfrac{2.2 \, lb}{1 \, kg}$

$$\frac{4 \, k\!\!\!/g}{1} \times \frac{2.2 \, \widehat{lb}}{1 \, k\!\!\!/g} = 8.8 \, lb$$

So, the infant weighs 8 lb + 0.8 lb

Next, change the 0.8 lb to ounces.

$$0.8 \, lb = ? \, ounces$$

You want to cancel the *pounds* and get the answer in *ounces*, so choose a fraction with *pounds* on the bottom and *ounces* on top. You need a fraction in the form of $\dfrac{? \, oz}{? \, lb}$

Because 1 *pound* = 16 *ounces*, the unit fraction you need is $\dfrac{16 \, oz}{1 \, lb}$

$$\frac{0.8 \, l\!\!\!/b}{1} \times \frac{16 \, \widehat{oz}}{1 \, l\!\!\!/b} = 12.8 \, oz \approx 13 \, oz$$

RATIO & PROPORTION

First change the weight to pounds.

Think of the problem this way:

$$4 \, kg = x \, lb$$
$$1 \, kg = 2.2 \, lb \quad \text{[known equivalent]}$$

One way to set up the proportion is

$$\frac{lb}{kg} = \frac{lb'}{kg'}$$

Substituting, you obtain

$$\frac{x \, lb}{4 \, kg} = \frac{2.2 \, lb}{1 \, kg}$$

Eliminate the units of measurement, cross multiply, and simplify

$$\frac{x}{4} \diagdown \frac{2.2}{1}$$

$$(4)(2.2) = (1)(x)$$
$$8.8 = x$$

The infant weighs 8.8 pounds (8 pounds + 0.8 pounds). To change the 0.8 pound to ounces, think of the problem as

$$0.8 \, lb = x \, oz$$
$$1 \, lb = 16 \, oz \quad \text{[known equivalent]}$$

One way to set up the proportion is

$$\frac{lb}{oz} = \frac{lb'}{oz'}$$

Substituting you obtain

$$\frac{0.8 \, lb}{x \, oz} = \frac{1 \, lb}{16 \, oz}$$

Eliminate the units of measurement, cross multiply, and simplify

$$\frac{0.8}{x} \diagdown \frac{1}{16}$$

$$(1)(x) = (0.8)(16)$$
$$x = 12.8 \approx 13$$

The infant weighs 8 pounds 13 ounces.

Length Conversions

EXAMPLE 5.8

Adam is 6 feet 3 inches tall. What is his height in centimeters?

DIMENSIONAL ANALYSIS

6 ft 3 in   means   6 ft + 3 in

First determine Adam's height in inches. To do this, convert 6 feet to inches

$$6 \text{ ft} = ? \text{ in}$$

You want to cancel feet and obtain the equivalent height in inches

$$6 \text{ ft} \times \frac{? \text{ in}}{? \text{ ft}} = ? \text{ in}$$

Because 1 ft = 12 in, the unit fraction is $\dfrac{12 \text{ in}}{1 \text{ ft}}$

$$6 \text{ ft} \times \frac{12 \text{ in}}{1 \text{ ft}} = 72 \text{ in}$$

Now, add the extra 3 inches

$$72 \text{ in} + 3 \text{ in} = 75 \text{ in}$$

Now convert 75 inches to centimeters

$$75 \text{ in} = ? \text{ cm}$$

You want to cancel inches and obtain the equivalent length in centimeters

$$75 \text{ in} \times \frac{? \text{ cm}}{? \text{ in}} = ? \text{ cm}$$

Because 1 in = 2.5 cm, the unit fraction is $\dfrac{2.5 \text{ cm}}{1 \text{ in}}$

$$75 \text{ in} \times \frac{2.5 \text{ cm}}{1 \text{ in}} = 187.5 \text{ cm}$$

NOTE

In Example 5.8, the 6 feet could have been changed to 72 inches by understanding that because 1 foot = 12 inches, then 6 times as many feet (6 ft) will equal six times as many inches (72 in). That is, 6 ft = 72 in.

RATIO & PROPORTION

6 ft 3 in   means   6 ft + 3 in

First, determine Adam's height in inches. To do this, convert 6 feet to inches.

Think of the problem this way:

$$6 \text{ ft} = x \text{ in}$$
$$1 \text{ ft} = 12 \text{ in} \quad \text{[known equivalent]}$$

One way to set up the proportion is

$$\frac{6 \, ft}{x \, in} = \frac{1 \, ft}{12 \, in}$$

Eliminate the units of measurement, cross multiply, and simplify

$$\frac{6 \, ft}{x \, in} = \frac{1 \, ft}{12 \, in}$$

$$(1)(x) = (6)(12)$$
$$x = 72$$

Now, add the extra 3 inches

$$72 \text{ in} + 3 \text{ in} = 75 \text{ in}$$

Adam is 75 inches tall.

To change 75 inches to centimeters, think of the problem as

$$75 \text{ in} = x \text{ cm}$$
$$1 \text{ in} = 2.5 \text{ cm} \quad \text{[known equivalent]}$$

One way to set up the proportion is

$$\frac{75 \, in}{x \, cm} = \frac{1 \, in}{2.5 \, cm}$$

Eliminate the units of measurement, cross multiply, and simplify

$$\frac{75 \, in}{x \, cm} = \frac{1 \, in}{2.5 \, cm}$$

$$(1)(x) = (75)(2.5)$$
$$x = 187.5 \approx 188$$

So, Adam is 188 centimeters tall.

EXAMPLE 5.9

A tumor has a diameter of 2 inches. What is the diameter of the tumor measured in millimeters?

DIMENSIONAL ANALYSIS

First change from *inches* to *centimeters*, and then from *centimeters* to *millimeters*.

$$2\,inches \rightarrow ?\,centimeters \rightarrow ?\,millimeters$$

You want to cancel the *inches* and get the answer in *centimeters*, so choose a fraction with *inches* on the bottom and *centimeters* on top.

Because 1 *inch* = 2.5 *centimeters*, the unit fraction you need is $\dfrac{2.5\,cm}{1\,in}$

$$\frac{2\,in}{1} \times \frac{2.5\,cm}{1\,in} = ?\,mm$$

Next, you want to cancel the *cm* and get the answer in *mm*, so choose a unit fraction with *cm* on the bottom and *mm* on top.

Because 1 *centimeter* = 10 *millimeters*, the unit fraction you need is $\dfrac{10\,mm}{1\,cm}$

$$\frac{2\,in}{1} \times \frac{2.5\,cm}{1\,in} \times \frac{10\,mm}{1\,cm} = 50\,mm$$

RATIO & PROPORTION

First use the equivalence 2.5 centimeters = 1 inch.
  Think of the problem this way:

$$2\,in = x\,cm$$
$$1\,in = 2.5\,cm \quad [\text{known equivalent}]$$

One way to set up the proportion is

$$\frac{in}{cm} = \frac{in'}{cm'}$$

Substituting, you obtain

$$\frac{2\,in}{x\,cm} = \frac{1\,in}{2.5\,cm}$$

Eliminate the units of measurement, cross multiply, and simplify

$$\frac{2}{x} \diagup\hspace{-0.9em}= \frac{1}{2.5}$$

$$(x)(1) = (2)(2.5)$$
$$x = 5$$

So, the diameter of the tumor is 5 centimeters. Now change to millimeters

$$5\,cm = ?\,mm$$

To convert *centimeters* to *millimeters* is a jump of *1 place to the right*.

meter	decimeter	centimeter	millimeter
m	dm	cm	mm

So, in 5 cm, move the decimal point *1 place to the right*.

$$5\,cm = 5.0\,cm = 5\,0.\,mm = 50.\,mm = 50\,mm$$

So, the tumor has a diameter of 50 millimeters.

Summary

In this chapter, quantities measured in one system of measurement were converted to equivalent quantities measured in a different system of measurement.

- It is important to memorize all the equivalences for volume, weight, and length between the metric and household systems of measurement.
- Both Dimensional Analysis and Ratio & Proportion can be used to perform conversions between the metric and household systems.

- The equivalences between systems are not exact; they are approximate.
- When performing conversions between two systems, your answers are not exact; they are approximate.
- When performing conversions between two systems, answers may differ somewhat, depending on which approximate equivalences are used.

Practice Sets

The answers to *Try These for Practice, Exercises,* and *Cumulative Review Exercises* are found in Appendix A. Ask your instructor for the answers to the *Additional Exercises*.

Try These for Practice

Test your comprehension after reading the chapter.

1. In order to do the exercises at the end of this chapter, you need to memorize all the equivalents presented so far. To test yourself, fill in the missing numbers in the following chart.

Metric System

(a) 1 L = _____ mL

(b) 1 kg = _____ g

(c) 1 g = _____ mg

(d) 1 mg = _____ mcg

(e) 1 cm = _____ mm

Household System

(f) 1 qt = _____ pt

(g) 1 pt = _____ cups

(h) 1 cup = _____ oz

(i) 1 glass = _____ oz

(j) 1 oz = _____ T

(k) 1 T = _____ t

(l) 1 lb = _____ oz

(m) 1 ft = _____ in

Workspace

Workspace

Mixed Systems

(n) 1 in ≈ _____ cm

(o) 1 kg ≈ _____ lb

(p) 1 t ≈ _____ mL

(q) 1 T ≈ _____ mL

(r) 1 oz ≈ _____ mL

(s) 1 cup ≈ _____ mL

(t) 1 glass ≈ _____ mL

(u) 1 pt ≈ _____ mL

(v) 1 qt ≈ _____ mL

(w) 1 oz = _____ T = _____ t ≈ _____ mL

(x) 1 qt = _____ pt = _____ cups = _____ oz ≈ _____ mL

2. Use the label in • **Figure 5.3** to determine how many teaspoons of Naproxen will contain 125 mg of the drug.

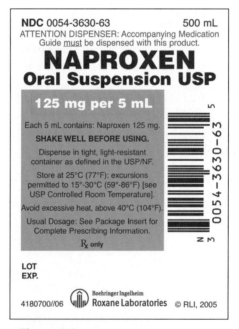

NDC 0054-3630-63   500 mL
ATTENTION DISPENSER: Accompanying Medication Guide <u>must</u> be dispensed with this product.

NAPROXEN
Oral Suspension USP

125 mg per 5 mL

Each 5 mL contains: Naproxen 125 mg.

SHAKE WELL BEFORE USING.

Dispense in tight, light-resistant container as defined in the USP/NF.

Store at 25°C (77°F); excursions permitted to 15°-30°C (59°-86°F) [see USP Controlled Room Temperature].

Avoid excessive heat, above 40°C (104°F).

Usual Dosage: See Package Insert for Complete Prescribing Information.

R̩ only

LOT
EXP.

4180700//06   Boehringer Ingelheim
Roxane Laboratories   © RLI, 2005

• **Figure 5.3**
Drug label for Naproxen.

3. The diameter of a wound is 50 mm. What is the diameter of the wound measured in inches?

4. The urinary output of a patient with an indwelling Foley catheter is observed to be 900 milliliters. What is this output measured in liters?

5. A patient must drink $1\frac{1}{2}$ ounces of a prescribed solution. If only a teaspoon is available, how many teaspoons of the solution should the patient drink?

Exercises

Reinforce your understanding in class or at home.

1. 4.7 mg = _____ mcg

2. 400 mL = _____ L

3. 60 mL ≈ _____ t

4. 4 T ≈ _____ mL

5. 50 lb ≈ _____ kg *(Round off to the nearest tenth)*

6. 50 kg ≈ _____ lb

7. 3.5 pt = _____ oz

8. 4 T = _____ oz

9. 7.5 cm ≈ _____ in

10. How many tablespoons are contained in the Lexapro container whose label is shown in •**Figure 5.4**?

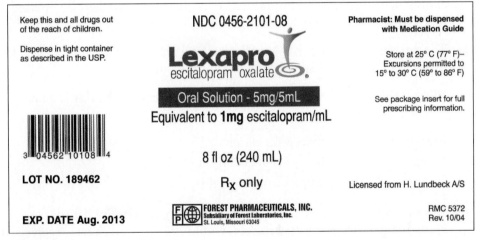

• **Figure 5.4**
Drug label for Lexapro.

11. A patient is 5 feet 9 inches tall. Find the height of the patient in centimeters.

12. Find the weight in grams of a 7 pound infant. (*Round off to the nearest gram*)

13. Harold weighs 250 pounds now. If Harold goes on a diet and loses 30 pounds, then how many kilograms will he weigh?

Workspace

14. Use • **Figure 5.5** to determine how many teaspoons of Namenda will contain 2 mg of the drug.

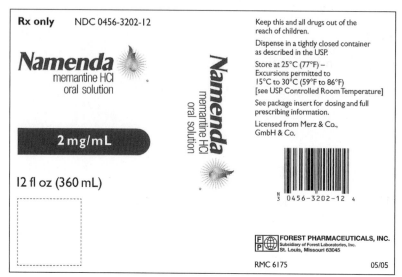

Rx only   NDC 0456-3202-12

Namenda
memantine HCl
oral solution

2 mg/mL

12 fl oz (360 mL)

Namenda
memantine HCl
oral solution

Keep this and all drugs out of the reach of children.

Dispense in a tightly closed container as described in the USP.

Store at 25°C (77°F) –
Excursions permitted to
15°C to 30°C (59°F to 86°F)
[see USP Controlled Room Temperature]

See package insert for dosing and full prescribing information.

Licensed from Merz & Co., GmbH & Co.

3 0456-3202-12 4

FOREST PHARMACEUTICALS, INC.
Subsidiary of Forest Laboratories, Inc.
St. Louis, Missouri 63045

RMC 6175   05/05

• **Figure 5.5**
Drug label for Namenda.

15. A nurse administers 30 mL of a drug by mouth t.i.d. to a patient. This patient is to be discharged, and the patient must continue to take the medication at home. How many tablespoons should the patient be advised to take daily?

16. The patient is required to take *Allegra (fexofenadine) 60 mg po b.i.d.* How many grams of this drug will the patient take in 3 days?

17. What is the patient's total fluid intake in milliliters for the day if he had the following fluid intake:

Breakfast: 8 oz milk; 8 oz water
Lunch: 6 oz juice; 3 T medication
Dinner: 6 oz soup; 12 oz soda; 4 oz jello

18. The order for a patient is *Robitussin syrup (guaifenesin) 10 mL po q4h.* How many ounces of Robitussin would the patient have received by 10 P.M. if the first dose was administered at noon?

19. The patient must receive *Cipro (ciprofloxacin hydrochloride) 500 mg b.i.d. × 10 d* for acute sinusitis. How many grams of Cipro will the patient have received in total after the 10 days?

20. A school nurse administers 2 *teaspoons* of Children's Tylenol to a child who has a fever. How many such doses are contained in an 8 *ounce* bottle of this medication?

Additional Exercises

Now, test yourself!

1. 4,500 mcg = _____ mg

2. 1.5 L = _____ mL

3. 4 t ≈ _____ mL

4. 15 mL ≈ _____ t

5. 45 kg ≈ _____ lb

6. 110 lb ≈ _____ kg

7. 48 oz = _____ pt

8. 3 oz = _____ T

9. 10 cm ≈ _____ in

10. 6 in ≈ _____ cm

11. A patient is 6 feet 2 inches tall. Find the height of the patient in centimeters.

12. Using the label in •**Figure 5.6**, determine the number of teaspoons of the fluconazole suspension that would contain 50 mg of the drug.

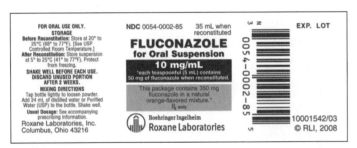

•**Figure 5.6**
Drug label for fluconazole.

13. A woman weighs 165 pounds. What is her weight in kilograms?

14. A patient takes 2 teaspoons of Robitussin (guaifenesin). How many milliliters of this cough suppressant did the patient take?

15. A nurse administers KCl 30 mL by mouth daily to Mrs. M. This patient is to be discharged, and she must continue to take the medication at home. How many tablespoons should she be advised to take daily?

16. Read the information in •**Figure 5.7** and determine the number of teaspoons of the bronchodilator metaproterenol you will administer if the label reads "10 mg/5 mL."

UNIVERSITY HOSPITAL

AUTHORIZATION IS HEPEBY GIVEN TO DISPENSE THE GENERIC OR CHEMICAL EQUIVALENT UNLESS OTHERWISE INDICATED BY THE WORDS — **NO SUBSTITUTE**

DATE ORDERED	TIME ORDERED	DOCTOR'S ORDERS (PLEASE WRITE IN CLEARLY AND SIGN)
10/1/10	2 PM	*metaproterenol sulfate syrup 10 mg PO t.i.d.*

DO NOT USE FOR ANTIBIOTIC ORDERS

PATIENT CERTIFCATION

3/12/32
Roman Catholic
Medicare

10/1/2013

712456
Martha Noonan
100 River St.
Rotland, VT
05701

Dr. Ali Vondé

PLEASE INDICATE BEEPER # →

• **Figure 5.7**
Physician's order sheet.

Workspace

17. A patient drank 12 ounces of orange juice. How many milliliters did the patient drink?

18. The label indicates that in the container there are 120 metered sprays, each of which contains 32 mcg of Rhinocort. Use this information to determine the total number of milligrams of this corticosteroid inhalant that are in the container.

19. Using the label in •**Figure 5.8**, determine the total number of milliliters of vaccine that are in the vial.

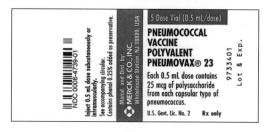

• **Figure 5.8**
Drug label for pneumococcal vaccine polyvalent pneumovax 23.

20. Read the label in •**Figure 5.9** and determine the number of micrograms in 1 tablet of his antihypertensive drug.

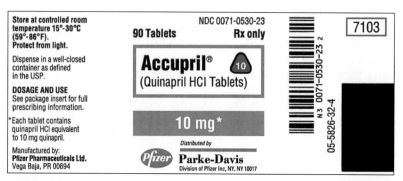

• **Figure 5.9**
Drug label for Accupril.

(Reg. Trademark of Pfizer Inc. Reproduced with permission.)

Cumulative Review Exercises

Reinforce your mastery of previous chapters.

1. 0.6 g = _____ mg

2. 5 oz = _____ T

3. 66 lb ≈ _____ kg

4. 6.4 mm = _____ cm

5. 90 mL ≈ _____ oz

6. 100 mg/day = _____ mg/week

7. 400 mg/day = _____ g/week

8. Azulfidine 1.5 g has been ordered every twelve hours. How many mg will the patient receive per day?

9. A therapy starts at 10:30 A.M. It continues for 5 hours. At what time will it finish (in military time)?

10. Premarin is ordered daily for your patient. The only available tablet strength is 625 mcg. How many milligrams would be contained in two of these Premarin tablets?

11. A wound has a diameter of 1.7 inches. What is this diameter measured in millimeters?

12. How many mL are contained in 2 t?

13. Find the weight in pounds of a patient who weighs 90 kg.

14. Find the height of a 6-foot-tall patient in centimeters.

15. Convert $\frac{4\,mL}{min}$ to an equivalent rate in $\frac{cups}{hour}$

Unit

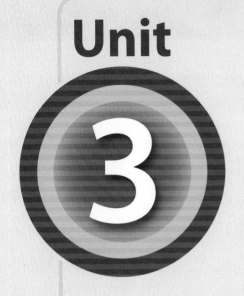

3

Oral and Parenteral Medications

CHAPTER 6

Oral Medications

CHAPTER 7

Syringes

CHAPTER 8

Solutions

CHAPTER 9

Parenteral Medications

Chapter

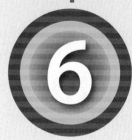

6 Oral Medications

Learning Outcomes

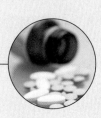

After completing this chapter, you will be able to

1. Use the Formula method to calculate dosages.
2. Calculate Simple (one-step) problems for oral medications in solid and liquid form.
3. Calculate Complex (multi-step) problems for oral medications in solid and liquid form.
4. Calculate doses for medications measured in milliequivalents.
5. Interpret drug labels in order to calculate doses for oral medication.
6. Calculate doses based on body weight.
7. Calculate body surface area (BSA).
8. Calculate doses based on body surface area (BSA).

In this chapter you will learn how to calculate doses of oral medications both in solid and liquid form. You will be introduced to *patient-specific* dosages that use the *size of the patient* (body weight or body surface area [BSA]) to determine the appropriate dose. You will also be introduced to another method for calculating dosages, the **Formula** method.

Simple (One-Step) Problems

In the calculations you have done in previous chapters, all the equivalents have come from standard tables, for example, 1t = 5 mL. In this chapter, the equivalent used will depend on the *strength of the drug* that is available; for example *1 tab = 15 mg*. In the following examples, the equivalent is found on the label of the drug container.

Medication in Solid Form

Oral medications are the most common type of prescription. As discussed in Chapter 2, oral medications come in many forms (tablets, capsules, caplets, and liquid), and drug manufacturers prepare oral medications in commonly prescribed dosages. Oral medications are often supplied in a variety of strengths.

Whenever possible, it is preferable to obtain the medication in the same strength as the dose ordered, or if that is not available, choose a strength that equals a multiple of the prescribed dose. For example, if the order requires 100 mg to be administered, tablets with a strength of 100 mg/tab would make dosage computation unnecessary, and 1 tablet would be administered. However, tablets with a strength of 50 mg/tab would make dosage computation necessary and 2 tablets would be administered.

It is best to *administer the fewest number of tablets or capsules possible*. For example, if a prescriber orders *ampicillin 750 mg po q12h* and you have both the 250-mg and 500-mg capsules available, then you would administer one 500-mg capsule and one 250-mg capsule rather than three 250-mg capsules.

In clinical settings, unit-dose medications are usually supplied by the pharmacist.

Formula Method

In Chapters 3, 4, and 5 three different methods for converting one unit of measurement to another were illustrated: *dimensional analysis, ratio & proportion*, and *moving the decimal point*. Now these three methods will be used to calculate dosages along with the *formula* method. The formula method is used only for *dosage calculation*; it is not used for *unit conversion*, which was the focus of the last three chapters.

$$\frac{D}{H} \times Q = X$$

The formula is commonly used to calculate dosages. To use this formula, you must be able to identify what the four symbols represent.

D stands for the DESIRED dose.

H stands for the amount of the drug on HAND.

Q stands for the QUANTITY containing the amount of the drug on hand.

X stands for the UNKNOWN amount to be administered.

If 50 mg of drug is to be administered to a patient and the strength of the drug is 25 mg per tablet, then the patient would receive 2 tablets. The formula method uses a shorthand for the elements of this illustration: the desired dose is 50 mg (*D*); the strength of the drug as 25 mg/tablet (*H/Q*) so the amount on hand is 25 mg (*H*) and the quantity containing the 25 mg is 1 tablet (*Q*); and finally the amount to be administered is 2 tablets (*X*).

Read the following chart and identify D, H, Q, and X for the formula method.

A. Coumadin (warfarin sodium) 5 mg PO daily. How many tablets will you give? The label states 2.5 mg/tab	D = H = Q = X =
B. Procardia (nifedipine) 20 mg PO T.I.D. How many capsules will you give? The label states 10 mg/cap	D = H = Q = X =
C. Amoxicillin 75 mg PO Q.I.D. How many milliliters will you give? The label states 125 mg/5 mL.	D = H = Q = X =
D. Lanoxin (digoxin) 5 mg PO daily. How many tablets will you give? The label states 250 mcg/tab	D = H = Q = X =
E. Potassium chloride 15 mEq PO daily. How many milliequivalents will you give? The label states 20 mEq/15 mL	D = H = Q = X =

Here are the answers:

A. Coumadin (warfarin sodium) 5 mg PO daily. How many tablets will you give? The label states 2.5 mg/tab	D = 5 mg H = 2.5 mg Q = 1 tab X =? tab
B. Procardia (nifedipine) 20 mg PO T.I.D. How many capsules will you give? The label states 10 mg/cap	D = 20 mg H = 10 mg Q = 1 cap X =? cap
C. Amoxicillin 75 mg PO Q.I.D. How many milliliters will you give? The label states 125 mg/5 mL.	D = 75 mg H = 125 mg Q = 5 mL X =? mL
D. Lanoxin (digoxin) 5 mg PO daily. How many tablets will you give? The label states 250 mcg/tab	D = 5 mg H = 250 mcg Q = 1tab X =? tab
E. Potassium chloride 15 mEq PO daily. How many milliequivalents will you give? The label states 20 mEq/15 mL	D = 15 mEq H = 20 mEq Q = 15 mL X = ? mL

For comparison purposes here is a typical oral medication problem which will be done by using the formula method, ratio & porportion, and dimensional analysis. Suppose the order is *Tegretol 400 mg po b.i.d.* The Tegretol on hand is in the form of 200-mg tablets. How many tablets will you administer?

Using the Formula Method

D: The desired dose is **400 mg.**

H & Q: To find H and Q, the strength of the drug $\frac{200\,mg}{1\,tablet}$ is thought of as $\frac{H}{Q}$. The amount of the drug on hand (H) is **200 mg**, and the quantity (Q) containing 200 mg of drug is **1 tablet.**

X: The unknown amount to be administered is **? tablets.**

Fill in the formula $\dfrac{D}{H} \times Q = X$

$$\frac{400\,mg}{200\,mg} \times 1\,tab = ?\,tab$$

Cancel $\dfrac{\overset{2}{\cancel{400}}\,mg}{\underset{1}{\cancel{200}}\,mg} \times 1\,tab = ?\,tab$

Multiply $2 \times 1\,tab = 2\,tab$

Using Ratio & Proportion

You want to convert the prescribed dose of 400 mg to the number of tablets to be administered.

  Think of the problem this way:

$$400\,mg = x\,tab \quad (dose)$$
$$200\,mg = 1\,tab \quad (strength)$$

One way to set up the proportion is

$$\frac{mg}{tab} = \frac{mg'}{tab'}$$

Substitute into the proportion

$$\frac{400\,mg}{x\,tab} = \frac{200\,mg}{1\,tab}$$

Eliminate the units of measurement, cross multiply, and simplify

$$\frac{400}{x} = \frac{200}{1}$$

$$(200)(x) = (400)(1)$$
$$200x = 400$$

Divide both sides of the equation by 200, the coefficient of x

$$\frac{200x}{200} = \frac{400}{200}$$

Simplify

$$\frac{\cancel{200}x}{\cancel{200}} = \frac{400}{200}$$

$$x = 2$$

Using Dimensional Analysis

You must convert the dose of 400 mg to tablets.

$$400\,mg = ?\,tab$$

Cancel the milligrams and obtain the equivalent amount in tablets

$$400\,mg \times \frac{?\,tab}{?\,mg} = ?\,\mathbf{tab}$$

Use the strength to obtain the unit fraction. Because $1\,tab = 200\,mg$, the fraction is $\dfrac{1\,tab}{200\,mg}$

$$\frac{400\,\cancel{mg}}{1} \times \frac{1\,tab}{200\,\cancel{mg}} = \mathbf{2\,tab}$$

Each of the above three methods gives the same answer of 2 tablets. In this chapter all of the examples can be solved by any one of these methods. The formula method, along with one of the other methods, will be illustrated in most of the remaining examples in this chapter.

EXAMPLE 6.1

The order reads *Cymbalta (duloxetine HCl) 60 mg PO daily*.

Read the drug label shown in •**Figure 6.1**. How many capsules of this antidepressant drug will you administer to the patient?

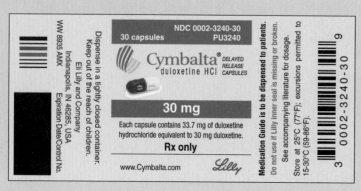

• **Figure 6.1**
Drug label for Cymbalta.

FORMULA METHOD

D   (desired dose)   = 60 mg

H   (dose on hand) = 30 mg

Q   (dosage unit)   = 1 cap

X   (unknown)   = ? cap

Fill in the formula $\dfrac{D}{H} \times Q = X$

$$\frac{60\,mg}{30\,mg} \times 1\,cap = ?\,cap$$

Cancel

$$\frac{\overset{2}{\cancel{60\,mg}}}{\underset{1}{\cancel{30\,mg}}} \times 1\,cap = ?\,cap$$

Multiply $2 \times 1\,cap = 2\,cap$

NOTE

D and *H* must always be the same unit of measurement, and *Q* and *X* must always be the same unit of measurement before you can use the formula method.

DIMENSIONAL ANALYSIS

Convert 60 mg to capsules

$$60\,mg = ?\,cap$$

Cancel the milligrams and calculate the equivalent amount in capsules

$$60\,mg \times \frac{?\,cap}{?\,mg} = ?\,cap$$

Because the label indicates that each capsule contains 30 mg, use the unit fraction $\dfrac{1\,cap}{30\,mg}$

$$\overset{2}{\cancel{60}}\ \cancel{mg} \times \frac{\boxed{1\,cap}}{\underset{1}{\cancel{30}\ \cancel{mg}}} = 2\,cap$$

NOTE

Throughout this textbook, when calculating dosages to be administered to the patient, do your calculations for *one dose* of medication, unless otherwise directed.

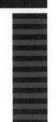

So, you would give 2 capsules by mouth once a day to the patient.

EXAMPLE 6.2

The prescriber orders *Geodon (ziprasidone) 40 mg PO b.i.d.* Read the drug label shown in • Figure 6.2 and determine how many capsules of this antipsychotic drug you would give to the patient.

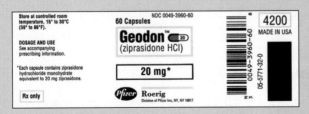

• **Figure 6.2**
Drug label for Geodon.
(Reg. trademark of Pfizer Inc. Reproduced with permission.)

FORMULA METHOD

D   (desired dose)   = 40 mg

H   (dose on hand) = 20 mg

Q   (dosage unit)   = 1 capsule

X   (unknown)   = ? cap

RATIO & PROPORTION

You want to change the prescribed dose of 40 milligrams to the number of capsules to be administered. The strength of the drug is 20 mg per cap.

Think of the problem this way:

$$40\,mg = x\,cap \quad (dose)$$
$$20\,mg = 1\,cap \quad (strength)$$

Fill in the formula

$$\frac{D}{H} \times Q = X$$

$$\frac{40\,mg}{20\,mg} \times 1\,cap = ?\,cap$$

Cancel

$$\frac{\overset{2}{\cancel{40}\,\cancel{mg}}}{\underset{1}{\cancel{20}\,\cancel{mg}}} \times 1\,cap = ?\,cap$$

Multiply

$$2 \times 1\,cap = 2\,cap$$

One way to set up the proportion is

$$\frac{mg}{cap} = \frac{mg'}{cap'}$$

Substitute into the proportion

$$\frac{40\,mg}{x\,cap} = \frac{20\,mg}{1\,cap}$$

Eliminate the units of measurement, cross multiply, and simplify

$$\frac{40}{x} = \frac{20}{1}$$

$$(20)(x) = (40)(1)$$

$$20x = 40$$

Divide both sides of the equation by 20, the coefficient of x

$$\frac{20x}{20} = \frac{40}{20}$$

Simplify

$$\frac{\cancel{20}x}{\cancel{20}} = \frac{40}{20}$$

$$x = 2$$

Because 2 capsules contain 40 mg of Geodon, you would give 2 capsules by mouth to the patient.

EXAMPLE 6.3

Read the label in •Figure 6.3. How many tablets of this narcotic analgesic will be needed for a dose containing 10 mg of hydrocodone bitartrate and 1,000 mg of acetaminophen?

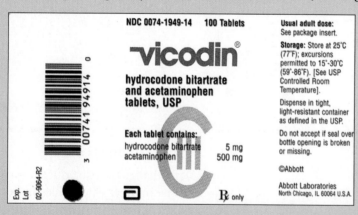

• Figure 6.3
Drug label for Vicodin.

Vicodin is a combination drug (see Figures 2.24 and 2.25 in Chapter 2) composed of hydrocodone bitartrate and acetaminophen. Therefore, for computational purposes, you need address only the first listed drug (hydrocodone bitartrate). Because the dose requires 10 mg of hydrocodone bitartrate, convert the 10 mg to the appropriate number of tablets.

However, before doing any calculations, you should check to see if the ratios of the amounts of the two drugs in Vicodin are equivalent in *both the* prescribed *dose* and on the *label*. The hydrocodone bitartrate-acetaminophen ratio in the *dose* is 10:1,000 or 1:100. The hydrocodone bitartrate-acetaminophen ratio on the *label* is 5:500 or 1:100. The ratios are equivalent, and you can now proceed with the calculations.

FORMULA METHOD

D (desired dose) = 10 mg

H (dose on hand) = 5 mg

Q (dosage unit)   = 1 tablet

X (unknown)   = ? tab

Fill in the formula $\dfrac{D}{H} \times Q = X$

$$\frac{10\,mg}{5\,mg} \times 1\,tab = ?\,tab$$

Cancel $\dfrac{\overset{2}{\cancel{10\,mg}}}{\underset{1}{\cancel{5\,mg}}} \times 1\,tab = ?\,tab$

Multiply $2 \times 1\,tab = 2\,tab$

DIMENSIONAL ANALYSIS

$$10\ mg = ?\ tab$$

Cancel the milligrams and obtain the equivalent amount in tablets

$$10\ \cancel{mg} \times \frac{?\ tab}{?\ \cancel{mg}} = ?\ tab$$

The label indicates that one tablet contains 5 mg of hydrocordone bitartrate.

Because 1 tab = 5 mg, the unit fraction is $\dfrac{1\ tab}{5\ mg}$

$$\overset{2}{\cancel{10}}\ \cancel{mg} \times \frac{1\ \text{(tab)}}{\underset{1}{\cancel{5}}\ \cancel{mg}} = 2\ tab$$

Because 2 tablets contain 10 mg of hydrocordone bitartrate and 1,000 mg of acetaminophen, 2 tablets would be needed for this dose.

EXAMPLE 6.4

The order is *Ryzolt (tramadol HCl) 300 mg PO daily*. The medication is available in three different strengths (•Figure 6.4). Determine how you would administer this dose using the fewest number of the available tablets.

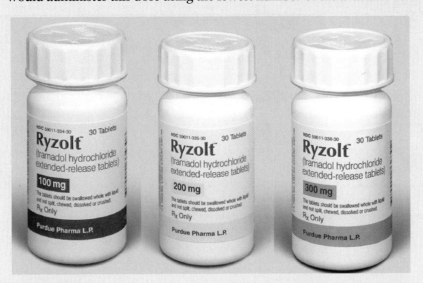

•**Figure 6.4**
Containers of Ryzolt of differing concentrations: 100, 200, and 300 mg/tablet.

The 300 mg dose could be administered in any of the following ways:

- One 300-mg tablet
- One 200-mg tablet and one 100-mg tablet
- Three 100-mg tablets

Because you want to administer the fewest number of tablets, you would choose to administer one 300-mg tablet.

NOTE

Some liquid oral medications are supplied with special calibrated droppers or oral syringes that are used *only* for these medications (e.g., digoxin and Lasix). Some medication cups do not accurately measure amounts less than 5 mL.

Medication in Liquid Form

Because pediatric and geriatric patients, as well as patients with neurological conditions, may be unable to swallow medication in tablet form, sometimes oral medications are ordered in liquid form. The label states how much drug is contained in a given amount of liquid.

For medications supplied in liquid form, you must calculate the volume of the liquid that contains the prescribed drug dosage. Medication cups, oral syringes, or calibrated droppers are used to measure the dose. See • Figure 6.5.

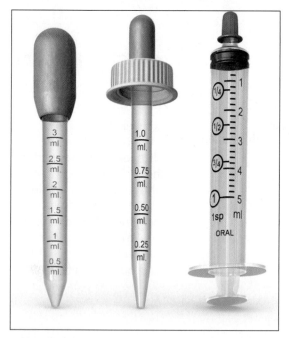

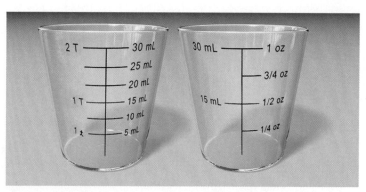

• **Figure 6.5**
Measuring drugs in liquid form (calibrated droppers, oral syringe, and measuring cups).

EXAMPLE 6.5

The prescriber orders *alprazolam oral solution 0.25 mg PO b.i.d.* Read the label in •Figure 6.6 and determine how many milliliters you will prepare.

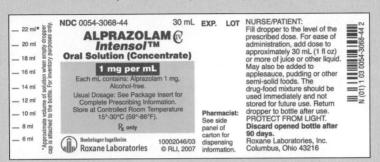

•Figure 6.6
Drug label for alprazolam.

FORMULA METHOD

D   (desired dose)   = 0.25 mg

H   (dose on hand) = 1 mg

Q   (dosage unit)   = 1 mL

X   (unknown)   = ? mL

Fill in the formula $\dfrac{D}{H} \times Q = X$

$$\frac{0.25\,mg}{1\,mg} \times 1\,mL = ?\,mL$$

Cancel $\dfrac{0.25\,\cancel{mg}}{1\,\cancel{mg}} \times 1\,ml = ?\,mL$

Multiply $0.25 \times 1\,mL = 0.25\,mL$

NOTE

The critical thinker would recognize that because the strength in Example 6.5 is 1 mg = 1 mL, this example does not require computation, that is, 0.25 mg = 0.25 mL.

RATIO & PROPORTION

You want to change the 0.25-mg dose prescribed to milliliters. The strength of the drug is 1 mg (of alprazolam) per mL.

Think of the problem this way:

$$0.25\,mg = x\,mL \quad \text{(dose)}$$
$$1\,mg = 1\,mL \quad \text{(strength)}$$

One way to set up the proportion is

$$\frac{mg}{mL} = \frac{mg'}{mL'}$$

Substitute into the proportion

$$\frac{0.25\,mg}{x\,mL} = \frac{1\,mg}{1\,mL}$$

Eliminate the units of measurement, cross multiply, and simplify

$$\frac{0.25}{x} = \frac{1}{1}$$

$$(1)(x) = (0.25)(1)$$
$$x = 0.25$$

So, follow the directions on the label, and add 0.25 mL of alprazolam to 30 mL of juice or other liquid.

EXAMPLE 6.6

The physician orders *Lexapro (escitalopram oxalate) 10 mg PO once daily*. Read the label in
•Figure 6.7 and determine the number of milliliters you would administer to the patient.

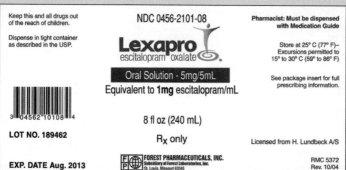

Keep this and all drugs out of the reach of children.

Dispense in tight container as described in the USP.

NDC 0456-2101-08

Lexapro
escitalopram oxalate

Oral Solution - 5mg/5mL
Equivalent to **1mg** escitalopram/mL

8 fl oz (240 mL)

Rₓ only

LOT NO. 189462

EXP. DATE Aug. 2013

Pharmacist: Must be dispensed with Medication Guide

Store at 25° C (77° F)–
Excursions permitted to
15° to 30° C (59° to 86° F)

See package insert for full prescribing information.

Licensed from H. Lundbeck A/S

FOREST PHARMACEUTICALS, INC.
Subsidiary of Forest Laboratories, Inc.
St. Louis, Missouri 63045

RMC 5372
Rev. 10/04

3 04562 10108 4

• Figure 6.7
Drug label for Lexapro.

FORMULA METHOD

D   (desired dose)   = 10 mg
H   (dose on hand) = 5 mg
Q   (dosage unit)   = 5 mL
X   (unknown)   = ? mL

Fill in the formula $\dfrac{D}{H} \times Q = X$

$$\dfrac{10\,mg}{5\,mg} \times 5\,mL = ?\,mL$$

Cancel $\dfrac{\overset{2}{\cancel{10\,mg}}}{\underset{1}{\cancel{5\,mg}}} \times 5\,ml = ?\,mL$

Multiply $2 \times 5\,mL = 10\,mL$

DIMENSIONAL ANALYSIS

Convert 10 milligrams to milliliters.

$$10\ mg = ?\ mL$$

Cancel the milligrams and calculate the equivalent amount in mL

$$10\ mg \times \dfrac{?\ mL}{?\ mg} = ?\ mL$$

Because the label indicates that every 5 mL of the solution contains 5 mg of Lexapro, use the unit fraction $\dfrac{5\ mL}{5\ mg}$

$$10\ mg \times \dfrac{5\ mL}{5\ mg} = 10\ mL$$

So, you would give 10 mL of this antidepressant by mouth once a day to the patient. See • **Figure 6.8.**

NOTE

In Example 6.6, the strength of 5 mg/5 mL is the same as 1 mg = 1 mL, as in Example 6.5. Therefore, this example also does not require computation, and 10 mg = 10 mL.

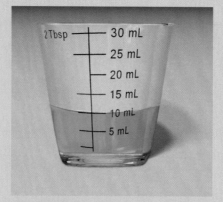

• Figure 6.8
Medication cup with 10 mg (10 mL) of Lexapro.

EXAMPLE 6.7

The physician orders *Omnicef (cefdinir) 500 mg PO q12h*. Read the label in • Figure 6.9. Determine the number of mL you would administer to the patient.

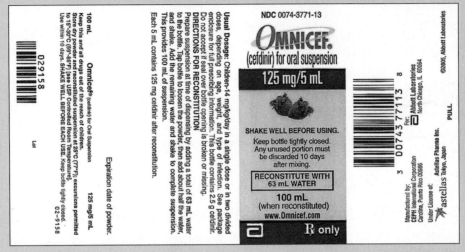

• Figure 6.9
Drug label for Omnicef.

FORMULA METHOD

D (desired dose) = 500 mg

H (dose on hand) = 125 mg

Q (dosage unit) = 5 mL

X (unknown) = ? mL

Fill in the formula $\dfrac{D}{H} \times Q = X$

$$\dfrac{500 \, mg}{125 \, mg} \times 5 \, mL = ? \, mL$$

Cancel

$$\dfrac{\overset{4}{\cancel{500 \, mg}}}{\underset{1}{\cancel{125 \, mg}}} \times 5 \, ml = ? \, mL$$

Multiply $4 \times 5 \, mL = 20 \, mL$

RATIO & PROPORTION

You want to change the 500 mg dose prescribed to milliliters. The strength of the drug is 12.5 mg per 5 mL.

Think of the problem this way:

$$500 \, mg = x \, mL \quad \text{(dose)}$$
$$125 \, mg = 5 \, mL \quad \text{(strength)}$$

One way to set up the proportion is

$$\dfrac{mg}{mL} = \dfrac{mg'}{mL'}$$

Substitute into the proportion

$$\dfrac{500 \, mg}{x \, mL} = \dfrac{125 \, mg}{5 \, mL}$$

Eliminate the units of measurement, cross multiply, and simplify

$$\dfrac{500}{x} = \dfrac{125}{5}$$

$$(125)(x) = (500)(5)$$

$$125x = 2{,}500$$

$$x = \dfrac{2{,}500}{125}$$

$$x = 20$$

So, you would give 20 mL of this antibiotic by mouth every 12 hours to the patient. See • **Figure 6.10**.

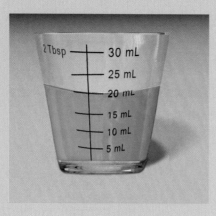

• **Figure 6.10**
Medication cup with 500 mg (20 mL) of Omnicef.

Medications Measured in Milliequivalents

Some drugs are measured in **milliequivalents**, which are abbreviated as *mEq*. A milliequivalent is an expression of the number of grams of a drug contained in one milliliter of solution. Pharmaceutical companies label electrolytes (sodium chloride, potassium chloride, and calcium chloride, for example) in milligrams as well as in milliequivalents.

EXAMPLE 6.8

Order: *potassium chloride 30 mEq PO daily in three divided doses*. Read the label in • Figure 6.11 and determine how many tablets of this electrolyte supplement you should administer.

NOTE

In Example 6.8, the order states "in three divided doses." This instructs the practitioner to separate the total daily dose into 3 equal parts over a 24-hour period. To ensure even distribution of the medication, the frequency of the doses should also be regular and consistent, so the drug is administered every 8 hours.

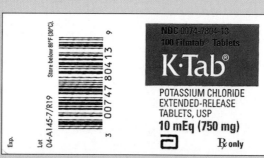

• **Figure 6.11**
Drug label for K-Tab.

FORMULA METHOD	RATIO & PROPORTION
D (desired dose) = 30 mEq	Think of the problem this way:
H (dose on hand) = 10 mEq	30 mEq = *x* tab (dose)
Q (dosage unit) = 1 tab	10 mEq = 1 tab (strength)
X (unknown) = ? tab	

Fill in the formula $\dfrac{D}{H} \times Q = X$

$$\dfrac{30\,mEq}{10\,mEq} \times 1\,tab = ?\,tab$$

Cancel

$$\dfrac{\overset{3}{\cancel{30\,mEq}}}{\underset{1}{\cancel{10\,mEq}}} \times 1\,tab = ?\,tab$$

Multiply $3 \times 1\,tab = 3\,tab$

One way to set up the proportion is

$$\dfrac{mEq}{tab} = \dfrac{mEq'}{tab'}$$

Substitute into the proportion

$$\dfrac{30\,mEq}{x\,tab} = \dfrac{10\,mEq}{1\,tab}$$

Eliminate the units of measurement, cross multiply, and simplify

$$\dfrac{30}{x} = \dfrac{10}{1}$$

$$10x = 30$$

$$x = 3$$

Because the order indicates "three divided doses," you would administer 1 tablet of K-Tab every 8 hours.

EXAMPLE 6.9

The prescriber ordered *potassium chloride 40 mEq po daily in two divided doses*. Read the label in • Figure 6.12 and determine the number of milliliters of this electrolyte supplement that you would administer.

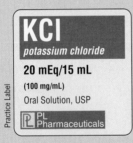

KCl
potassium chloride
20 mEq/15 mL
(100 mg/mL)
Oral Solution, USP

PL PL Pharmaceuticals

Practice Label

• **Figure 6.12**
Drug label for Potassium Chloride.
(For educational purposes only)

ALERT

Potassium chloride is a high-alert drug. Follow the manufacturer's directions for diluting.

FORMULA METHOD

D   (desired dose) $= 40\,mEq$

H   (dose on hand) $= 20\,mEq$

Q   (dosage unit) $= 15\,mL$

X   (unknown) $= ?\,mL$

Fill in the formula $\dfrac{D}{H} \times Q = X$

$$\dfrac{40\,mEq}{20\,mEq} \times 15\,mL = ?\,mL$$

DIMENSIONAL ANALYSIS

You want to change the 40 mEq prescribed to milliliters.

$$40\,mEq = ?\,mL$$

Cancel the mEq and calculate the equivalent amount in mL.

$$\dfrac{40\,mEq}{1} \times \dfrac{?\,mL}{?\,mEq} = ?\,mL$$

Cancel	$\dfrac{\overset{2}{\cancel{40}\,\cancel{mEq}}}{\underset{1}{\cancel{20}\,\cancel{mEq}}} \times 15\,mL = ?\,mL$	Because the label indicates that every 15 mL of the solution contains 20 mEq of potassium chloride, use the unit fraction $\dfrac{15\ mL}{20\ mEq}$
Multiply	$2 \times 15\,mL = 30\,mL$	$\dfrac{40\ \cancel{mEq}}{1} \times \dfrac{15\ mL}{20\ \cancel{mEq}} = 30\ mL$

Because the 30 mL must be administered in "two divided doses," you would administer 15 mL to the patient.

Complex (Multistep) Problems

Sometimes dosage calculations will require that multiplication by unit fractions be repeated one or more times. Recall that we examined complex problems in Chapter 3.

For example, if each tablet of a drug contains 1.25 mg, how many tablets would contain 0.0025 gram? This problem will be done below using three different approaches.

USING DIMENSIONAL ANALYSIS

For complex problems, it helps to organize the information you will need for the computation as follows:

Given quantity   0.0025 g [*single unit of measurement*]
Strength   1 tab = 1.25 mg [*equivalence*]
Quantity you want to find   ? tab [*single unit of measurement*]

Because you want to find a *single unit of measurement* (? tablets), you must start with a *single unit of measurement* (0.0025 g). The *equivalence* (1 tab = 1.25 mg) will be used to form a unit fraction. So, the problem is

$$0.0025\ g = ?\ tab$$

You do not know the direct equivalence between grams and tablets. This is a **complex** problem because you need to first convert 0.0025 grams to milligrams, and then convert the milligrams to tablets.

$$0.0025\ g \longrightarrow ?\ mg \longrightarrow ?\ tab$$

First, you want to cancel *grams (g)*. To do this you must use an equivalence containing *grams* to make a unit fraction with *grams* in the denominator. Because the equivalence is 1 g = 1,000 mg, the unit fraction is $\dfrac{1,000 \text{ mg}}{1 \text{ g}}$

$$0.0025 \text{ g} \times \frac{1,000 \text{ mg}}{1 \text{ g}} = ? \text{ tab}$$

After the *grams* are cancelled, only *milligrams* remain on the left side. Now you need to change the *milligrams* to *tablets*. Because the strength is 1.25 mg = 1 tab, the unit fraction is $\dfrac{1 \text{ tab}}{1.25 \text{ mg}}$

$$0.0025 \text{ g} \times \frac{1,000 \text{ mg}}{1 \text{ g}} \times \frac{1 \text{ tab}}{1.25 \text{ mg}} = ? \text{ tab}$$

After cancelling the milligrams, only tablets remain on the left side. Now complete your calculation by multiplying the numbers.

$$0.0025 \text{ g} \times \frac{1,000 \text{ mg}}{1 \text{ g}} \times \frac{1 \text{ tab}}{1.25 \text{ mg}} = \frac{2.5 \text{ tab}}{1.25} = 2 \text{ tab}$$

USING RATIO & PROPORTION AND MOVING THE DECIMAL POINT

You want to change 0.0025 g to tablets. The strength of the tablets is 1.25 mg per tab.

Think of the problem this way:

$$0.0025 \;\boxed{\text{g}}\; = x \text{ tab} \quad \text{(dose)}$$
$$1.25 \;\boxed{\text{mg}}\; = 1 \text{ tab} \quad \text{(strength)}$$

Notice that the g and mg do not match. Therefore, a conversion must be done before you can set up a proportion. In this case, change 0.0025 g to an equivalent amount of milligrams.

kilogram	gram	milligram	microgram
kg	g	mg	mcg

Move the decimal point *3 places to the right*

$$0.0025 \text{ g} = 0.0\,0\,2\,5 \text{ g} = 0002.5 \text{ mg} = 2.5 \text{ mg}$$

Now, think of the problem this way:

$$2.5 \text{ mg} = x \text{ tab} \quad \text{(dose)}$$
$$1.25 \text{ mg} = 1 \text{ tab} \quad \text{(strength)}$$

One way to set up the proportion is

$$\frac{2.5\,mg}{x\,tab} = \frac{1.25\,mg}{1\,tab}$$

Eliminate the units of measurement, cross multiply, and simplify

$$\frac{2.5}{x} = \frac{1.25}{1}$$

$$1.25x = 2.5$$

$$x = 2$$

USING MOVING THE DECIMAL POINT AND THE FORMULA METHOD

D (desired dose) = 0.0025 g
H (dose on hand) = 1.25 mg
Q (dosage unit) = 1 tab
X (unknown) = ? tab

D and H are not in the same units of measurement. To use the formula method the units of measurement of D and H must match. Also, the units of measurement of Q and X must match.

This is a complex problem because first you need to convert 0.0025 grams to an equivalent amount of milligrams before you can apply the formula. You can this by moving the decimal point *3 places to the right*.

kilogram	gram	milligram	microgram
kg	g	mg	mcg

$$0.0025\,g = 0.\,0\,0\,2\,5\,g = 000.25\,mg = 2.5\,mg$$

Now, both D and H match; they are in milligrams, and you have:

D (desired dose) = 2.5 mg
H (dose on hand) = 1.25 mg
Q (dosage unit) = 1 tab
X (unknown) = ? tab

Fill in the formula $\dfrac{D}{H} \times Q = X$

$$\frac{2.5\,mg}{1.25\,mg} \times 1\,tab = ?\,tab$$

Cancel

$$\frac{2.5 \, \overset{2}{\cancel{mg}}}{\underset{1}{\cancel{1.25}} \, mg} \times 1 \, tab = ? \, tab$$

Multiply $\quad\quad\quad 2 \times 1 \, tab = 2 \, tab$

So, two 1.25 mg tablets contains 0.0025 grams.

EXAMPLE 6.10

How many 300-mg Ziagen (abacavir sulfate) tablets contain 0.9 g of Ziagen?

FORMULA METHOD

D   (desired dose)   = 0.9 g

H   (dose on hand)   = 300 mg

Q   (dosage unit)   = 1 tab

X   (unknown)   = ? tab

D and H do not match. This is a complex problem because you first need to convert 0.9 g to an equivalent amount of milligrams.

kilogram	gram	milligram	microgram
kg	g	mg	mcg

Move the decimal point *3 places to the right*

$0.9 \, g = 0.900 \, g = 0.900 \, g = 0900. \, mg = 900 \, mg$

D   (desired dose)   = 900 mg

H   (dose on hand)   = 300 mg

Q   (dosage unit)   = 1 tab

X   (unknown)   = ? tab

Now, D and H match.

Fill in the formula $\quad \dfrac{D}{H} \times Q = X$

$$\frac{900 \, mg}{300 \, mg} \times 1 \, tab = ? \, tab$$

Cancel

$$\frac{\overset{3}{\cancel{900}} \, \cancel{mg}}{\underset{1}{\cancel{300}} \, \cancel{mg}} \times 1 \, tab = ? \, tab$$

Multiply $\quad\quad\quad 3 \times 1 \, tab = 3 \, tab$

RATIO & PROPORTION

You want to change 0.9 g to tablets. The strength of the tablets is 300 mg per tab.

Think of the problem this way:

0.9	g	= x tab (dose)
300	mg	= 1 tab (strength)

Notice that the g and mg do not match. Therefore, a conversion must be done before you can set up a proportion. In this case, change 0.09 g to an equivalent amount of milligrams.

kilogram	gram	milligram	microgram
kg	g	mg	mcg

Move the decimal point *3 places to the right*

$0.9 \, g = 0.900 \, g = 0.900 \, g = 0900. \, mg = 900 \, mg$

Now, think of the problem this way:

$900 \, mg = x \, tab \quad$ (dose)

$300 \, mg = 1 \, tab \quad$ (strength)

One way to set up the proportion is

$$\frac{900 \, mg}{x \, tab} = \frac{300 \, mg}{1 \, tab}$$

Eliminate the units of measurement, cross multiply, and simplify

$$\frac{900}{x} = \frac{300}{1}$$

$$300 \, x = 900$$

$$x = 3$$

So, three 300-mg tablets contain 0.9 g of Ziagen.

EXAMPLE 6.11

Read the label in • Figure 6.13 to determine the number of Diflucan tablets that would contain a dose of 0.4 g.

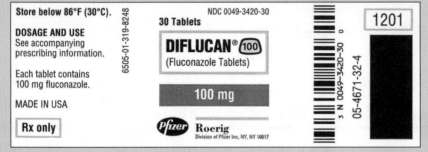

• **Figure 6.13**
Drug label for Diflucan.

(Reg. trademark of Pfizer Inc. Reproduced with permission.)

FORMULA METHOD

D (desired dose) = 0.4 g
H (dose on hand) = 100 mg
Q (dosage unit) = 1 tab
X (unknown) = ? tab

You need to first convert 0.4 g to an equivalent amount of milligrams.

kilogram	gram	milligram	microgram
kg	g	mg	mcg

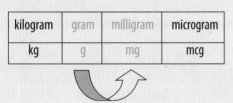

Move the decimal point *3 places to the right*
0.4 g = 0.400 g = 0. 4 0 0 g = 0400.mg = 400mg

Fill in the formula $\dfrac{D}{H} \times Q = X$

$$\dfrac{400\,mg}{100\,mg} \times 1\,tab = ?\,tab$$

Cancel $\dfrac{400\,\cancel{mg}}{100\,\cancel{mg}} \times 1\,tab = ?\,tab$

Multiply $4 \times 1\,tab = 4\,tab$

DIMENSIONAL ANALYSIS

Given quantity: 0.4 g
Strength: 1 tab = 100 mg
Quantity you want to find: ? tab

In this problem you want to convert 0.4 gram to milligrams and then convert milligrams to tablets.

$$0.4\,g \longrightarrow ?\,mg \longrightarrow ?\,tab$$

You can do this on one line as follows

$$0.4\,g \times \dfrac{?\,mg}{?\,g} \times \dfrac{?\,tab}{?\,mg} = ?\,tab$$

Because 1,000 mg = 1 g, the first unit fraction is $\dfrac{1,000\,mg}{1\,g}$

Because 100 mg = 1 tab, the second unit fraction is $\dfrac{1\,tab}{100\,mg}$

$$0.4\,\cancel{g} \times \dfrac{\overset{10}{\cancel{1,000}}\,\cancel{mg}}{1\,\cancel{g}} \times \dfrac{1\,\text{(tab)}}{\underset{1}{\cancel{100}}\,\cancel{mg}} = 4\,tab$$

So, you should give 4 tablets of this antifungal drug by mouth once a day to the patient.

EXAMPLE 6.12

The order is *Tikosyn (dofetilide) 0.5 mg PO b.i.d.* Read the label shown in •Figure 6.14. Calculate how many capsules of this antiarrythmic drug should be given to the patient. Although there are two strengths on the label (mcg and mg), calculate the problem using microgram strength.

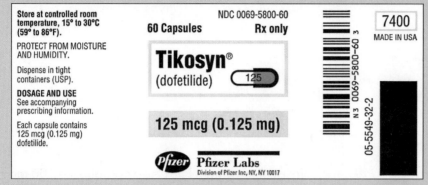

Store at controlled room temperature, 15° to 30°C (59° to 86°F).

PROTECT FROM MOISTURE AND HUMIDITY.

Dispense in tight containers (USP).

DOSAGE AND USE
See accompanying prescribing information.

Each capsule contains 125 mcg (0.125 mg) dofetilide.

NDC 0069-5800-60

60 Capsules   **Rx only**

Tikosyn®
(dofetilide)   `125`

125 mcg (0.125 mg)

Pfizer **Pfizer Labs**
Division of Pfizer Inc, NY, NY 10017

7400
MADE IN USA

N3 0069-5800-60 3

05-5549-32-2

•**Figure 6.14**
Drug label for Tikosyn.
(Reg. trademark of Pfizer Inc. Reproduced with permission.)

NOTE

Although Example 6.12 would be simpler using milligrams, we will do the calculation using micrograms to practice complex problems. For safety purposes, drug manufacturers often place both microgram and milligram concentrations on drug labels.

FORMULA METHOD

D   (desired dose) $= 0.5\,mg$

H   (dose on hand) $= 125\,mcg$

Q   (dosage unit) $= 1\,cap$

X   (unknown) $= ?\,cap$

You need to first convert 0.5 milligrams to an equivalent amount of micrograms.

kilogram	gram	milligram	microgram
kg	g	mg	mcg

Move the decimal point *3 places to the right*

$0.5\,g = 0.500\,g = \mathbf{0.5\,0\,0\,g} = 0500.\,mcg = 500\,mcg$

Fill in the formula $\dfrac{D}{H} \times Q = X$

$$\frac{500\,mcg}{125\,mcg} \times 1\,cap = ?\,cap$$

RATIO & PROPORTION

Think of the problem this way:

$$0.5 \;\boxed{mg} \;= x\,cap \;\; (dose)$$
$$125 \;\boxed{mcg} \;= 1\,cap \;\;(strength)$$

Notice that the mg and mcg do not match. Therefore, a conversion must be done before you can set up a proportion. In this case, change 0.5 mg to an equivalent amount of micrograms.

kilogram	gram	milligram	microgram
kg	g	mg	mcg

Move the decimal point *3 places to the right*

$0.5\,mg = 0.500\,mg = \mathbf{0.5\,0\,0}\;mg = \mathbf{0500.}\,mcg = 500\,mcg$

Now, think of the problem this way:

$$500\,mcg = x\,cap \;\; (dose)$$
$$125\,mcg = 1\,cap \;\; (strength)$$

One way to set up the proportion is

$$\frac{500\,mcg}{x\,cap} = \frac{125\,mcg}{1\,cap}$$

Cancel $\dfrac{\overset{4}{\cancel{500\,mcg}}}{\underset{1}{\cancel{125\,mcg}}} \times 1\,cap = ?\,cap$

Multiply $\quad 4 \times 1\,cap = 4\,cap$

Eliminate the units of measurement, cross multiply, and simplify

$$\dfrac{500}{x} = \dfrac{125}{1}$$

$$125\,x = 500$$

$$x = 4$$

So, you should give 4 capsules by mouth twice a day to the patient.

EXAMPLE 6.13

The order is *Daypro (oxaprozin) 1.8 g PO once daily each morning.* The drug is supplied as 600 mg per caplet. How many caplets of this anti-inflammatory drug should be given to the patient?

FORMULA METHOD

D (desired dose) = 1.8 g
H (dose on hand) = 600 mg
Q (dosage unit) = 1 cap
X (unknown) = ? cap

You need to first convert 1.8 g to an equivalent amount of milligrams.

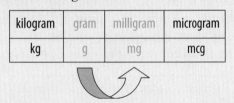

kilogram	gram	milligram	microgram
kg	g	mg	mcg

Move the decimal point *3 places to the right*
$1.8\,g = 1.800\,g = \mathbf{1.\,8\,0\,0\,g} = 1800.\,mg = 1{,}800\,mg$

Fill in the formula $\quad \dfrac{D}{H} \times Q = X$

$$\dfrac{1800\,mg}{600\,mg} \times 1\,cap = ?\,cap$$

Cancel $\quad \dfrac{\overset{3}{\cancel{1800\,mg}}}{\underset{1}{\cancel{600\,mg}}} \times 1\,cap = ?\,cap$

Multiply $\quad 3 \times 1\,cap = 3\,cap$

DIMENSIONAL ANALYSIS

Given quantity: 1.8 g
Strength: 1 cap = 600 mg
Quantity you want to find: ? cap

In this problem you want to convert 1.8 grams to milligrams and then convert milligrams to caplets.

$$1.8\,g \longrightarrow ?\,mg \longrightarrow ?\,cap$$

You can do this on one line as follows

$$1.8\,g \times \dfrac{?\,mg}{?\,g} \times \dfrac{?\,cap}{?\,mg} = ?\,cap$$

Because 1,000 mg = 1 g, the first unit fraction is $\dfrac{1{,}000\,mg}{1\,g}$

Because 1 cap = 600 mg, the second unit fraction is $\dfrac{1\,cap}{600\,mg}$

$$1.8\,\cancel{g} \times \dfrac{1{,}000\,\cancel{mg}}{1\,\cancel{g}} \times \dfrac{1\,\boxed{cap}}{600\,\cancel{mg}} = \dfrac{18\,cap}{6} = 3\,cap$$

So, you should give 3 caplets by mouth to the patient once a day in the morning.

EXAMPLE 6.14

The physician orders *Norvir (ritonavir) 0.6 g PO b.i.d.* Read the label in •Figure 6.15 and determine the number of mL of this protease inhibitor your patient would receive.

NDC 0074-1940-63

Norvir®
Ritonavir
Oral Solution

80 mg per mL

240 mL

Do Not Refrigerate

ALERT: Find out about
medicines that should NOT
be taken with NORVIR.

**Note to Pharmacist: Do not cover
ALERT box with pharmacy label.**

04-A347-2/R5

Rx only   Abbott

• Figure 6.15
Drug label for Norvir.

FORMULA METHOD

D (desired dose)   = 0.6 g
H (dose on hand) = 80 mg
Q (dosage unit)   = 1 mL
X (unknown)   = ? mL

You need to first convert 0.6 g to an equivalent amount of milligrams.

kilogram	gram	milligram	microgram
kg	g	mg	mcg

Move the decimal point *3 places to the right*

$0.6 \, g = 0.600 \, g = \mathbf{0.6\,0\,0} \, g = 600. \, mg = 600 \, mg$

Fill in the formula $\dfrac{D}{H} \times Q = X$

$$\frac{600 \, mg}{80 \, mg} \times 1 \, mL = ? \, mL$$

RATIO & PROPORTION

Think of the problem this way:

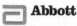

0.6 | g | = x mL (dose)
80 | mg | = 1 mL (strength)

Notice that the g and mg do not match. Therefore, a conversion must be done before you can set up a proportion. In this case, change 0.6 g to an equivalent amount of milligrams.

kilogram	gram	milligram	microgram
kg	g	mg	mcg

Move the decimal point *3 places to the right*

$0.6 \, g = 0.600 \, g = \mathbf{0.6\,0\,0} \, g = 600. \, mg = 600 \, mg$

Now, think of the problem this way:

$600 \, mg = x \, mL$ (dose)
$80 \, mg = 1 \, mL$ (strength)

Cancel

$$\frac{\overset{15}{\cancel{600}\,mg}}{\underset{2}{\cancel{80}\,mg}} \times 1\,mL = ?\,mL$$

Multiply

$$\frac{15}{2} \times 1\,mL = 7.5\,mL$$

One way to set up the proportion is

$$\frac{600\,mg}{x\,mL} = \frac{80\,mg}{1\,mL}$$

Eliminate the units of measurement, cross multiply, and simplify

$$\frac{600}{x} = \frac{80}{1}$$

$$80x = 600$$

$$x = 7.5$$

So, you would give 7.5 mL by mouth to the patient.

EXAMPLE 6.15

The order is *indomethacin 75 mg PO daily in 3 divided doses*. Read the label in • Figure 6.16 and determine the number of teaspoons of this anti-inflammatory drug you should administer.

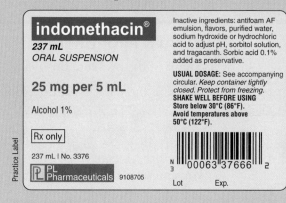

indomethacin®

237 mL
ORAL SUSPENSION

25 mg per 5 mL

Alcohol 1%

Rx only

237 mL | No. 3376

PL Pharmaceuticals   9108705

Practice Label

Inactive ingredients: antifoam AF emulsion, flavors, purified water, sodium hydroxide or hydrochloric acid to adjust pH, sorbitol solution, and tragacanth. Sorbic acid 0.1% added as preservative.

USUAL DOSAGE: See accompanying circular. *Keep container tightly closed. Protect from freezing.* **SHAKE WELL BEFORE USING Store below 30°C (86°F). Avoid temperatures above 50°C (122°F).**

N 3   00063 37666   2

Lot   Exp.

• **Figure 6.16**
Drug label for indomethacin.
(For educational purposes only)

FORMULA METHOD

D (desired dose) = 75 mg
H (dose on hand) = 25 mg
Q (dosage unit)   = 5 mL
X (unknown)   = ? t

Q and X are in different units. Because 5 mL = 1 t, make Q = 1 t.

Fill in the formula $\dfrac{D}{H} \times Q = X$

$$\frac{75\,mg}{25\,mg} \times 1\,t = ?\,t$$

DIMENSIONAL ANALYSIS

Given quantity: 75 mg
Strength: 25 mg per 5 mL
The quantity you want to find: ? t

In this problem you want to convert 75 milligrams to milliliters and then convert mL to teaspoons.

$$75\,mg \longrightarrow ?\,mL \longrightarrow ?\,t$$

You can do this on one line as follows

$$75\,mg \times \frac{?\,mL}{?\,mg} \times \frac{?\,t}{?\,mL} = ?\,t$$

Because 25 mg = 5 mL, the first unit fraction is $\dfrac{5\,mL}{25\,mg}$

Cancel	$\dfrac{\overset{3}{\cancel{75}\,mg}}{\underset{1}{\cancel{25}\,mg}} \times 1\,t = ?\,t$		Because 5 mL = 1 t, the second unit fraction is $\dfrac{1\,t}{5\,mL}$
Multiply	$3 \times 1\,t = 3\,t$		$75\,\cancel{mg} \times \dfrac{\cancel{5\,mL}}{25\,\cancel{mg}} \times \dfrac{\cancel{1\,t}}{\cancel{5\,mL}} = 3\,t$

Because the order specifies "3 divided doses," the 3 t must be divided into 3 equal amounts over 24 hours. Therefore, each dose would be 1 teaspoon (25 mg), and you would give 1 teaspoon of indomethacin by mouth to the patient.

Dosages Based on the Size of the Patient

Sometimes the amount of medication prescribed is based on the patient's size. A patient who is larger will receive a larger dose of the drug, and a patient who is smaller will receive a smaller dose of the drug. The size of a patient is measured by either *body weight* or *body surface area (BSA)*. In general, when the order is based on the size of the patient, if you multiply the *size of the patient* by the *order*, you will obtain the *dose*. This can be expressed by the formula:

$$Size\ of\ patient \times Order = Dose$$

Dosages Based on Body Weight

EXAMPLE 6.16

Order: *Dilantin (phenytoin) 15 mg/kg loading dose PO, then 300 mg/d.* For the loading dose, how many mg of this anticonvulsant would you administer to a patient who weighs 80 kg?

Body weight: 80 kg

Order: 15 mg/kg

Find: ? mg

NOTE

The expression 15 mg/kg means that the patient is to receive 15 milligrams of the drug for each kilogram of body weight. Therefore, you will use the equivalent 15 mg (of drug) = 1 kg (of body weight).

FORMULA METHOD

You want to "change" the body weight of the patient (80 kg) to milligrams of drug. The order is 15 mg/kg, so use the formula

$$Size\ of\ patient \times Order = Dose$$

$$80\,\cancel{kg} \times \dfrac{15\,mg}{1\,\cancel{kg}} = 1{,}200\,mg$$

RATIO & PROPORTION

Think of the problem this way:

$$80\,kg\,(body\ weight) = x\,mg\,(drug) \quad (dose)$$
$$1\,kg\,(body\ weight) = 15\,mg\,(drug) \quad (order)$$

One way to set up the proportion is

$$\dfrac{80\,kg}{x\,mg} = \dfrac{1\,kg}{15\,mg}$$

$$x = 1{,}200$$

Therefore, the patient should receive 1,200 mg of Dilantin for the loading dose.

EXAMPLE 6.17

Order: *Didronel (etidronate disodium) 20 mg/kg/d PO for 3 months.* **The patient who has Paget's disease weighs 81 kg. How many 400-mg tablets would you administer?**

Body weight:	81 kg [single unit of measurement]
Order:	20 mg/kg per day [equivalence]
Strength:	1 tab = 400 mg [equivalence]
Quantity you want to find:	? tab [single unit of measurement]

FORMULA METHOD

You want to "change" the body weight of the patient (81 kg) to milligrams of drug. The order is 20 mg/kg/day, so use the formula

$$\text{Size of patient} \times \text{Order} = \text{Dose}$$

$$81\,kg \times \frac{20\,mg}{1\,kg} = 1{,}620\,mg$$

D (desired dose) = 1,620 mg
H (dose on hand) = 400 mg
Q (dosage unit)   = 1 tab
X (unknown)   = ? tab

Fill in the formula $\dfrac{D}{H} \times Q = X$

$$\frac{1620\,mg}{400\,mg} \times 1\,tab = ?\,tab$$

Cancel $\dfrac{1620\,\overline{mg}}{400\,\overline{mg}} \times 1\,tab = ?\,tab$

Multiply $\dfrac{1620}{400} \times 1\,tab = 4.05$

DIMENSIONAL ANALYSIS

When drugs are prescribed based on body weight, you start the problem with the weight of the patient. You first change the single unit of measurement, kilograms (kg of body weight), to another single unit of measurement, milligrams (mg of drug), and then convert the milligrams to tablets.

81 kg (of body weight) ⟶ ? mg (of drug)
⟶ ? tab

$$81\text{ kg (of body weight)} \times \frac{?\text{ mg (of drug)}}{?\text{ kg (of body weight)}}$$

$$\times \frac{?\text{ tab}}{?\text{ mg (of drug)}} = ?\text{ tab}$$

Because the order is for 20 mg per kg, the first unit fraction is $\dfrac{20\text{ mg}}{1\text{ kg}}$

Because each tablet contains 400 mg, the second unit fraction is $\dfrac{1\text{ tab}}{400\text{ mg}}$

You can do this on one line as follows:

$$81\,kg \times \frac{20\,\overline{mg}}{1\,kg} \times \frac{1\,tab}{400\,\overline{mg}} = 4.05\,tab$$

The patient should receive 4 tablets of Didronel by mouth daily.

EXAMPLE 6.18

The physician orders *Biaxin (clarithromycin) 7.5 milligrams per kilogram PO q12h.* If the drug strength is 250 milligrams per 5 mL, how many mL of this antibiotic drug should be administered to a patient who weighs 70 kilograms?

Body weight	70 kg
Order	7.5 mg/kg
Strength	250 mg/5 mL
Find	? ml

FORMULA METHOD

You want to "change" the body weight of the patient (70 kg) to milligrams of drug. The order is 7.5 mg/kg, so use the formula

$$Size\ of\ patient \times Order = Dose$$

$$70\,kg \times \frac{7.5\,mg}{1\,kg} = 525\,mg$$

Therefore, the patient should receive 525 mg

D (desired dose) = 525 mg
H (dose on hand) = 250 mg
Q (dosage unit)   = 5 mL
X (unknown)   = ? mL

Fill in the formula $\frac{D}{H} \times Q = X$

$$\frac{525\,mg}{250\,mg} \times 5\,mL = ?\,mL$$

Cancel $\frac{\overset{21}{\cancel{525}}\,mg}{\underset{10}{\cancel{250}}\,mg} \times 5\,mL = ?\,mL$

Multiply $2.1 \times 5\,mL = 10.5\,mL$

RATIO & PROPORTION

The patient's weight is 70 kg and the order is for 7.5 mg/kg. Multiply the *size of the patient* by the *order* to determine how many milligrams of Biaxin to give the patient.

$$70\,kg \times \frac{7.5\,mg}{kg} = 525\,mg$$

So, the patient must receive 525 mg of Biaxin.
Now, convert the 525 mg of Biaxin to milliliters. The strength of the solution is 250 mg/5 mL. Think of the problem this way:

$$525\,mg = x\,mL \quad (dose)$$
$$250\,mg = 5\,mL \quad (strength)$$

One way to set up the proportion is

$$\frac{525\,mg}{x\,mL} = \frac{250\,mg}{5\,mL}$$

$$250x = 2{,}626$$
$$x = 10.5$$

The patient should receive 10.5 mL of Biaxin by mouth every 12 hours.

Dosages Based on Body Surface Area (BSA)

NOTE

Use a search engine, such as Google, to search the Web for "Body Surface Area Calculators" to obtain links to online BSA calculators.

In some cases, **body surface area (BSA)** may be used rather than **weight** in determining appropriate drug dosages. This is particularly true when calculating dosages for children, those receiving cancer therapy, burn patients, and patients requiring critical care. A patient's BSA can be estimated by using formulas.

BSA Formulas

Body surface area can be approximated by formula using either a handheld calculator or an online Web site. BSA, which is measured in square meters (m²), can be determined by using either of the following two mathematical formulas:

Formula for metric units:

$$BSA = \sqrt{\frac{weight\ in\ kilograms \times height\ in\ centimeters}{3{,}600}}$$

Formula for household units:

$$BSA = \sqrt{\frac{weight\ in\ pounds \times height\ in\ inches}{3{,}131}}$$

NOTE

In Example 6.19, the metric formula for BSA was used, and in Example 6.20, the household formula for BSA was used. However, each formula provided the BSA measured in square meters (m^2). In this book, we will round off BSA to two decimal places.

EXAMPLE 6.19

Find the BSA of an adult who is 183 cm tall and weighs 92 kg.

Because this example has metric units (kilograms and centimeters), we use the following formula:

$$BSA = \sqrt{\frac{\text{weight in kilograms} \times \text{height in centimeters}}{3,600}}$$

$$= \sqrt{\frac{92 \times 183}{3,600}}$$

At this point we need a calculator with a square-root key.

$$= \sqrt{4.6767}$$

$$= 2.16256$$

Therefore, the BSA of this adult is 2.16 m^2.

EXAMPLE 6.20

What is the BSA of a man who is 4 feet 10 inches tall and weighs 142 pounds?

First you convert 4 feet 10 inches to 58 inches.

Because the example has household units (pounds and inches), we use the following formula:

$$BSA = \sqrt{\frac{\text{weight in pounds} \times \text{height in inches}}{3,131}}$$

$$= \sqrt{\frac{142 \times 58}{3,131}}$$

$$= \sqrt{2.6305}$$

$$= 1.62187$$

Therefore, the BSA of this adult is 1.62 m^2.

EXAMPLE 6.21

The physician orders 40 mg/m^2 of a drug PO once daily. How many milligrams of the drug would you administer to an adult patient weighing 88 kg with a height of 150 cm?

The first step is to determine the BSA of the patient.

Using the formula, you get

$$BSA = \sqrt{\frac{88 \times 150}{3,600}}$$

$$= \sqrt{3.6667}$$

$$= 1.91 \, m^2$$

BSA: 1.91 m²
Order: 40 mg/m²
Find: ? mg

The patient's BSA is 1.91 *m²*, and the order is for 40 *mg/m²*. Multiply the *size of the patient* by the *order* to determine how many milligrams of the drug to give the patient.

$$1.91 \ \text{m}^2 \times \frac{40 \ \text{mg}}{\text{m}^2} = 76.4 \ \text{mg}$$

You would administer 76.4 mg of the drug to the patient.

EXAMPLE 6.22

The prescriber ordered 30 mg/m² of a drug PO stat for a patient who has a BSA of 1.65 m². The "safe dose range" for this drug is 20 to 40 mg per day. Calculate the prescribed dose in milligrams and determine if it is within the safe range.

BSA: 1.65 m²
Order: 30 mg/m²
Find: ? mg

The patient's BSA is 1.65 *m²*, and the order is for 30 *mg/m²*. Multiply the *size of the patient* by the *order* to determine how many milligrams of the drug to give the patient.

$$1.65 \ \text{m}^2 \times \frac{30 \ \text{mg}}{\text{m}^2} = 49.5 \ \text{mg}$$

The safe dose range is 20–40 mg per day.

So, the dose prescribed, 49.5 mg, is higher than the upper limit (40 mg) of the daily "safe dose range." It is an overdose. Therefore, the prescribed dose is not safe, and you may not administer this drug. You must consult with the prescriber.

EXAMPLE 6.23

Order: *Etopophos (etoposide) 200 mg/m² PO for five consecutive days.* How many scored 50-mg capsules of this antineoplastic drug would you administer to a patient who has a BSA of 1.49 m² and who has testicular cancer?

BSA: 1.49 m² [single unit of measurement]
Order: 200 mg/m² per day [equivalence]
Strength: 1 cap = 50 mg [equivalence]
Find: ? cap [single unit of measurement]

The patient's BSA is 1.49 m^2, and the order is for 200 mg/m^2. First, multiply the *size of the patient* by the *order* to determine how many milligrams of the drug to give the patient, and then use the strength to change mg to cap.

$$1.49 \; \cancel{m^2} \times \frac{200 \; \cancel{mg}}{\cancel{m^2}} \times \frac{cap}{50 \; \cancel{mg}} = 5.96 \; cap$$

So, you would administer 6 capsules to the patient daily for five days in a row.

Summary

In this chapter, you learned the computations necessary to calculate dosages of oral medications in liquid and solid form. You also learned about the equipment used to accurately measure liquid medication.

- It is crucial to ensure that every medication administered is within the recommended safe dosage range.

Calculating doses for oral medications in solid and liquid form

- The label states the strength of the drug (e.g., 10 mg/tab, 15 mg/mL).
- Sometimes oral medications are ordered in liquid form for special populations such as pediatrics, geriatrics, and patients with neurological conditions.
- Some medication cups cannot accurately measure volumes less than 5 mL.
- Special calibrated droppers or oral syringes that are supplied with some liquid oral medications may be used to administer *only those medications*.
- Some drugs, such as electrolytes, are measured in milliequivalents (mEq).

Calculating dosages using the formula method

- The formula $\frac{D}{H} \times Q = X$ can be used to calculate dosages.
- Always include the units of measurement when setting up the formula.

- *D and H* must always have the same units of measurement, and *Q and X* must have the same units of measurement.
- If the desired dose ordered is in a different unit of measurement than the dose on hand, convert them to the same unit of measurement before using the formula.

Calculating doses based on body weight

- Dosages based on body weight are generally measured in milligrams per kilogram (mg/kg).
- Start calculations with the weight of the patient.
- Multiply the size of the patient (kg) by the order to obtain the dose.
- Size of the Patient × Order = Dose
- Medications may be prescribed by body weight in special populations such as pediatrics and geriatrics.

Calculating doses based on body surface area

- Body surface area (BSA) is measured in square meters (m^2).
- Start calculations with the BSA of the patient.
- Multiply the size of the patient (m^2) by the order to obtain the dose.
- Size of the Patient × Order = Dose
- BSA is estimated by using a formula.
- BSA may be utilized to determine dosages for special patient populations such as those receiving cancer therapy, burn therapy, and for patients requiring critical care.

Case Study 6.1

Read the case study and answer the questions. Answers can be found in Appendix A.

A 58 year old male who has a history of angina, type II diabetes mellitus, hypertension, and hyperlipidemia has had a cardiac catheterization. He is 6 feet tall and weighs 325 pounds, and has a very stressful job in the financial business. His vital signs are stable, there is no bleeding from the catheterization site, and he is awaiting his discharge. Review his discharge orders, and use the labels to answer the questions if required.

Discharge Orders

- 2,200 calorie ADA diet
- Follow-up with PMD in one week
- Janumet (sitagliptin/metformin HCl) 50/1,000 mg PO B.I.D.
- lansoprazole 30 mg PO daily before breakfast
- Xanax (alprazolam) 2 mg PO prn anxiety
- Lipitor (atorvastatin calcium) 40 mg PO daily
- Lovaza (omega-3-acid ethyl esters) 2 g PO B.I.D.
- lisinopril/hydrochlorothiazide 20/12.5 mg PO daily
- Tricor (fenofibrate) 48 mg PO daily
- Amaryl (glimepiride) 2 mg PO daily with breakfast
- Plavix (clopidogrel bisulfate) 75 mg PO daily
- Coreg (carvedilol) 12.5 mg PO B.I.D.
- Sumaycin (tetracycline HCl) 500 mg PO B.I.D.

1. Select the appropriate label and calculate how many tablets of sitagliptin/metformin the patient must take for each dose.
2. How many capsules of omega-3-acid ethyl esters contain the dose?
3. How many tablets of atorvastatin will the patient take each day?
4. Calculate the number of tablets of carvedilol the patient will take per day.
5. How many tablets of alprazolam may the patient take per dose?
6. What is the dose of clopidogrel in grams?
7. How many tablets of fenofibrate will the patient take in four weeks?
8. The strength of the glimepiride is 1 mg/tab. How many tablets contain the dose?
9. How many capsules of lansoprazole contain the dose?
10. The strength of the tetracycline is 250 mg/cap. How many capsules will the patient take per day?
11. Calculate the patient's BSA.

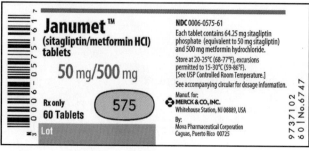

(a)

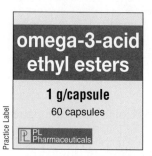

(b) **(For educational purposes only)**

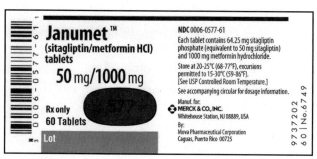

(c)

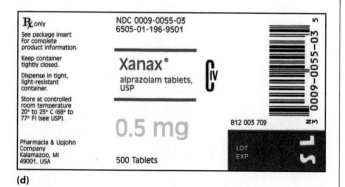

(d)

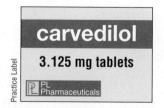

(e) **(For educational purposes only)**

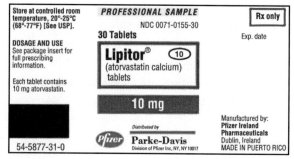

(f) **(For educational purposes only)**

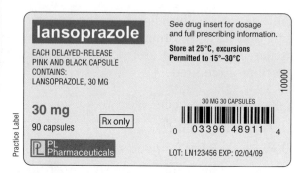

(g)

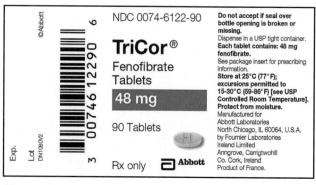

(h)

Drug Labels for Case Study 6.1

Practice Reading Labels

Using the following labels, identify the strength of the medication and calculate the doses indicated. The answers are found in Appendix A.

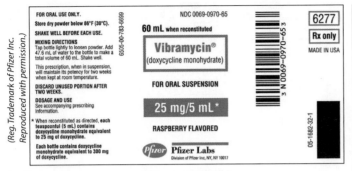

1. Strength: _____
   Vibramycin (doxycycline monohydrate)
   100 mg = _____ mL

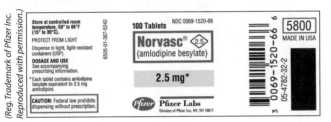

2. Strength: _____
   Norvasc (amlodipine besylate)
   10 mg = _____ tab

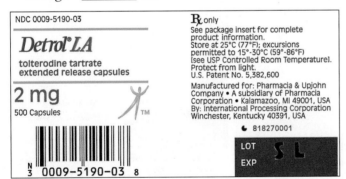

3. Strength: _____
   Detrol (tolterodine) 4 mg = _____ cap

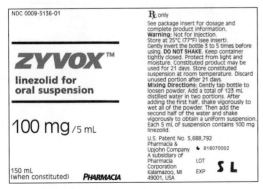

4. Strength: _____
   Zyvox (linezolid) 400 mg = _____ mL

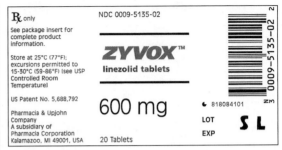

5. Strength: _____
   Zyvox (linezolid)
   0.6 g = _____ tab

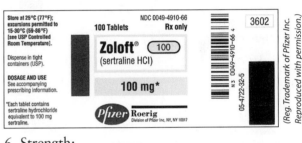

6. Strength: _____
   Zoloft (sertraline HCl)
   200 mg = _____ tab

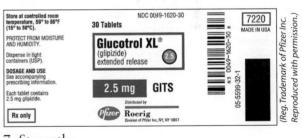

7. Strength: _____
   Glucotrol XL (glipizide)
   10 mg = _____ tab

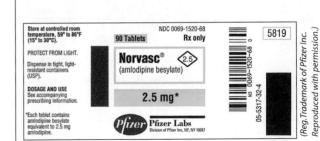

8. Strength: _____
   Norvasc (amlodipine besylate)
   5 mg = _____ tab

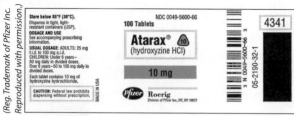

9. Strength: _____
   Atarax (hydroxyzine HCl)
   50 mg = _____ tab

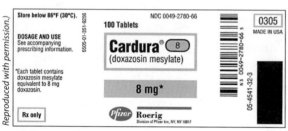

10. Strength: _____
    Cardura (doxazosin mesylate)
    16 mg = _____ tab

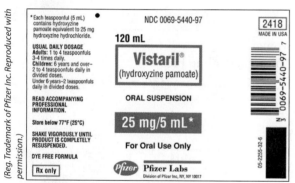

11. Strength: _____
    Vistaril (hydroxyzine pamoate)
    75 mg = _____ mL

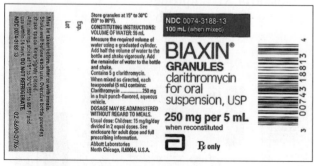

12. Strength: _____
    Biaxin (clarithromycin)
    375 mg = _____ mL

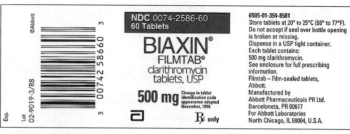

13. Strength: _____
    Biaxin (clarithromycin)
    500 mg = _____ tab

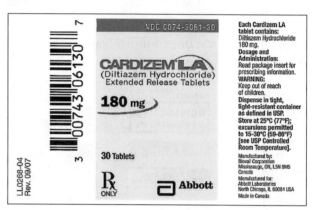

14. Strength: _____
    Cardizem LA (diltiazem HCl)
    180 mg = _____ tab

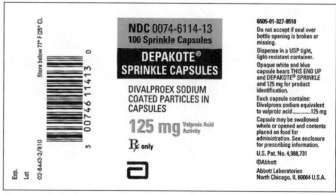

15. Strength: _____
    Depakote (divalproex sodium)
    250 mg = _____ cap

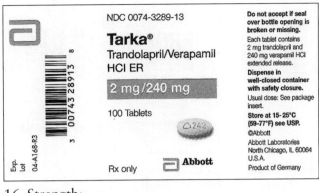

16. Strength: _____
    Tarka (trandolapril/verapamil)
    4/480 mg = _____ tab

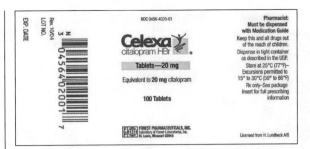

20. Strength: _____
    Celexa (citalopram)
    40 mg = _____ tab

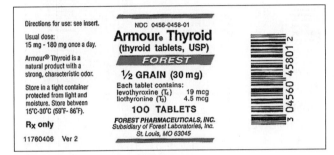

17. Strength: _____
    Armour Thyroid (thyroid tablets)
    60 mg = _____ tab

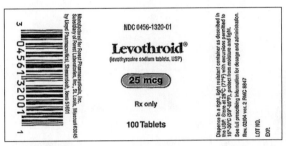

21. Strength: _____
    Levothroid (levothyroxine sodium)
    100 mcg = _____ tab

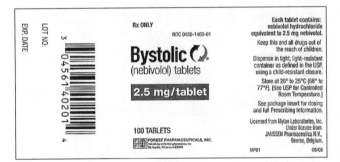

18. Strength: _____
    Bystolic (nebivolol) 5 mg = _____ tab

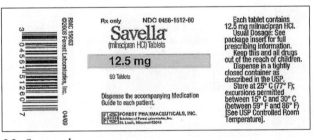

22. Strength: _____
    Savella (milnacipran HCl)
    50 mg = _____ tab

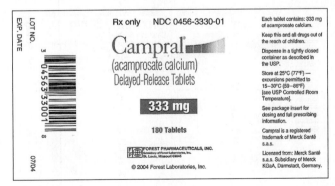

19. Strength: _____
    Campral (acamprosate calcium)
    666 mg = _____ tab

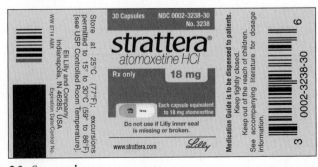

23. Strength: _____
    Strattera (atomoxetine HCl)
    54 mg = _____ cap

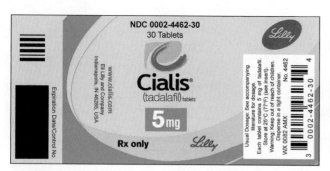

24. Strength: _____
    Cialis (tadalafil) 20 mg = _____ tab

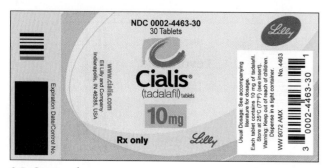

25. Strength: _____
    Cialis (tadalafil) 20 mg = _____ tab

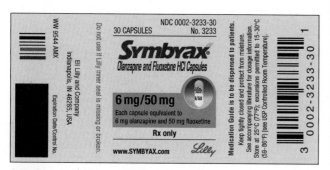

26. Strength: _____
    Symbyax (olanzapine and fluoxetine)
    6/50 mg = _____ cap

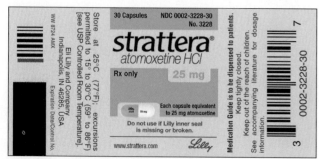

27. Strength: _____
    Strattera (atomoxetine HCl)
    50 mg = _____ cap

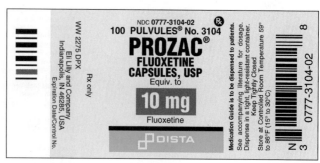

28. Strength: _____
    Prozac (fluoxetine) 20 mg = _____ cap

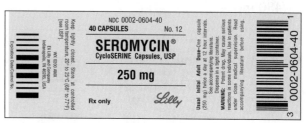

29. Strength: _____
    Seromycin (CycloSERINE)
    500 mg = _____ cap

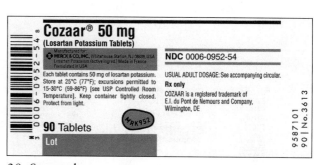

30. Strength: _____
    Cozaar (losartan potassium)
    100 mg = _____ tab

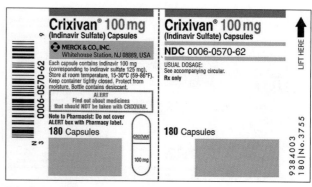

31. Strength: _____
    Crixivan (indinavir sulfate)
    400 mg = _____ cap

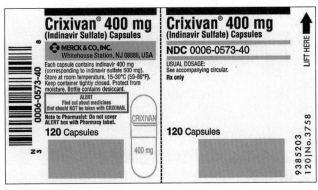

32. Strength: _____
   Crixivan (indinavir sulfate)
   400 mg = _____ cap

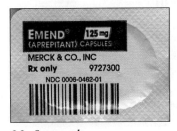

33. Strength: _____
   Emend (aprepitant) 375 mg = _____ cap

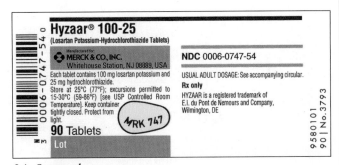

34. Strength: _____
   Hyzaar (losartan potassium/hydrochlorothiazide)
   200/50 mg = _____ tab

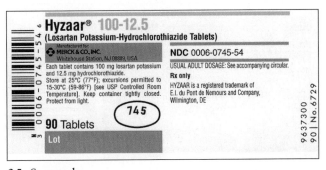

35. Strength: _____
   Hyzaar (losartan potassium/hydrochlorothiazide)
   400/50 mg = _____ tab

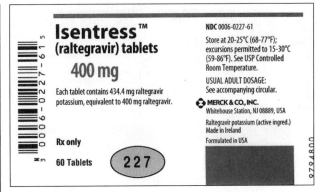

36. Strength: _____
   Isentress (raltegravir) 400 mg = _____ tab

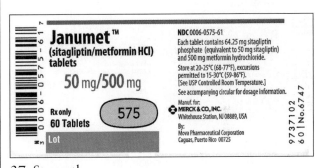

37. Strength: _____
   Janumet (sitagliptin/metformin HCl)
   100/1,000 mg = _____ tab

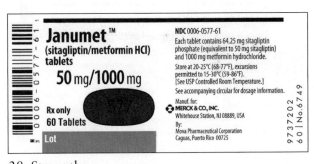

38. Strength: _____
   Janumet (sitagliptin/metformin HCl)
   150/3,000 mg = _____ tab

39. Strength: _____
   Mevacor (lovastatin) 60 mg = _____ tab

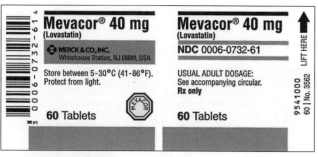

40. Strength: _____

Mevacor (lovastatin) 40 mg = _____ tab

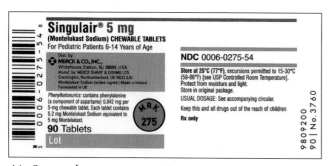

41. Strength: _____

Singulair (montelukast sodium)
10 mg = _____ tab

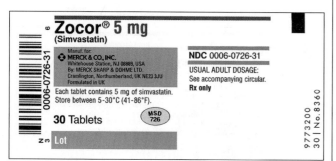

42. Strength: _____

Zocor (simvastatin) 20 mg = _____ tab

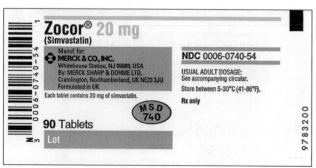

43. Strength: _____

Zocor (simvastatin) 40 mg = _____ tab

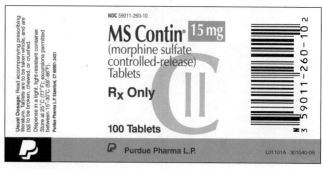

44. Strength: _____

MS Contin (morphine sulfate)
30 mg = _____ tab

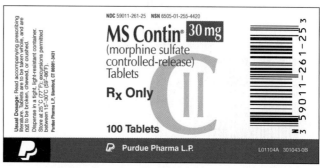

45. Strength: _____

MS Contin (morphine sulfate)
30 mg = _____ tab

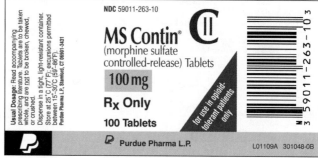

46. Strength: _____

MS Contin (morphine sulfate)
200 mg = _____ tab

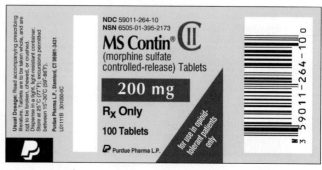

47. Strength: _____

MS Contin (morphine sulfate)
200 mg = _____ tab

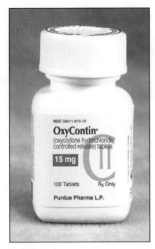

48. Strength: _____
    OxyContin (oxycodone HCl)
    45 mg = _____ tab

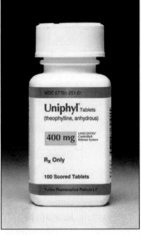

50. Strength: _____
    Uniphyl (theophylline, anhydrous)
    400 mg = _____ tab

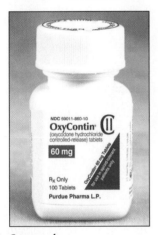

49. Strength: _____
    OxyContin (oxycodone HCl)
    180 mg = _____ tab

Practice Sets

The answers to *Try These for Practice,* *Exercises,* and *Cumulative Review Exercises* are found in Appendix A. Ask your instructor for the answers to the *Additional Exercises.*

Note: Remember that throughout this text when you are asked to calculate the amount of drug to administer, it is assumed to be the amount "per administration"—unless specified otherwise.

Try These for Practice

Test your comprehension after reading the chapter.

1. Use the formula to estimate the body surface area of a person who is 160 cm tall and weighs 83 kg.

2. Order: *Anadrol-50 (oxymetholone) 200 mg po daily.* The recommended dose for this anabolic steroid is 1–5 mg/kg/d. Is the prescribed order in the recommended range for a patient who has aplastic anemia and weighs 75 kg?

Workspace

Workspace

3. The prescribed order is *120 mg/m²/d × 14 days PO*. How many grams will the patient who has a BSA of 1.4 m² receive in total after this two-week regimen?

4. See •**Figure 6.17** to determine the number of capsules of Cymbalta (duloxetine hydrochloride) that you would administer each day after the first week to a patient who has fibromyalgia.

ROUTE & DOSAGE
Depression Adult: PO 40–60 mg/d in one or two divided doses
Generalized Anxiety/Diabetic Neuropathy Adult: PO 60 mg once daily
Fibromyalagia Adult: PO 30 mg/d in × 1 wk then 60 mg/d

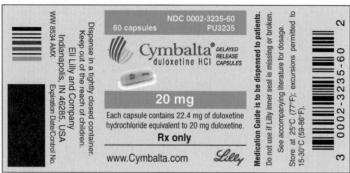

•**Figure 6.17**
Exerpt from a drug guide and the drug label for Cymbalta.

5. Order: *paregoric 10 mL PO prn after loose bowel movement, maximum 4 times daily*. The strength of this antidiarrheal drug is 2 mg/5 mL. How many milligrams will the patient receive?

Exercises

Reinforce your understanding in class or at home.

1. Order: *Depakene (valproic acid) 750 mg/day po in three divided doses*. Read the label in •**Figure 6.18**. How many capsules of this anticonvulsant will you administer to the patient who has mania?

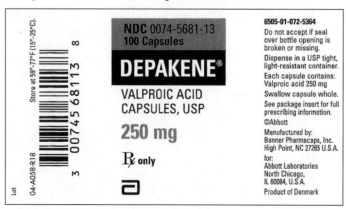

•**Figure 6.18**
Drug label for Depakene.

2. Order: *Xanax (alprazolam) 1.5 mg po t.i.d.* How many 0.5 mg tablets of this antianxiety drug will you administer to the patient who suffers from panic attacks?

3. Order: *amoxicillin oral suspension 500 mg po q8h.* The concentration of the amoxicillin solution is 125 mg/5 mL. How many milliliters of this antibiotic will you administer to the patient who has a mild infection?

4. Order: *potassium chloride 80 mEq po in two divided doses daily.* The concentration of the potassium chloride is 40 mEq/15 mL. How many milliliters of this electrolytic replacement solution will you administer to the patient who has hypokalemia?

5. Order: *furosemide 50 mg po b.i.d.* Read the label in •**Figure 6.19.** How many teaspoons of this diuretic will you administer to the patient who has high blood pressure?

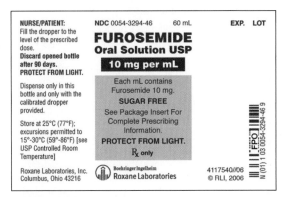

NURSE/PATIENT:
Fill the dropper to the level of the prescribed dose.
Discard opened bottle after 90 days.
PROTECT FROM LIGHT.

Dispense only in this bottle and only with the calibrated dropper provided.

Store at 25°C (77°F); excursions permitted to 15°-30°C (59°-86°F) [see USP Controlled Room Temperature]

Roxane Laboratories, Inc.
Columbus, Ohio 43216

NDC 0054-3294-46   60 mL   EXP. LOT

FUROSEMIDE
Oral Solution USP
10 mg per mL

Each mL contains Furosemide 10 mg.
SUGAR FREE
See Package Insert For Complete Prescribing Information.
PROTECT FROM LIGHT.
R_x only

Boehringer Ingelheim
Roxane Laboratories

4117540//06
© RLI, 2006

• **Figure 6.19**
Drug label for furosemide.

6. Order: *Xyrem (sodium oxybate) 2.25 g po given at bedtime while in bed and repeat 4 hours later.* How many milliliters of this CNS depressant will you administer to the patient who has cataplexy if the strength of the Xyrem solution is 500 mg/mL?

7. Basketball player Shaquille O'Neal stands 7 feet 1 inch in height and weighs 325 pounds. Estimate his body surface area.

8. Entertainer Madonna weighs 52 kg and is 160 cm in height. Estimate her body surface area.

9. A drug is ordered *6 mg/kg po b.i.d.* How many tablets will a patient receive if he weighs 148 pounds and the strength of the tablet is 200 mg/tab?

10. A drug is ordered *200 mg/m² po b.i.d.* How many mL will a patient receive if her BSA is 1.34 m², and the concentration of the solution is 5 mg/mL?

11. Order: *ERY-TAB (erythromycin) 333 mg po q8h.* Read the label in •**Figure 6.20.** How many tablets of this macrolide antibiotic will you administer to the patient who has a severe infection?

Workspace

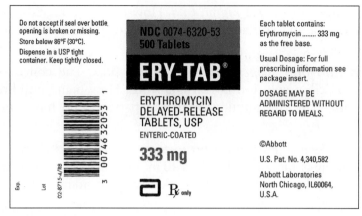

● **Figure 6.20**
Drug label for ERY-TAB.

12. Order: *Kaletra (lopinavir/ritonavir) 800/200 mg po daily.* Read the label in
●**Figure 6.21.** How many mL of this antiretroviral agent will you administer
to the patient who has HIV infection?

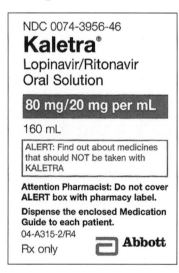

● **Figure 6.21**
Drug label for Kaletra.

13. Order: *metformin hydrochloride 750 mg po b.i.d. with meals.* Read the
label in ●**Figure 6.22.** How many tablets of this antidiabetic drug will you
administer to the patient?

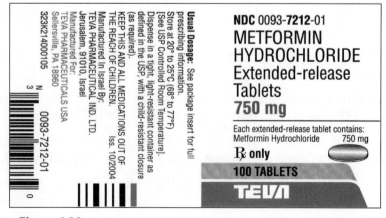

● **Figure 6.22**
Drug label for metformin HCl.

14. Order: *phenobarbitol sodium 400 mg po in two divided doses daily.* The recommended dosage of this anticonvulsant is 1–3 mg/kg/d. Is the prescribed dose safe for the patient who weighs 203 pounds?

15. Read the label in • **Figure 6.23** and determine the number of grams of OxyContin (oxycodone HCl) that are contained in the entire bottle.

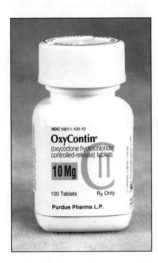

• **Figure 6.23**
Container of OxyContin.

16. Estimate the body surface area of a patient who is 5 feet tall and weighs 60 kg.

17. A drug is ordered *50 mg/m² po b.i.d.* How many mL will a patient receive if her BSA is 1.44 m² and the concentration of the solution is 2 mg/mL?

18. Order: *Lexapro (escitalopram oxalate)10 mg po daily.* Read the label in • **Figure 6.24** and determine the number of milliliters of this antidepressant that a geriatric patient who has generalized anxiety will receive in a week.

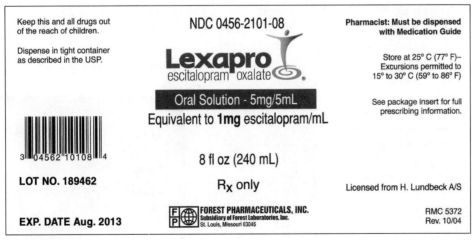

• **Figure 6.24**
Drug label for Lexapro.

19. Order: *digoxin 0.75 mg po stat.* How many 0.25 mg tablets of this antiarrhythmic drug will you administer to the patient?

20. Order: *Percocet (oxycodone/acetaminophen) 5/650 mg po prn pain q6h.* How many 2.5/325 mg tablets of this opioid analgesic will you administer to the patient?

Workspace

Additional Exercises

Now, test yourself!

1. *Paxil (paroxetine HCl) 50 mg PO daily* has been ordered for your patient. Only 10-mg, 20-mg, and 30-mg strength tablets are available. Which combination of tablets contains the exact dosage using the smallest number of tablets?

2. The physician prescribes *500 mcg of Baraclude (entecavir) per day* via NG (nasogastric tube) for a patient with chronic hepatitis B virus infection. The oral solution contains 0.05 mg of entecavir per milliliter. How many mL of this antiviral medication would you deliver?

3. Order: *Prilosec (omeprazole) 40 mg PO once daily for 4 weeks.* The available strength is 10 mg per capsule. Determine the number of capsules of this antacid drug that you would administer to the patient over the entire treatment period.

4. The prescriber ordered *Precose (acarbose) 75 mg PO t.i.d. with meals.* The medication is available in 25-mg tablets. How many tablets of this a glucosidase inhibitor (antidiabetic agent) will you give your patient in 24 hours?

5. *Toprol-XL (metoprolol succinate) extended release tablets 200 mg PO daily* has been prescribed for a patient. The label reads 200 mg per tablet. Calculate the number of tablets of this antihypertensive drug the patient would have received after 7 days.

6. *Keftab (cephalexin) 50 mg/kg PO in two equally divided doses* is prescribed for a patient who weighs 40 kilograms. If each tablet contains 500 mg, how many tablets of this cephalosporin antibiotic will the patient receive per dose?

7. *Zyvox (linezolid) 600 mg PO q12h* has been prescribed for an elderly patient who is diagnosed with pneumonia. Read the label in •**Figure 6.25**.
   (a) Calculate the number of milliliters of this antibacterial suspension you would administer.
   (b) Indicate the dose on the medication cup shown in Figure 6.25.

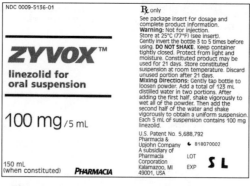 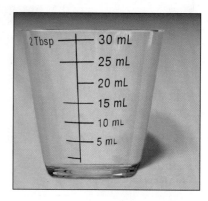

• **Figure 6.25**
Drug label for Zyvox and medication cup.

8. A patient is scheduled to receive 0.015 g of a drug by mouth every morning. The drug is available as 7.5-mg tablets. How many tablets would you administer?

9. A patient who is diagnosed with rheumatoid arthritis is ordered *Voltaren (diclofenac sodium) 50 mg PO t.i.d.* Your drug reference book states that the dose should not exceed 225 mg daily. Is the prescribed dose safe?

10. An elderly patient who has depression is ordered *Aventyl (nortriptyline HCl) 25 mg PO t.i.d.* The label reads Aventyl Oral Solution 10 mg/5mL. How many mL will you administer?

11. *Antivert (meclizine HCl) 25 mg PO once daily for three days* has been ordered for a patient who has a history of motion sickness who is planning extensive traveling. Read the information on the label in •**Figure 6.26** and calculate the number of scored tablets that the patient will receive when the prescription is completed at the end of the three days.

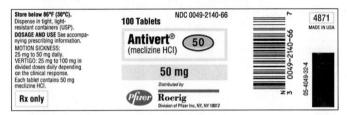

• **Figure 6.26**
Drug label for Antivert.

(Reg. trademark of Pfizer Inc. Reproduced with permission.)

12. The physician orders *7.5 mg of Tranxene SD (clorazepate dipotassium) PO t.i.d.* for an elderly patient who is diagnosed with extreme anxiety. This drug is available in 15 mg scored tablets. How many tablets would the patient receive in 24 hours?

13. A patient develops a mild skin reaction to a transfusion of a unit of packed red blood cells and is given 75 milligrams of Benadryl (diphenhydramine HCl) PO stat. The only drug strength available is 25-mg capsules. How many capsules will you give?

14. The physician orders *two Tylenol #3 (codeine 30 mg, acetaminophen 300 mg) PO every 6 hours.* How many milligrams of acetaminophen will the patient have received by the end of the day?

15. The physician orders *Detrol LA (tolterodine tartrate) 4 mg PO daily* for a patient with an overactive bladder. Read the label in •**Figure 6.27** and determine how many capsules you will give this patient.

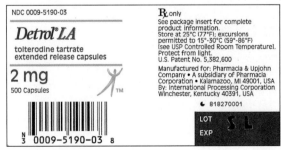

• **Figure 6.27**
Drug label for Detrol LA.

16. A patient who has difficulty sleeping is medicated for insomnia with 0.25 g of a drug PO at bedtime. The drug is available as 500 mg per scored tablet. How many tablets will you administer to your patient?

Workspace

17. The physician orders *Coumadin (warfarin sodium) 6.5 mg PO* every other day from Monday through Sunday. How many milligrams of Coumadin will your patient receive in the week?

18. A physician is treating a patient for *H. influenzae*. He writes the following prescription:

    Vantin (cefpodoxime proxetil) 200 mg PO q12h for 14 days

    Read the label in •**Figure 6.28**.
    (a) Calculate the number of milliliters you will give this patient.
    (b) Indicate the dose on the medication cup in Figure 6.28.

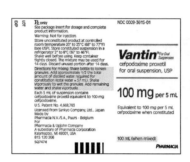
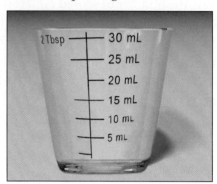

• **Figure 6.28**
Drug label for Vantin and medication cup.

19. The physician orders *Deltasone (prednisone) 60 mg/m²* PO *daily* as part of the treatment protocol for a patient with leukemia.
    (a) How many milligrams of this steroid drug would you administer if the patient is 5 feet 6 inches tall and weighs 140 pounds?
    (b) The drug is supplied in 50 mg per tablet. How many tablets will you administer?

20. The antibiotic, Zithromax (azithromycin), is ordered to treat a patient who has a diagnosis of chronic obstructive pulmonary disease (COPD). The order is:

    Zithromax (azithromycin) 500 mg PO as a single dose on day one,
    followed by 250 mg once daily on days 2 through 5

    How many milligrams will the patient receive by the completion of the prescription?

Cumulative Review Exercises

Review your mastery of previous chapters.

1. 2 T = ? mL

2. 88 lb = ? kg

3. 2 pt = ? oz

4. 1 cm = ? mm

5. Order: *Zithromax (azithromycin) 500 mg po daily × 3 days*. The concentration of the Zithromax solution is 200 mg/5 mL. How many milliliters of this antibiotic will you administer to the patient who has a bacterial infection?

6. Order: *Zyprexa (olanzapine) 7.5 mg po daily.* How many 2.5-mg tablets of this antipsychotic drug would you administer?

7. Order: *Vistaril (hydroxyzine pamoate) 75 mg po q.i.d.* The concentration is 25 mg/5 mL. How many teaspoons of this antianxiety drug will you administer to the patient?

8. Order: *amoxicillin 3 g and probenecid 1 g po stat.* How many 500-mg tablets of amoxicillin would you administer to a patient who has gonorrhea?

9. Actor Tom Cruise is 5 ft 7 in and weighs 150 lb. Estimate his body surface area.

10. Harold is 165 cm and 89 kg, while John is 160 cm and 95 kg. Who has the larger BSA?

11. Order: *Flagyl (metronidazole) 7.5 mg/kg po q6h.* How many mg of this amebicide would you administer to a patient who weighs 150 lb?

12. Order: *codeine sulfate 10 mg po q4h prn pain.* The strength of the codeine sulfate is 15 mg/5 mL. How many mL of this narcotic drug will you administer to the patient?

13. Convert *0.5 mL/min* to an equivalent rate in *mL/h.*

14. Order: *Micro-K (potassium chloride) 16 mEq po stat.* How many 8-mEq tablets would you administer?

15. Write 10:30 P.M. in military time.

nursing.pearsonhighered.com
Prepare for success with animated examples, practice questions, challenge tests, and interactive assignments.

Workspace

Chapter

7 Syringes

Learning Outcomes

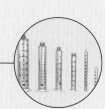

After completing this chapter, you will be able to

1. Identify the parts of a syringe and needle.
2. Identify various types of syringes.
3. Read the calibrations on syringes of various sizes.
4. Select the appropriate syringe to administer prescribed doses.
5. Measure single insulin dosages.
6. Measure combined insulin dosages.

I n this chapter, you will learn how to use various types of syringes to measure medication dosages. You will also discuss the difference between the types of insulin and how to measure single insulin dosages and combined insulin dosages.

Syringes are made of plastic or glass, designed for one-time use, and are packaged either separately, or together with needles of appropriate sizes. After use, syringes must be discarded in special puncture-resistant containers. See ●**Figure 7.1**.

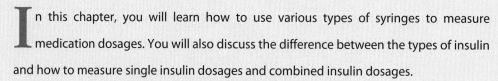

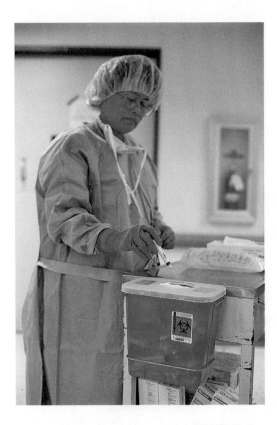

● **Figure 7.1**
Puncture-resistant container for needles, syringes, and other "sharps."

Parts of a Syringe

A syringe consists of a barrel, plunger, and tip.

● **Barrel:** a hollow cylinder that holds the medication. It has calibrations (markings) on the outer surface.

● **Plunger:** fits in the barrel and is moved back and forth. Pulling back on the plunger draws medication or air into the syringe. Pushing in the plunger forces air or medication out of the syringe.

● **Tip:** the end of the syringe that holds the needle. The needle slips onto the tip or can be twisted and locked in place (Luer-Lok™).

The inside of the barrel, plunger, and tip must always be sterile.

Needles

Needles are made of stainless steel and come in various lengths and diameters. They are packaged with a protective cover that keeps them from being contaminated. The parts of a needle are the **hub**, which attaches to the syringe; the **shaft**, the long part of the needle that is embedded in the hub; and the **bevel**, the slanted portion of the tip. The **length** of the needle is the distance from the point to the hub. Needles most commonly used in medication administration range from $\frac{3}{8}$ inch to 2 inches. The **gauge** of the needle refers to the thickness of the inside of the needle and varies from 18 to 28 (the larger the gauge, the thinner the needle). The parts of a syringe and needle are shown in ● **Figure 7.2**.

ALERT

The patient's size, the type of tissue being injected, and the viscosity of the medication will determine the size of the needle to be used. The inside of the barrel, plunger, tip of the syringe, and the needle should never come in contact with anything unsterile.

Parts of a 10 mL Luer-Lok™ Hypodermic Syringe and Needle

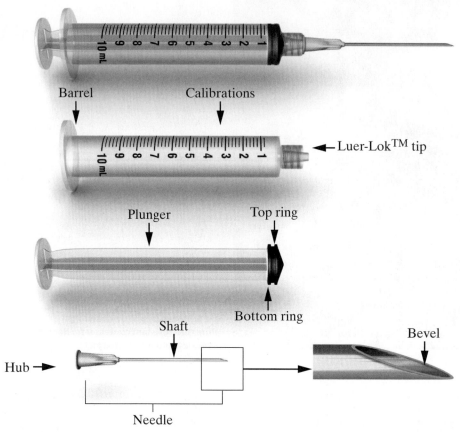

• **Figure 7.2**
Parts of a syringe and needle.

Commonly Used Sizes of Hypodermic Syringes

The two major types of syringes are hypodermic and oral. In 1853, doctors Charles Pravaz and Alexander Wood were the first to develop a syringe with a needle that was fine enough to pierce the skin. This is known as a **hypodermic syringe.** Use of oral syringes will be discussed in Chapter 12.

Hypodermic syringes are calibrated (marked) in cubic centimeters (cc), milliliters (mL), or units. Practitioners often refer to syringes by the volume of cubic centimeters they contain, for example, a 3-cc syringe. Although some syringes are still labeled in cubic centimeters, manufacturers are now phasing in syringes labeled in milliliters. In this text, we will generally use mL instead of cc.

The smaller capacity syringes (0.5, 1, 2, $2\frac{1}{2}$, and 3 mL) are used most often for intradermal, subcutaneous, or intramuscular injections of medication. The larger sizes (5, 6, 10, and 12 mL) are commonly used to draw blood or prepare medications for intravenous administration. Syringes 20 mL and larger are used to inject large volumes of solutions. A representative sample of commonly used syringes is shown in •**Figure 7.3.**

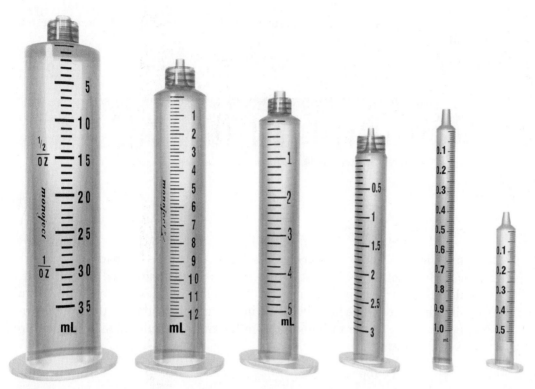

• Figure 7.3
A sample of commonly used hypodermic syringes (35 mL, 12 mL, 5 mL, 3 mL, 1 mL, and 0.5 mL).

A 35 mL syringe is shown in **• Figure 7.4**. Each line on the barrel represents 1 mL, and the longer lines represent 5 mL.

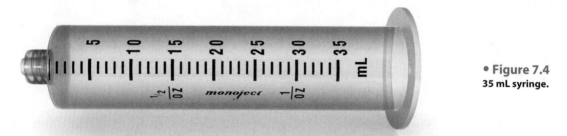

• Figure 7.4
35 mL syringe.

A 12 mL syringe is shown in **• Figure 7.5**. Each line on the barrel represents 0.2 mL, and the longer lines represent 1 mL.

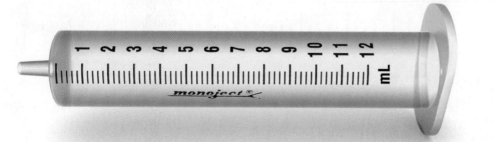

• Figure 7.5
12 mL syringe.

A 5 mL syringe is shown in •**Figure 7.6**. Each line on the barrel represents 0.2 mL, and the longer lines represent 1 mL.

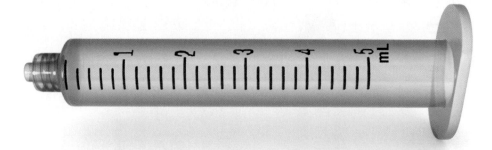

• **Figure 7.6**
5 mL syringe.

In •**Figure 7.7**, a 3 mL syringe is shown. There are 10 spaces between the largest markings. This indicates that the syringe is measured in tenths of a milliliter. So, each of the lines is 0.1 mL. The longer lines indicate half and full milliliter measures. The liquid volume in a syringe is read from the *top ring*, **not** the bottom ring or the raised section in the middle of the plunger. Therefore, this syringe contains 0.9 mL.

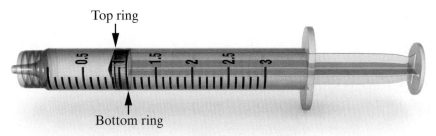

• **Figure 7.7**
Partially filled 3 mL syringe.

EXAMPLE 7.1

How much liquid is in the partially filled 12 mL syringe shown in •**Figure 7.8?**

The top ring of the plunger is at the second line after the 5 mL line. Because each line measures 0.2 mL, the second line measures 0.4 mL. Therefore, the amount in the syringe is 5.4 mL.

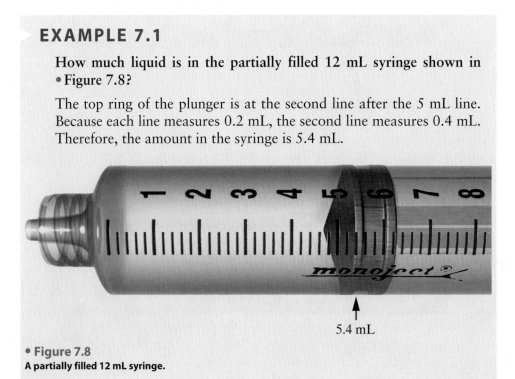

• **Figure 7.8**
A partially filled 12 mL syringe.

EXAMPLE 7.2

How much liquid is in the 5 mL syringe shown in •Figure 7.9?

The top ring of the plunger is at the third line after 4 mL. Because each line measures 0.2 mL, the third line measures 0.6 mL. Therefore, the amount of liquid in the syringe is 4.6 mL.

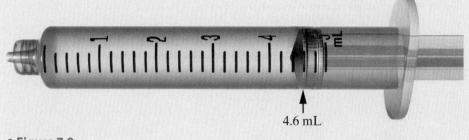

4.6 mL

• Figure 7.9
A partially filled 5 mL syringe.

EXAMPLE 7.3

How much liquid is in the 3 mL syringe shown in •Figure 7.10?

The top ring of the plunger is at the second line after 1 mL. Because each line measures 0.1 mL, the two lines measure 0.2 mL. Therefore, the amount in the syringe is 1.2 mL.

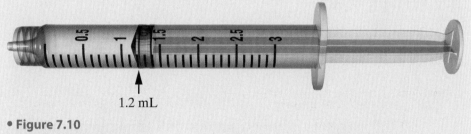

1.2 mL

• Figure 7.10
A partially filled syringe.

When small volumes of 1 milliliter or less are required, a low-volume syringe provides the greatest accuracy. The 1 mL syringe, also called a tuberculin syringe, shown in •**Figure 7.11** is calibrated in hundredths of a milliliter. Because there are 100 lines on the syringe, each line represents 0.01 mL. The 0.5 mL syringe shown in •**Figure 7.12** has 50 lines and each line also represents 0.01 mL. For doses of 0.5 mL or less, this syringe should be used. These syringes are used for intradermal injection of very small amounts of substances in tests for tuberculosis, allergies, as well as for intramuscular injections of small quantities of medication.

ALERT

The calibrations on the 1 mL syringe are very small and close together. Use caution when drawing up medication in this syringe.

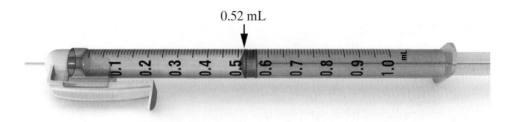

● **Figure 7.11**
A partially filled 1 mL safety tuberculin syringe.

The top ring of the plunger in Figure 7.11 is at the second line after 0.5 mL. Therefore, the amount in the syringe is 0.52 mL.

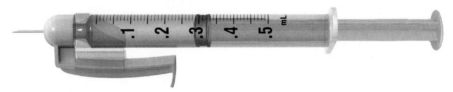

● **Figure 7.12**
A partially filled 0.5 mL safety syringe.

The top ring of the plunger in Figure 7.12 is at the first line before 0.3 mL (0.30 mL). Therefore, the syringe contains 0.29 mL.

NOTE

Because 0.5 mL and 1 mL tuberculin syringes can accurately measure amounts to hundredths of a milliliter, the volume of fluid to be measured in these syringes is rounded to the nearest hundredth; for example, 0.358 mL is rounded off to 0.36 mL. The 3 mL syringe can accurately measure amounts to tenths of a milliliter. The volume of fluid to be measured in this syringe is rounded to the nearest tenth of a milliliter; for example, 2.358 mL is rounded off to 2.4 mL.

EXAMPLE 7.4

How much liquid is shown in the portion of the 1 mL tuberculin syringe shown in ● Figure 7.13?

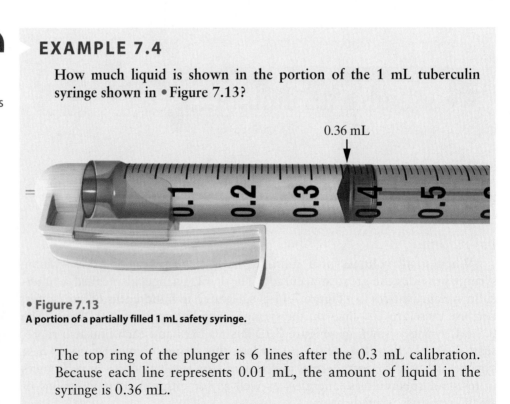

● **Figure 7.13**
A portion of a partially filled 1 mL safety syringe.

The top ring of the plunger is 6 lines after the 0.3 mL calibration. Because each line represents 0.01 mL, the amount of liquid in the syringe is 0.36 mL.

Insulin

Insulin is a hormone used to treat patients who have insulin-dependent diabetes mellitus (IDDM). Diabetes is fast becoming the epidemic of the 21st century.

Insulin is a high-risk medication. Therefore, a thorough understanding of the various types of insulins and insulin syringes is essential in preventing medication errors. Depending on its form, insulin can be administered via subcutaneous injection, intravenous route, or continuously via an insulin pump.

Insulin dosage is determined by the patient's daily blood-glucose readings, frequently referred to as a "fingerstick." A blood-glucose monitor is small and can quickly analyze a drop of blood and display the amount of blood glucose measured in milligrams per deciliter (mg/dL). See • **Figure 7.14**.

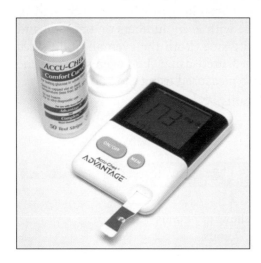

• **Figure 7.14**
Blood-Glucose Monitor.

Insulin is supplied as a premixed liquid measured in standardized units of potency rather than by weight or volume. These standardized units are called **USP** *units*, which are often shortened to *units*. The most commonly prepared concentration of insulin is 100 units per milliliter, which is referred to as *units 100 insulin* and is abbreviated as U-100. Although a 500 units/mL concentration of insulin (U-500) is also available, it is used only for the rare patient who is markedly insulin-resistant. U-40 insulin is used in some countries; however in the United States, insulin is standardized at U-100.

Insulin Syringes

Insulin syringes are used for the subcutaneous injection of insulin and are calibrated in *units* rather than *milliliters*.

Insulin syringes are calibrated for the administration of standard U-100 insulin only. Therefore, insulin syringes should not be used for administering nonstandard strengths of insulin. To ensure patient safety, an order for nonstandard insulin should contain the number of units as well as its volume in milliliters. For example, if the order were "*Regular Insulin U-500, 100 units, inject 0.2 mL subcutaneously stat,*" then 0.2 mL of U-500 insulin would be administered using a 1 mL tuberculin syringe.

Insulin syringes have three different capacities: the standard 100 unit capacity, and the **Lo-Dose** 50 unit or 30 unit capacities.

• **Figure 7.15** shows a *single-scale standard* 100 unit insulin syringe calibrated in 2-unit increments. Any odd number of units (e.g., 23, 35) is measured halfway between the even calibrations. These calibrations and spaces are very small, so this is not the syringe of choice for a person with impaired vision.

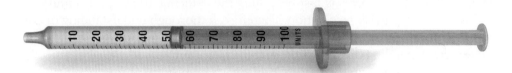

● **Figure 7.15**
A single-scale standard 100 unit insulin syringe with 52 units of insulin.

The dual-scale version of the 100 unit insulin syringe is easier to use. ●**Figure 7.16** shows a *dual-scale* 100 unit insulin syringe, also calibrated in 2-unit increments. However, it has a scale with *even* numbers on one side and a scale with *odd* numbers on the opposite side. Both the even and odd sides are shown. Even numbered doses are measured using the "even" side of the syringe, whereas odd numbered doses are measured using the "odd" side.

Each line on the barrel represents 2 units.

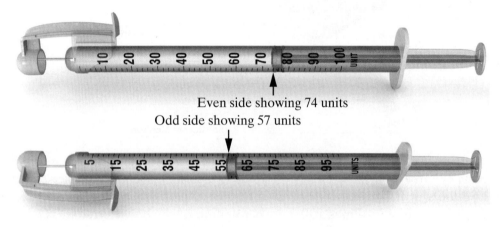

Even side showing 74 units
Odd side showing 57 units

● **Figure 7.16**
Two views of the same dual-scale standard 100 unit insulin safety syringe.

For small doses of insulin (50 units or fewer) Lo-Dose insulin syringes more accurately measure these doses, and should be used. A 50-unit Lo-Dose insulin syringe, shown in ●**Figure 7.17**, is a single-scale syringe with 50 units. It is calibrated in 1-unit increments.

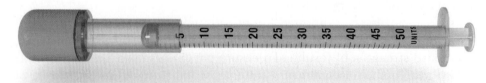

● **Figure 7.17**
A 50-unit Lo-Dose insulin syringe with protective cap.

A 30-unit Lo-Dose insulin syringe, shown in ●**Figure 7.18**, is a syringe with a capacity of 30 units. It is calibrated in 1-unit increments and is used when the dose is less than 30 units.

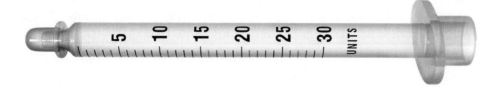

• **Figure 7.18**
A 30-unit Lo-Dose insulin syringe.

Types of Insulin

Insulin is available in 100 units/mL multidose vials. The major route of administration of insulin is by subcutaneous injection. *Insulin is never given intramuscularly*. It can also be administered with an insulin pen that contains a cartridge filled with insulin or with a Continuous Subcutaneous Insulin Infusion (CSII) pump. The CSII pump is used to administer a programmed dose of a rapid-acting 100 units insulin at a set rate of units per hour.

The *source* (animal or human) and *type* (rapid-, short-, intermediate-, or long-acting) are indicated on the insulin label. Today, the most commonly used *source* is human insulin. Insulin from a human source is designated on the label as recombinant DNA (rDNA origin). The *type* of insulin relates to both the *onset and duration of action*. See • **Figure 7.19** for examples of drug labels for various types of insulin.

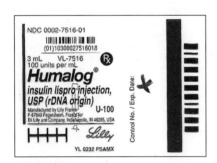

(a) rapid-acting

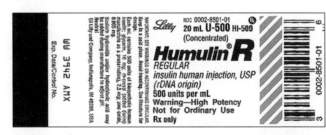

(b) short-acting

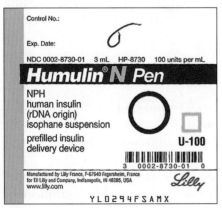

(c) intermediate-acting

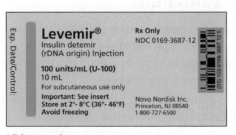

(d) long-acting

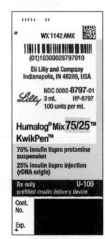

(e) premixed combination

• **Figure 7.19**
Drug labels for various types of insulin.

Healthcare providers must be familiar with the various **types of insulin**, as summarized in **Table 7.1.** Insulins are classified according to how fast they begin to work, when they reach maximum effect, and how long their effects last:

- **onset of action:** the length of time before insulin reaches the bloodstream and begins to lower blood glucose,

- **peak of action:** the time period when the insulin is the most effective in lowering blood glucose,

- **duration of action:** the period of time that the insulin continues to lower blood glucose.

Table 7.1 Types of Insulin

Type	Examples	Approximate Time	
Rapid-acting	Apidra (insulin glulisine)	Onset:	5–20 min
	Humalog (insulin lispro)	Peak:	0.5–3 h
	Novolog (insulin aspart)	Duration:	3–5 h
Short-acting	Novolin R (insulin regular)	Onset:	0.5–1 h
	Humulin R (insulin regular)	Peak:	2–3 h
		Duration:	5–8 h
Intermediate-acting	Novolin N (insulin isophane NPH)	Onset:	0.5–1 h
	Humulin N (insulin isophane NPH)	Peak:	2–3 h
		Duration:	10–16 h
Long-acting	Lantus (insulin glargine)	Onset:	2–8 h
	Levemir (insulin detemir)	Peak:	none
		Duration:	5–24 h
Premixed	Novolog 50/50	Onset:	5–60 min
Combinations	Novolog 70/30	Peak:	dual
	Humalog 75/25	Duration:	10–16 h

This table was adapted from AACE Diabetes Mellitus Guidelines, Endocr Pract. 2007.

Because each person responds differently to insulin, the prescriber will determine which insulin schedule is best for the particular patient.

Insulin Pens

An insulin pen is an insulin delivery system that looks like a pen, uses an insulin cartridge, and has disposable needles. Compared to the traditional syringe and vial, a pen device is easier to use, provides greater dose accuracy, and is more satisfactory to patients.

Some pens are disposed of after one use, whereas others have replaceable insulin cartridges. All pens use needles that minimize the discomfort of injection because they are extremely short and very thin.

The parts of an insulin pen are shown in •**Figure 7.20.** The dose selector knob is used to "dial" the desired dose of insulin. Once the pen has been "primed" (cleared of any air in the cartridge) and the dose set, the insulin is injected by

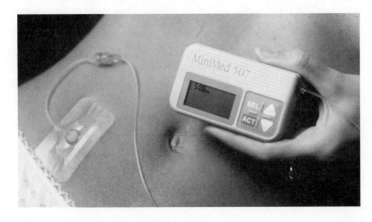

NovoFine needle

Lenvemir FlexPen
Pen cap

Rubber
stopper Cartidge Cartidge
scale
Pointer Dose Push
selector button

Big outer
needle cap
Inner
needle
cap Needle
Protective
tab

• Figure 7.20
Insulin pen.

See Video demo of the FlexPen at http://
www.levemir-us.com/
about-levemir-FlexPen-demo
.asp?WLac=LevemirFlexPen

pressing on the injection button. Because preparing a dose with a pen involves dialing a mechanical device and not looking at the side of a syringe, insulin users with reduced visual acuity can be more assured of accurate dosing. Some pens have a "memory," which records the date, time, and amount of doses administered.

Insulin Pumps

An insulin pump, shown in •**Figure 7.21**, is a beeper-like, external, battery-powered device that delivers rapid-acting insulin continuously for 24 hours a day through a **cannula** (a small hollow tube) inserted under the skin. The pump contains an insulin cartridge that is attached to tubing with a cannula or needle on the end. The needle is inserted under the skin of the abdomen, and it can remain in place for two to three days. The insulin is delivered through this "infusion set." This eliminates the need for multiple daily injections of insulin.

> **ALERT**
>
> Insulin is a *high-alert medication.* Be sure to check your institution's policy regarding administration. For example, some agencies may require insulin doses to be checked by two nurses.

• Figure 7.21
An insulin pump.

The pump can be programmed to deliver a basal rate and/or a bolus dose. **Basal** insulin is delivered continuously over 24 hours to keep blood glucose levels in range between meals and overnight. The basal rate can be programmed to deliver different rates at different times. **Bolus** doses can be delivered at mealtimes to provide control for additional food intake. The insulin pump currently on the market is the closest approximation to an artificial pancreas.

> **EXAMPLE 7.5**
>
> What is the dose of insulin in the single-scale 100-unit insulin syringe shown in •Figure 7.22?

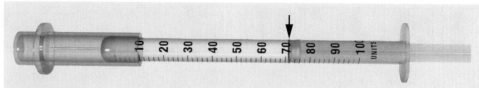

• Figure 7.22
A single-scale 100-unit insulin syringe.

The top ring of the plunger is one line after 70. Because each line represents 2 units, the dose is 72 units of insulin.

EXAMPLE 7.6

What is the dose of insulin in the dual-scale 100 unit insulin syringe shown in •Figure 7.23?

100-Unit Dual-scale Syringe

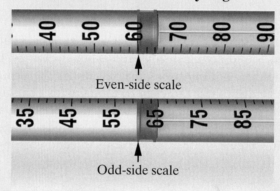

Even-side scale

Odd-side scale

• Figure 7.23
Two views of a dual-scale insulin syringe.

The top ring of the plunger is between calibrations and is slightly more than 2 lines after 55 on the odd side scale. Notice how difficult it would be to determine where 60 units would measure using the odd side scale of the syringe. However, on the even side scale, the plunger falls exactly on the 60. So, the dose is 60 units.

EXAMPLE 7.7

What is the dose of insulin in the 50-unit insulin syringe shown in •Figure 7.24?

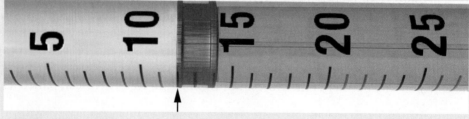

• Figure 7.24
A 50-unit insulin syringe.

The top ring of the plunger is at 12. Because each line represents 1 unit, the dose is 12 units.

EXAMPLE 7.8

What is the dose of insulin in the 30 unit insulin syringe shown in ● Figure 7.25?

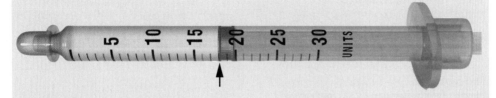

● **Figure 7.25**
A 30-unit Lo-Dose insulin syringe.

The top ring of the plunger is three lines after 15. Because each line represents one unit, the dose is 18 units of insulin.

EXAMPLE 7.9

The physician prescribed 8 units of regular insulin subcutaneously stat. Read the labels in ● Figure 7.26 to determine the correct insulin, and place an arrow at the appropriate level of measurement on the insulin syringe in ● Figure 7.27.

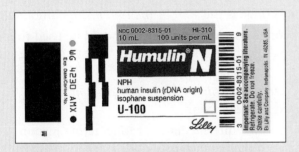

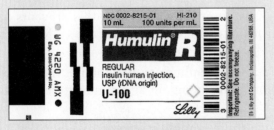

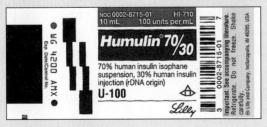

● **Figure 7.26**
Labels for Example 7.9.

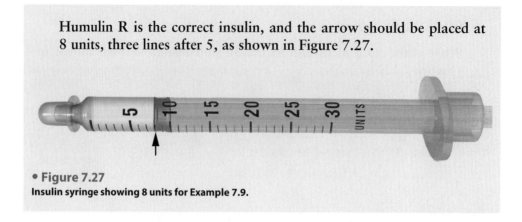

Humulin R is the correct insulin, and the arrow should be placed at 8 units, three lines after 5, as shown in Figure 7.27.

• **Figure 7.27**
Insulin syringe showing 8 units for Example 7.9.

Measuring Two Types of Insulin in One Syringe

Individuals who have insulin-dependent diabetes mellitus (IDDM) often must have two different types of insulin administered at the same time. This combination is usually composed of a *rapid-acting* insulin with either an *intermediate-* or *long-acting* insulin; this can be accomplished by using an appropriate premixed combination drug. However, often the different insulin types are mixed in a single syringe just before administration, and the important points to remember in this process are:

- The *total volume* in the syringe is the *sum of the two insulin* amounts.

- The smallest capacity syringe containing the dose should be used to measure the insulins because the enlarged scale is easier to read and therefore more accurate.

- The *amount of air equal to the amount of insulin to be withdrawn* from each vial must be injected into each vial.

- You must inject the air into the intermediate- or long-acting insulin before you inject the air into the regular insulin.

- The *regular* (rapid-acting) insulin is drawn up *first*; this prevents contamination of the regular insulin with the intermediate- or long-acting insulin.

- The intermediate- or long-acting insulins can precipitate; therefore, they must be mixed well before drawing up and administered without delay.

- Only insulins from the same source should be mixed together, for example, Humulin R and Humulin N are both human insulin and can be mixed.

- If you draw up too much of the intermediate- or long-acting insulin, you must discard the entire medication and start over.

The steps of preparing two types of insulin in one syringe are shown in Example 7.10.

NOTE

When you are mixing two types of insulin, think: "Clear, then Cloudy."

EXAMPLE 7.10

The prescriber ordered 10 units Humulin R insulin and 30 units Humulin N insulin subcutaneously, 30 minutes before breakfast. Explain how you would prepare to administer this in one injection. •Figures 7.28 and •7.29.

The total amount of insulin is 40 units (10 + 30). To administer this dose, use a 50 unit Lo-Dose syringe. Inject 30 units of air into the Humulin N vial and 10 units of air into the Humulin R vial. Withdraw 10 units of the Humulin R (rapid-acting) first and then withdraw 30 units of the Humulin N (intermediate-acting).

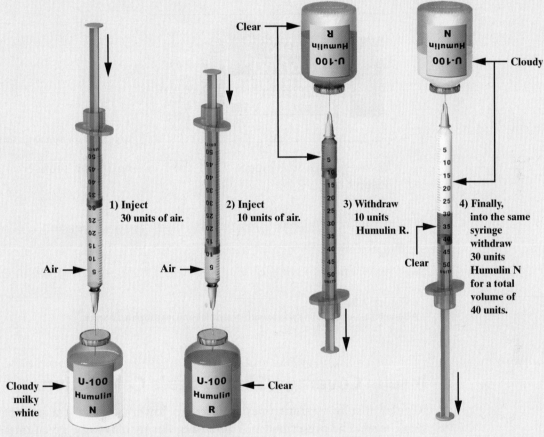

• Figure 7.28
Mixing two types of insulin in one syringe.

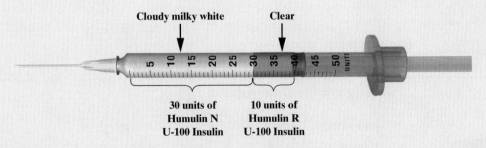

• Figure 7.29
Combination of 30 units Humulin N and 10 units of Humulin R.

Premixed Insulin

Using premixed insulin (see Table 7.1) eliminates errors that may occur when mixing two types of insulin in one syringe (Figure 7.28).

EXAMPLE 7.11

Order: Give 35 units of Humalog Mix 50/50 insulin subcutaneously 30 minutes before breakfast. Use the label shown in • Figure 7.30 and place an arrow at the appropriate calibration on the syringe.

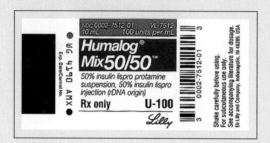

• Figure 7.30
Drug label for Humalog Mix 50/50.

In the syringe in • **Figure 7.31**, the top ring of the plunger is at the 35-unit line.

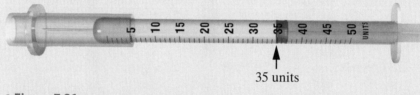

35 units

• Figure 7.31
A 50-unit Lo-Dose insulin syringe with protective cap measuring 35 units.

Insulin Coverage/Sliding Scale Calculations

Regular insulin is sometimes ordered to lower ("cover") a patient's blood sugar level. The prescriber may order regular insulin to be given on a "sliding scale" schedule that is related to the patient's current blood glucose level as measured by a fingerstick.

EXAMPLE 7.12

Order: *fingersticks Q.I.D., ac breakfast, lunch, dinner, and at bedtime. Give regular insulin as follows*:

glucose less than 150 mg/dL	*—no insulin*
glucose of 150–200 mg/dL	*—2 units*
glucose of 201–250 mg/dL	*—3 units*
glucose of 251–300 mg/dL	*—5 units*
glucose of more than 300 mg/dL	*—give 6 units and contact the prescriber stat*

ALERT

More than 15 units of regular insulin for coverage is usually too much. Contact the physician.

Use the "sliding scale" to determine how much insulin you will give the patient if the glucose level before lunchtime is:

(a) 125 mg/dL

(b) 278 mg/dL

(c) 350 mg/dL

(a) You need to compare the patient's level with the information provided in the sliding scale. Because 125 mg/dL is less than 150 mg/dL, you would not administer any insulin.

(b) Because 278 mg/dL is between 251 and 300 mg/dL, you would administer 5 units of regular insulin immediately.

(c) Because 350 mg/dL is more than 300 mg/dL, you would give 6 units of regular insulin and contact the prescriber stat.

Prefilled Syringes

A prefilled, single-dose syringe contains the usual dose of a medication. Some prefilled glass cartridges are available for use with a special plunger called a Tubex or Carpuject syringe (•**Figure 7.32**). If a medication order is for the exact amount of drug in the prefilled syringe, the possibility of measurement error by the person administering the drug is decreased.

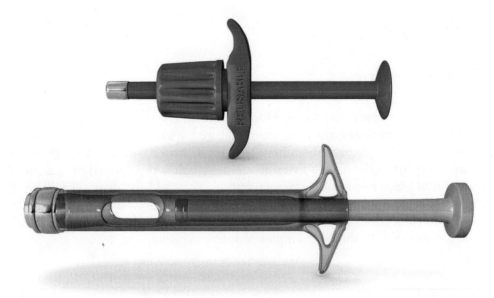

• **Figure 7.32**
Carpuject and Tubex prefilled cartridge holders.

EXAMPLE 7.13

The prefilled syringe cartridge shown in •Figure 7.33 is calibrated so that each line measures 0.1 mL and it has a capacity of 2.5 mL. How many milliliters are indicated by the arrow shown in Figure 7.33?

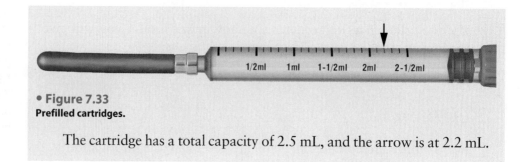

• Figure 7.33
Prefilled cartridges.

The cartridge has a total capacity of 2.5 mL, and the arrow is at 2.2 mL.

EXAMPLE 7.14

How much medication is in the prepackaged cartridge shown in
• Figure 7.34?

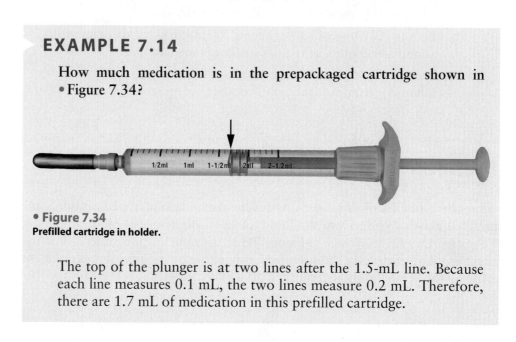

• Figure 7.34
Prefilled cartridge in holder.

The top of the plunger is at two lines after the 1.5-mL line. Because
each line measures 0.1 mL, the two lines measure 0.2 mL. Therefore,
there are 1.7 mL of medication in this prefilled cartridge.

Safety Syringes

NOTE

To view an animation of the
operation of a safety syringe,
go to http://www.bd.com/
hypodermic/products/
integra/

To prevent the transmission of blood-borne infections from contaminated
needles, many syringes are now manufactured with various types of safety
devices. For example, a syringe may contain a protective sheath (a) that can
be used to protect the needle's sterility. This sheath is then pulled forward and
locked into place to provide a permanent needle shield for disposal following
injection. Others may have a needle that automatically retracts (b) into the
barrel after injection. Each of these devices reduces the chance of needle stick
injury. • Figure 7.35 shows examples of safety syringes.

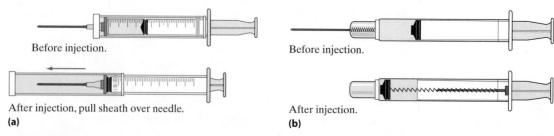

Before injection.

After injection, pull sheath over needle.
(a)

Before injection.

After injection.
(b)

• Figure 7.35
Safety syringes with (a) an active safety device and (b) a passive safety device.

Needleless Syringes

A needleless syringe is a type of safety syringe designed to prevent needle punctures. It may be used to extract medication from a vial (see • **Figure 7.36**), to add medication to intravenous (IV) tubing for medication administration (see • **Figure 7.37**), or to administer medication by mouth (see • **Figure 7.38**).

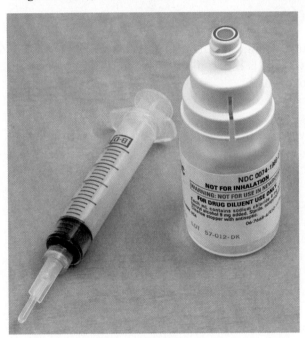

• **Figure 7.36**
A needleless syringe and vial.

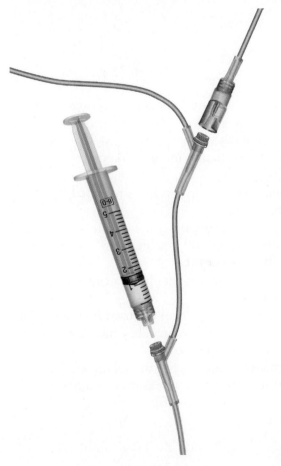

• **Figure 7.37**
A needleless syringe and IV tubing.

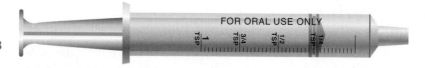

• **Figure 7.38**
Oral syringe.

Dosing Errors with Syringes

Care must be taken when filling a syringe. Being off by even a small amount on the syringe scale can be critical. This is especially true when a syringe contains a relatively small portion of its capacity.

For example, say a 3 mL syringe should correctly be filled to the prescribed 2.8 mL, and by mistake it is filled to 2.9 mL (one extra tick on the scale). This results in about a 4% overdose [Change/Old = 0.1/2.8]. On the other hand, if a 3 mL syringe should correctly be filled to 1 mL, and by mistake it is filled to 1.1 mL (one extra tick), this results in a more serious 10% overdose [Change/Old = 0.1/1].

Rounding your final calculations may lead to concerns. For example, say your computation yields a correct dose of 0.985 mL. If you correctly round off this result, and administer 0.99 mL, you have increased the dose by about 0.5% [Change/original = 0.005/0.985]. On the other hand, if your computation yields 0.045 mL, and you correctly round off this result and administer 0.05 mL, you have increased the dose by about 11% [Change/original = 0.005/0.045]. With pediatric and high-alert drugs, sometimes *rounding down* is used to avoid the possibility of overdose; consult the rounding protocols at your facility.

Summary

In this chapter, the various types of syringes were discussed. You learned how to measure the amount of liquid in various syringes. The types of insulin, how to measure a single dose, and how to mix two insulins in one syringe were explained. Prefilled, single-dose, and safety syringes were also presented.

- Milliliters (mL), rather than cubic centimeters (cc), are the preferred unit of measure for volume.
- All syringe calibrations must be read at the top ring of the plunger.
- Large-capacity hypodermic syringes (5, 12, 20, 35 mL) are calibrated in increments from 0.2 mL to 1 mL.
- Small-capacity hypodermic syringes (2, $2\frac{1}{2}$, 3 mL) are calibrated in tenths of a milliter (0.1 mL).
- The 0.5 mL and 1 mL hypodermic (tuberculin) syringes are calibrated in hundredths of a milliliter. They are the preferred syringes for use in measuring a dose of 1 millimeter or less.

- The calibrations on hypodermic syringes differ; therefore, be very careful when measuring medications in syringes.
- Amounts less than 1 mL are rounded to two decimal places.
- Amounts more than 1 mL are rounded to one decimal place.
- Insulin syringes are designed for measuring and administering U-100 insulin. They are calibrated for 100 units per mL.
- Standard insulin syringes have a capacity of 100 units.
- Lo-Dose insulin syringes are used for measuring small amounts of insulin. They have a capacity of 50 units or 30 units.
- For greater accuracy, use the smallest capacity syringe possible to measure and administer doses. However, avoid filling a syringe to its capacity.

- When measuring two types of insulin in the same syringe, Regular insulin is always drawn up in the syringe first. Think: *first clear, then cloudy.*
- The total volume when mixing insulins is the sum of the two insulin amounts.
- Insulin syringes are for measuring and administering insulin only. Tuberculin syringes are used to measure and administer other medications that are less than 1 mL. Confusion of the two can cause a medication error.
- The prefilled single-dose syringe cartridge is to be used once and then discarded.
- Syringes intended for injections should not be used to measure or administer oral medications.
- Use safety syringes to prevent needle stick injuries.

Case Study 7.1

Read the Case Study and answer the questions. Answers can be found in Appendix A.

A 55-year-old female with a medical history of obesity, hypertension, hyperlipidemia, and diabetes mellitus comes to the emergency department complaining of anorexia, nausea, vomiting, fever, chills, and severe sharp right upper quadrant pain that radiates to her back and right shoulder. She states that her pain is 9 (on a 0–10 pain scale). Vital signs are: T 100.2°F, BP 148/94; P 104; R 24. The diagnostic workup confirms gallstones and she is admitted for a cholecystectomy (removal of gall bladder).

Pre-Op Orders:
- NPO
- V/S q4h
- Demerol (meperidine hydrochloride) 75 mg IM stat
- IV D5/RL @ 125 mL/h

- Insert NG (nasogastric) tube to low suction
- Pre-op meds: Demerol (meperidine hydrochloride) 75 mg and Phenergan (promethazine) 25 mg IM 30 minutes before surgery
- Cefuroxime 1.5 g IV 30 minutes before surgery

Post-Op Orders:
- Discontinue NG tube
- NPO
- V/S q4h
- IV D5/RL @ 125 mL/h
- Compazine (prochlorperazine) 4 mg IM q4h prn nausea
- Demerol (meperidine hydrochloride) 75 mg and Vistaril (hydroxyzine) 25 mg IM q3h prn pain
- Merrem (meropenem) 1g IVPB q8h

1. The label on the meperidine for the stat dose reads 100 mg/mL.
   (a) Draw a line indicating the stat dose on each of the following syringes given.
   (b) Which syringe will most accurately measure this dose?

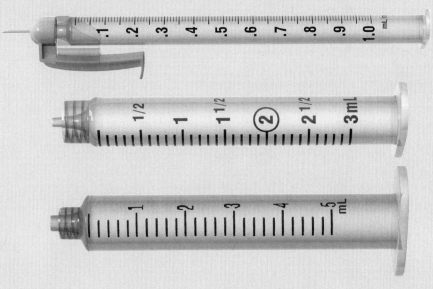

2. Calculate the pre-op dose of the Phenergan and Demerol to be administered 30 minutes before surgery. Phenergan is available in 25 mg/mL vials. Demerol is available in 2.5 mL capacity prefilled syringes, each containing 1 mL of Demerol. The Demerol prefilled syringes have strengths of 10 mg/mL, 25 mg/mL, and 75 mg/mL.
   (a) How many milliliters of Phenergan will you prepare?
   (b) Which prepackaged syringe of Demerol will you use?
   (c) Indicate, on the appropriate syringe given, the dose of each of these drugs that you will administer.

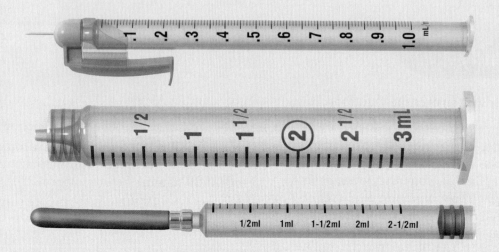

3. The label on the cefuroxime vial states: "add 9 mL of diluent to the 1.5 g vial." Draw a line on the appropriate syringe given indicating the amount of diluent you will add to the vial.

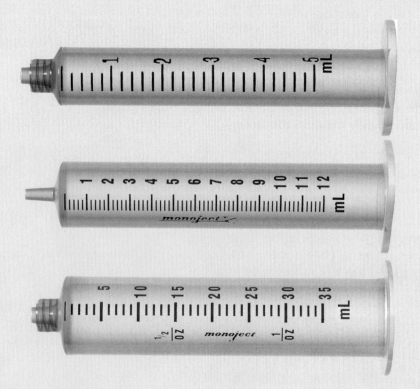

4. The patient is complaining of severe nausea. The Compazine vial is labeled 5 mg/mL. Draw a line on the appropriate syringe given indicating the dose of Compazine.

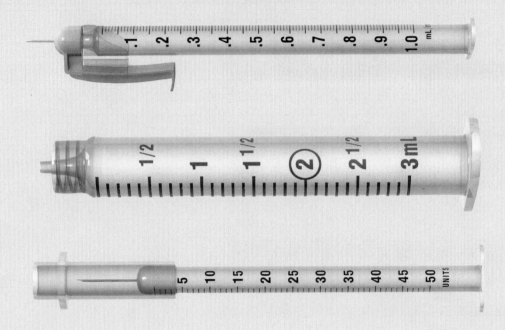

5. The patient is complaining of severe incisional pain of 10 (on a 0–10 pain scale) and has had no pain medication since her surgery. Calculate the dose of the Demerol and Vistaril order. The Vistaril is available in a concentration of 25 mg/mL. The Demerol is available as 100 mg/mL.
   (a) How many milliliters of Vistaril will you use?
   (b) How many milliliters of Demerol do you need?
   (c) How will you prepare these medications so that you can give the patient a single injection?
   (d) Indicate on the appropriate syringe given the number of milliliters you will administer.

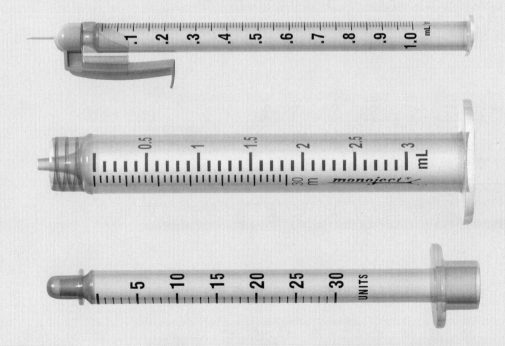

6. The label on the Merrem states 50 mg/mL.
   (a) How many mL will you need?
   (b) Draw a line on the appropriate syringe given indicating the dose of Merrem.

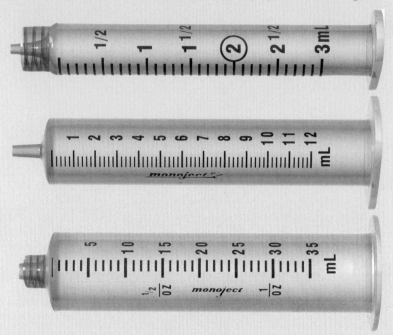

7. The patient has progressed to a regular diet and is ordered Humulin N 13 units and Humulin R 6 units subcutaneous 30 minutes ac breakfast, and Humulin N 5 units and Humulin R 5 units subcutaneous 30 minutes ac dinner.
   (a) How many units will the patient receive before breakfast?
   (b) Indicate on the appropriate syringe given the number of units of each insulin required before breakfast.

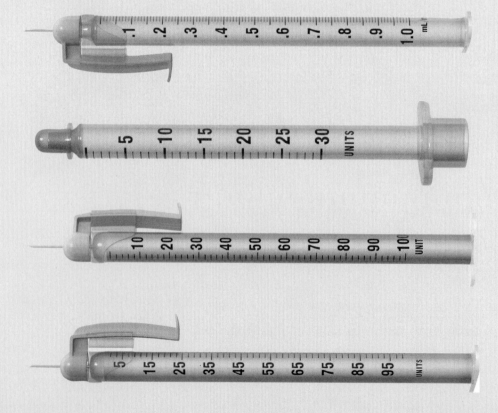

Practice Sets

The answers to *Try These for Practice*, *Exercises*, and *Cumulative Review Exercises* are found in Appendix A. Ask your instructor for the answers to the *Additional Exercises*.

Try These for Practice

Test your comprehension after reading the chapter.

In Problems 1 through 4, identify the type of syringe shown in the figure. Place an arrow at the appropriate level of measurement on the syringe for the volume given.

1. _____ syringe; 0.91 mL

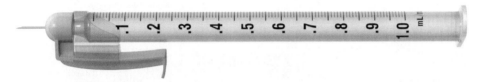

2. _____ syringe; 3.4 mL

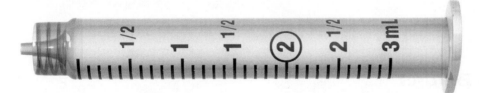

3. _____ syringe; 1.3 mL

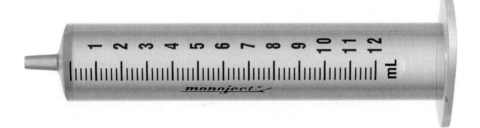

4. _____ syringe; 2.8 mL

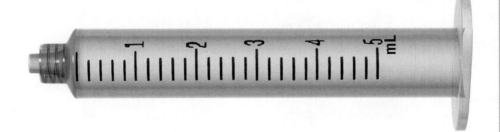

5. Order: *Meperidine 150 mg IM q4h prn severe pain*
   Read the label and calculate the number of milliliters to administer. Draw an arrow to show the dose on the most appropriate of the safety syringes.

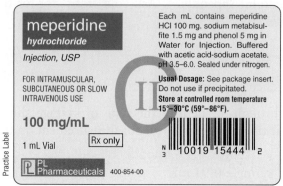

For educational purposes only

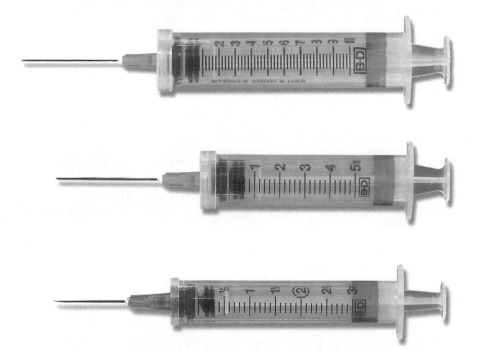

Exercises

Reinforce your understanding in class or at home.

In problems 1 through 14, identify the type of syringe shown in the figure. Then, for each quantity, place an arrow at the appropriate level of measurement on the syringe.

1. _____ syringe; 0.73 mL

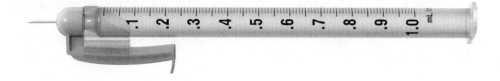

2. _____ syringe; 24 units

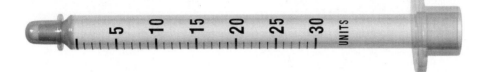

3. _____ syringe; 2.4 mL

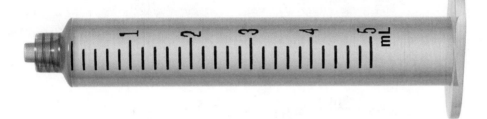

4. _____ syringe; 1.7 mL

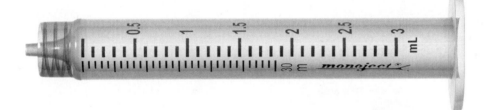

5. _____ syringe; 22 mL

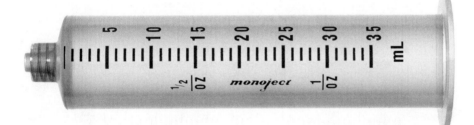

6. _____ syringe; 10.8 mL

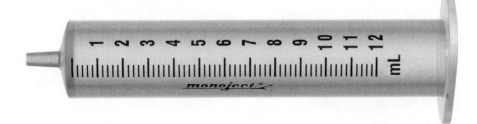

Workspace

Workspace

7. _____ syringe; 34 units

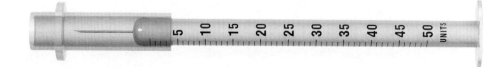

8. _____ syringe; 78 units

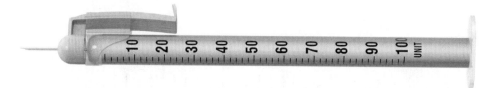

9. _____ syringe; 0.43 mL

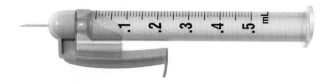

10. _____ syringe; 81 units

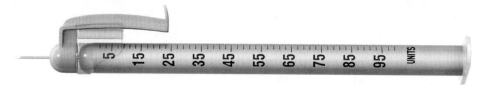

11. _____ syringe; 8.6 mL

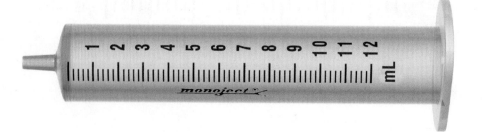

12. _____ syringe; 0.56 mL

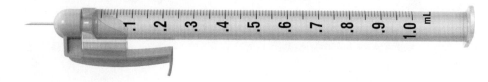

Workspace

13. _____ syringe; 9.2 mL

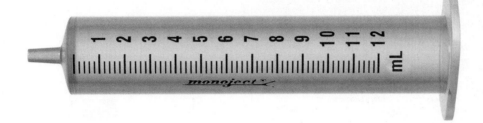

14. _____ syringe; 33 mL

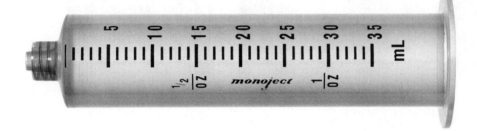

In problems 15 through 20, read the order, use the appropriate label in • **Figure 7.39**, calculate the dosage if necessary, and place an arrow at the appropriate level of measurement on the syringe.

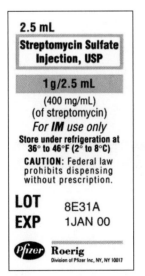

(a)

2.5 mL

Streptomycin Sulfate Injection, USP

1 g/2.5 mL

(400 mg/mL)
(of streptomycin)
*For **IM** use only*
Store under refrigeration at 36° to 46°F (2° to 8°C)
CAUTION: Federal law prohibits dispensing without prescription.

LOT   8E31A
EXP   1JAN 00

Pfizer **Roerig**
Division of Pfizer Inc, NY, NY 10017

(b)

NAFCILLIN SODIUM

(naf-sill'in)
Classifications: BETA-LACTAM ANTI-BIOTIC; PENICILLIN
Therapeutic: ANTISTAPHYLOCOCCAL PENICILLIN

Staphylococcal Infections
Adult: **IV** 500 mg–1 g q4h (max: 12 g/day) **IM** 500 mg q4–6h
Child: **IV** 50–200 mg/kg/day divided q4–6h (max: 12 g/day) **IM** *Weight greater than 40 kg, 500 mg q4–6h; weight less than 40 kg, 25 mg/kg b.i.d.*
Neonate: **IV** 50–100 mg/kg/day divided q6–12h **IM** 25–50 mg/kg b.i.d.

(c)

NALBUPHINE HYDROCHLORIDE

(nal'byoo-feen)
Nubain
Classifications: ANALGESIC; NARCOTIC (OPIATE) AGONIST-ANTAGONIST
Therapeutic: NARCOTIC ANALGESIC

Moderate to Severe Pain
Adult: **IV/IM/Subcutaneous** 10 mg/70 kg q3–6h prn (max: 160 mg/day)

Surgery Anesthesia Supplement
Adult: **IV** 0.3–3 mg/kg, then 0.25–0.5 mg/kg as required

• **Figure 7.39**
Drug labels and drug guide information for Exercises 15–20.

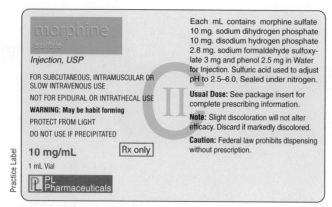

Each mL contains morphine sulfate 10 mg. sodium dihydrogen phosphate 10 mg. disodium hydrogen phosphate 2.8 mg. sodium formaldehyde sulfoxylate 3 mg and phenol 2.5 mg in Water for Injection. Sulfuric acid used to adjust pH to 2.5–6.0. Sealed under nitrogen.

Usual Dose: See package insert for complete prescribing information.

Note: Slight discoloration will not alter efficacy. Discard if markedly discolored.

Caution: Federal law prohibits dispensing without prescription.

morphine sulfate

Injection, USP

FOR SUBCUTANEOUS, INTRAMUSCULAR OR SLOW INTRAVENOUS USE

NOT FOR EPIDURAL OR INTRATHECAL USE

WARNING: May be habit forming

PROTECT FROM LIGHT

DO NOT USE IF PRECIPITATED

10 mg/mL

1 mL Vial

Rx only

PL Pharmaceuticals

Practice Label

(d)   (For educational purposes only)

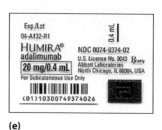

Exp./Lot
04-A132-R1

HUMIRA®
adalimumab
20 mg/0.4 mL
For Subcutaneous Use Only

NDC 0074-9374-02
U.S. License No. 0043   Rx only
Abbott Laboratories
North Chicago, IL 60064, USA

0.4 mL

(01)10300749374026

(e)

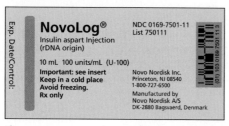

Exp. Date/Control:

NovoLog®
Insulin aspart Injection (rDNA origin)

10 mL 100 units/mL (U-100)

Important: see insert
Keep in a cold place
Avoid freezing.
Rx only

NDC 0169-7501-11
List 750111

Novo Nordisk Inc.
Princeton, NJ 08540
1-800-727-6500
Manufactured by
Novo Nordisk A/S
DK-2880 Bagsvaerd, Denmark

(f)

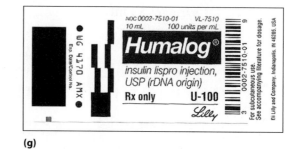

NDC 0002-7510-01   VL-7510
10 mL   100 units per mL

Humalog®

insulin lispro injection, USP (rDNA origin)

Rx only   U-100

Lilly

WG 4170 AMX

Exp. Date/Control No.

For subcutaneous use.
See accompanying literature for dosage.
Eli Lilly and Company, Indianapolis, IN 46285, USA

(g)

● **Figure 7.39**
(Continued)

Workspace

15. Order: *morphine sulfate 15 mg subcut q4h prn pain.*

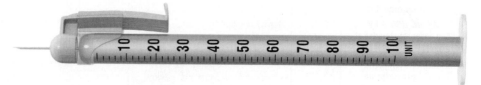

16. The patient weighs 220 pounds. The order is *insulin aspart 0.5 units/kg subcut daily 10 min ac.*

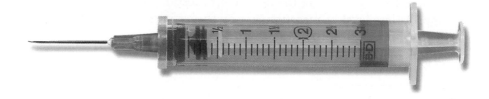

17. Order: *Streptomycin 800 mg IM daily*

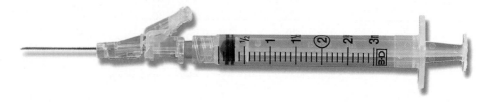

18. Order: *Humira 20 mg subcut stat*

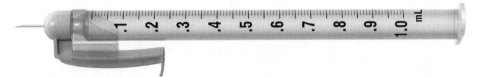

19. Nafcillin sodium is ordered IM for an adult patient. The strength of the nafcillin sodium on hand is 250 mg/mL. Is the amount shown by the arrow on the syringe a safe dose to administer?

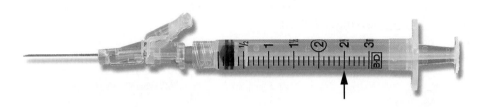

20. Indicate, by placing an arrow on the syringe, the dose of nalbuphine HCl to be administered IM for severe pain. The strength available is 10 mg/mL, and the adult patient weighs 105 kg.

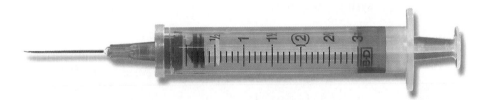

Additional Exercises

Now, test yourself!

In problems 1–15, identify the type of syringe shown in the figure. Then, for each quantity, place an arrow at the appropriate level of measurement on the syringe.

1. _____ syringe; 52 units

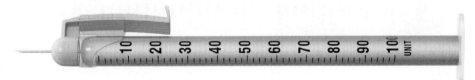

2. _____ syringe; 24 units

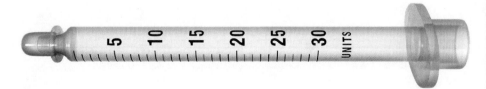

Workspace

3. _____ syringe; 2.6 mL

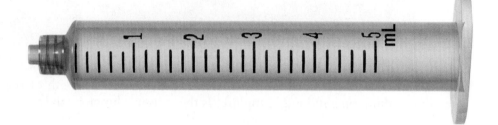

4. _____ syringe; 2.8 mL

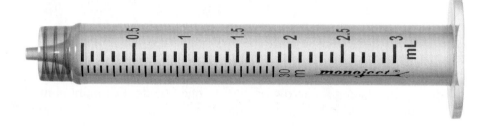

5. _____ syringe; 6.2 mL

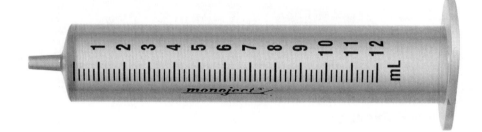

6. _____ syringe; 23 mL

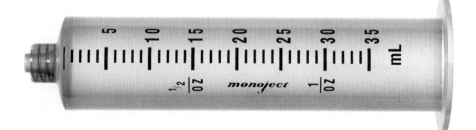

7. _____ syringe; 21 units

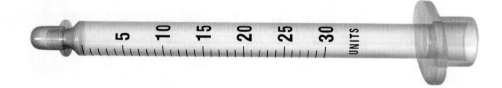

8. _____ syringe; 62 units

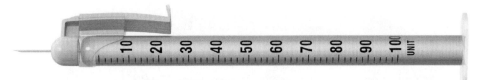

9. _____ syringe; 0.17 mL

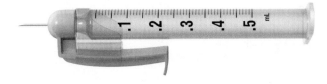

10. _____ syringe; 21 units

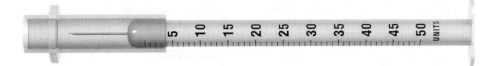

11. _____ syringe; 3.4 mL

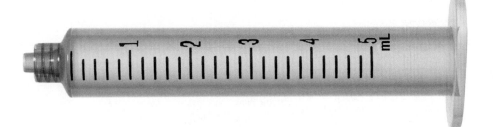

12. _____ syringe; 17 units

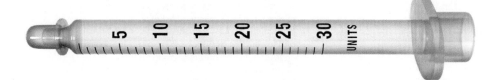

13. _____ syringe; 6.8 mL

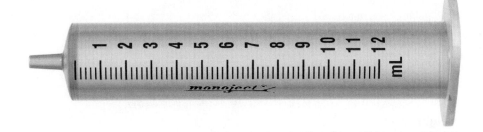

Workspace

14. _____ syringe; 23 mL

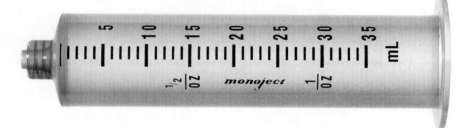

15. _____ syringe; 0.29 mL

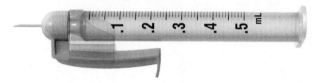

In problems 16 through 20, consult the labels in •**Figure 7.40** to answer the questions, then place arrows at the appropriate level of measurement on the syringes.

(a)

FENTANYL CITRATE

(fen'ta-nil)

Actiq Oralet, Duragesic, Fentora, Ionsys, Onsolis, Sublimaze

Classifications: ANALGESIC; NARCOTIC (OPIATE AGONIST)

Therapeutic: NARCOTIC ANALGESIC

Prototype: Morphine

Pregnancy Category: C (B for fentanyl injection)

Controlled Substance: Schedule II

AVAILABILITY 0.05 mg/mL injection; 100 mcg, 200 mcg, 300 mcg, 400 mcg lozenges; 200 mcg, 400 mcg, 600 mcg, 800 mcg, 1200 mcg, 1600 mcg lozenges on a stick; 12 mcg/h, 25 mcg/h, 50 mcg/h, 75 mcg/h, 100 mcg/h transdermal patch; 100 mcg, 200 mcg, 300 mcg, 400 mcg, 600 mcg, 800 mcg buccal tablet; 0.2 mg, 0.4 mg. 0.6 mg, 0.8 mg, 1.2 mg buccal film

Adjunct for Regional Anesthesia

Adult: **IM/IV** 50–100 mcg

General Anesthesia

Adult: **IV** 2–20 mcg/kg, additional doses of 25–100 mcg as required

Child: **IV** 2–3 mcg/kg as needed

Postoperative Pain

Adult: **IM/IV** 50–100 mcg q1–2h prn

Child: **IM** 1.7–3.3 mcg/kg q1–2h prn

Chronic Pain

Adult: **Transdermal** Individualize and regularly reassess doses of transdermal fentanyl; for patient not already receiving an opioid, the initial dose is 25 mcg/h patch q3days; for patients already on opioids, see package insert for conversions **Stick lozenge (Actiq)** Place in mouth between cheek and lower gum and suck on lozenge; should be consumed over 15-min period

(b)

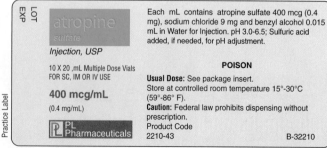

LOT
EXP

atropine
sulfate

Injection, USP

10 X 20 ,mL Multiple Dose Vials
FOR SC, IM OR IV USE

400 mcg/mL

(0.4 mg/mL)

PL Pharmaceuticals

Practice Label

Each mL contains atropine sulfate 400 mcg (0.4 mg), sodium chloride 9 mg and benzyl alcohol 0.015 mL in Water for Injection. pH 3.0-6.5; Sulfuric acid added, if needed, for pH adjustment.

POISON

Usual Dose: See package insert.
Store at controlled room temperature 15°-30°C (59°-86° F).
Caution: Federal law prohibits dispensing without prescription.
Product Code
2210-43   B-32210

For educational purposes only

•**Figure 7.40**
Drug labels for Additional Exercises 16–20.

Workspace

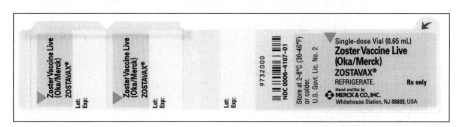

(c)

HYDROMORPHONE HYDROCHLORIDE

(hye-droe-mor'fone)

Dilaudid, Dilaudid-HP

Classifications: NARCOTIC (OPIATE) AGONIST; ANALGESIC
Therapeutic: NARCOTIC ANALGESIC; ANTITUSSIVE
Prototype: Morphine
Pregnancy Category: C; D in prolonged use or high doses at term
Controlled Substance: Schedule II

AVAILABILITY 2 mg, 4 mg, 8 mg tablets; 5 mg/5 mL oral liquid; 1 mg/mL, 10 mg/mL injection

ACTION & *THERAPEUTIC EFFECT*

Has more rapid onset and shorter duration of action than morphine, and is reported to have less hypnotic effect. *An effective narcotic analgesic that controls mild to moderate pain. Also has antitussive properties.*

ROUTE & DOSAGE

Moderate to Severe Pain
Adult: **PO** 2–4 mg q4–6h prn in naïve patients **Subcutaneous/IM/IV** 0.75–2 mg q4–6h depending on patient response
Child: **PO** 0.03–0.08 mg/kg q4–6h (max: 5 mg/dose) **IV** 0.015 mg/kg q4–6h prn

(d)

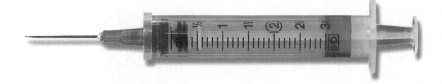

(e)

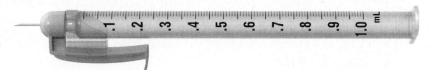

(f)

• **Figure 7.40**
(Continued)

16. Order: atropine sulfate 0.5 mg IM 30–60 min before surgery

17. Order: a single dose of Zoster Vaccine

Workspace

18. You withdraw one-half of the solution from the Varicella Virus Vaccine vial. Indicate by placing an arrow on the syringe the number of milliliters of vaccine in the syringe.

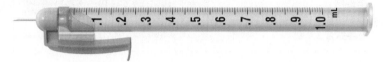

19. Fentanyl citrate has been ordered for an adult with postoperative pain. The strength of the drug is 0.05 mg/mL. Is the dose indicated by the arrow on the syringe in the safe dose range?

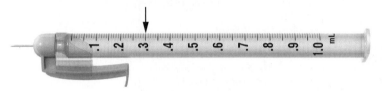

20. An adult has an order for Dilaudid for moderate pain to be administered subcutaneously. The strength of the Dilaudid is 10 mg/mL. Indicate with two arrows the safe dose range in milliliters on the syringe.

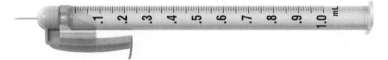

Cumulative Review Exercises

Review your mastery of previous chapters.

1. Prescriber's order: *Administer Humulin R (regular insulin [rDNA origin]) subcutaneously as per the following blood glucose results:*

For glucose less than 160 mg/dL	*— no insulin*
glucose 160 mg/dL–220 mg/dL	*— give 2 units*
glucose 221 mg/dL–280 mg/dL	*— give 4 units*
glucose 281 mg/dL–340 mg/dL	*— give 6 units*
glucose 341 mg/dL–400 mg/dL	*— give 8 units*
glucose greater than 400 mg/dL	*— notify MD stat*

   How many units will you administer if the patient's glucose level at lunchtime is
   (a) *152 mg/dL*
   (b) *174 mg/dL*
   (c) *343 mg/dL*

2. If 20 *mg* of a drug is ordered b.i.d., how many *mg* will the patient receive per day?

3. If 20 *mg* of a drug is ordered daily in two divided doses, how many *mg* will the patient receive per day?

Workspace

4. Order: *Celebrex 100 mg po q12h.* How many *grams* of this anti-inflamatory drug will the patient receive in one week?

5. Change *0.5 mL per minute* to an equivalent rate in *ounces per hour.*

6. *0.56 mg = ? mcg*

7. Find the height to the nearest *centimeter* of a patient who is 4 *feet* 11 *inches* tall.

8. Find the weight, to the nearest tenth of a *kilogram*, of a patient who weighs 155 *pounds.*

9. A certain drug is available in two concentrations: *25 mg/5 mL* and *250 mcg/mL.* Which concentration is the stronger?

10. Order: *potassium chloride 30 mEq po daily.* The strength of the potassium chloride is 10 *mEq/tab.* How many tablets will you administer?

11. Order: *Cytovene (ganciclovir) 5 mg/kg IV q12h for 14 d.* The patient weighs 110 *pounds.* How many *grams* of this antiviral drug will the patient receive over the 14-day period?

12. Using the formula, find the BSA of a patient who is *5 feet* tall and weighs 140 *pounds.*

13. Order: *Natulan (procarbazine HCl) 50 mg/m^2/d po.* How many *mg* of this antineoplastic drug would be administered daily to a patient whose BSA is 1.5 *m^2*?

14. What is the most appropriate syringe that would be used to administer 67 *units* of insulin subcut?

15. Your initial calculations indicate that you need to administer 0.66666 *mL* of a drug IM to a geriatric patient. To what volume would you round off, and what size syringe would you use?

Chapter

8 Solutions

Learning Outcomes

After completing this chapter, you will be able to

1. Describe the strength of a solution as a ratio, as a fraction, and as a percent.
2. Determine the amount of solute in a given amount of solution.
3. Determine the amount of solution that would contain a given amount of solute.
4. Do the calculations necessary to prepare solutions from pure drugs.
5. Do the calculations necessary to prepare solutions for irrigations, soaks, and nutritional feedings.

lidocaine hydrochloride
Topical Solution USP
4%

In this chapter you will learn about solutions. Although solutions are generally prepared by the pharmacist, healthcare providers should understand the concepts involved, and be able to prepare solutions.

Drugs are manufactured in both pure and diluted forms. A pure drug contains only the drug and nothing else. A pure drug can be diluted by dissolving a quantity of pure drug in a liquid to form a *solution*. The pure drug (either dry or liquid) is called the *solute*. The liquid added to the pure drug to form the solution is called the *solvent* or *diluent*.

Determining the Strength of a Solution

To make a cup of coffee, you might dissolve 2 teaspoons of instant coffee granules in a cup of hot water. The instant coffee granules (*solute*) are added to the hot water (*solvent*) to form the cup of coffee (*solution*). If instead of 2 teaspoons of instant coffee granules, you add either 1 or 3 teaspoons of instant coffee granules to the cup of hot water, the coffee solution will taste quite different. The **strength or concentration** of the coffee could be described in terms of *teaspoons per cup* (*t/cup*). Thus, a coffee solution with a strength of *1 t/cup* is a *"weaker"* solution than a coffee solution with a strength of *2 t/cup*, and a strength of *3 t/cup* is *"stronger" than a strength of 2 t/cup.*

Important terms for the elements of a solution:

- The **solute** is the solid or liquid to be dissolved or diluted. Some solutes are: various powdered drugs, chemical salts, and liquid nutritional supplements.

- The **solvent** (**diluent**) is the liquid that dissolves the solid solute or dilutes the liquid solute. Two commonly used solvents are sterile water and normal saline.

- The **solution** is the liquid resulting from the combination of the solute and solvent.

The strength of a drug is stated on the label. Liquid drugs are solutions. The strength of these solutions compares the *amount of drug* (*solute*) in the solution to the *volume of solution*. Some examples of drug strengths or concentrations are: *Lanoxin 500 mcg/2 mL, KCl 2 mEq/mL, Garamycin 80 mg/2 mL,* and *heparin 10,000 units/mL.*

Suppose a vial is labeled *furosemide 5 mg/mL.* This means that there are 5 milligrams of furosemide in each milliliter of the solution. If a second vial is labeled *furosemide 10 mg/mL,* then this second solution is "stronger" than the first because there are 10 mg of furosemide in each milliliter of the solution. If an order is *furosemide 10 mg po stat,* then to receive 10 mg of the drug, the patient would receive either 2 mL of the "weaker" first solution, or 1 mL of the "stronger" second solution.

Strengths of Solutions as Ratios, Fractions, and Percents

Sometimes the strength of a solution is specified *without using explicit units of measurement like milligrams or milliliters* but by comparing the number of parts of *solute* to the number of parts of *solution.* This method of stating strength is generally expressed by using either *ratios, fractions,* or *percents.* Some examples of these strengths are *epinephrine 1:1,000 (ratio), Enfamil $\frac{1}{2}$ strength (fraction),* and *0.9% NaCl (percent).*

$$\text{STRENGTH} = \frac{\text{SOLUTE}}{\text{SOLUTION}}$$

If a solution contains *1 part solute* in *2 parts of solution*, the strength could be expressed in the form of the *ratio 1:2* (read "1 to 2"), the *fraction $\frac{1}{2}$ strength* or, (because $\frac{1}{2} = 50\%$) the *percentage 50%.* See ● **Figure 8.1.**

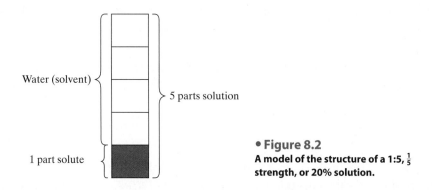

• Figure 8.1
A model of the structure of a 1:2, $\frac{1}{2}$ strength, or 50% Enfamil solution.

The ratio *1:5* means that there is 1 part *solute* in 5 parts *solution*. This solution is also referred to as a $\frac{1}{5}$ strength solution or as a *20%* solution. See **• Figure 8.2**.

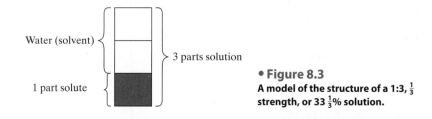

• Figure 8.2
A model of the structure of a 1:5, $\frac{1}{5}$ strength, or 20% solution.

A $\frac{1}{3}$ strength solution can be expressed as a *1:3* solution. This has 1 part *solute* for 3 parts *solution*. Because $\frac{1}{3} = 33\frac{1}{3}\%$, this is a $33\frac{1}{3}\%$ solution. See **• Figure 8.3**.

• Figure 8.3
A model of the structure of a 1:3, $\frac{1}{3}$ strength, or $33\frac{1}{3}\%$ solution.

A *60%* solution can be referred to (in fractional form) as a 60/100 solution, and after reducing this fraction becomes $\frac{3}{5}$. In ratio form this strength would be *3:5*. This solution has 3 parts *solute* for 5 parts *solution*. See **• Figure 8.4**.

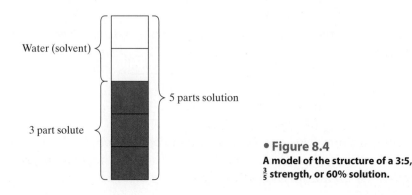

• Figure 8.4
A model of the structure of a 3:5, $\frac{3}{5}$ strength, or 60% solution.

EXAMPLE 8.1

Fill in the missing items in each line by following the pattern of the first line.

The solution contains:	The strength of the solution is		
	ratio	fraction	percent
1 part solute in 2 parts solution	1:2	$\frac{1}{2}$	50%
	1:4		
		$\frac{1}{5}$	
			3%
			5%
		$\frac{2}{5}$	
1 part solute in 1,000 parts solution			

Here are the answers.

The solution contains:	The strength of the solution is		
	ratio	fraction	percent
1 part solute in 2 parts solution	1:2	$\frac{1}{2}$	50%
1 part solute in 4 parts solution	1:4	$\frac{1}{4}$	25%
1 part solute in 5 parts solution	1:5	$\frac{1}{5}$	20%
3 parts solute in 100 parts solution	3:100	$\frac{3}{100}$	3%
1 part solute in 20 parts solution	1:20	$\frac{1}{20}$	5%
2 parts solute in 5 parts solution	2:5	$\frac{2}{5}$	40%
1 part solute in 1,000 parts solution	1:1,000	$\frac{1}{1,000}$	0.1%

Liquid Solutes

For a solute that is in liquid form, the ratio *1:40* means there is 1 milliliter of solute in every 40 milliliters of solution. So 40 milliliters of a *1:40* acetic acid solution means that 1 milliliter of pure acetic acid is diluted with water to make a total of 40 milliliters of solution. You would prepare this solution by placing 1 milliliter of pure acetic acid in a graduated cylinder and adding water until the level in the graduated cylinder reaches 40 milliliters. • Figure 8.5.

A 1% solution means that there is 1 part of the solute in 100 parts of solution. So you would prepare 100 mL of a 1% creosol solution by placing

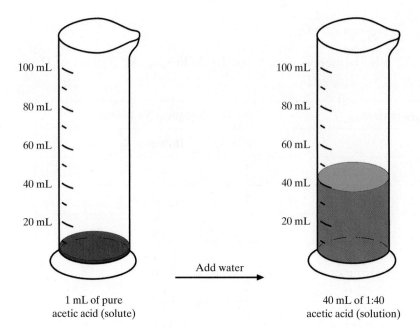

• **Figure 8.5**
Preparing a 1:40 solution from a liquid solute.

1 mL of pure
acetic acid (solute)

Add water

40 mL of 1:40
acetic acid (solution)

1 milliliter of pure creosol in a graduated cylinder and adding water until the level in the graduated cylinder reaches 100 mL. • **Figure 8.6**.

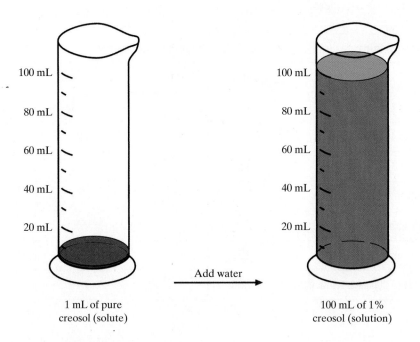

• **Figure 8.6**
Preparing a 1% solution from a liquid solute.

1 mL of pure
creosol (solute)

Add water

100 mL of 1%
creosol (solution)

EXAMPLE 8.2

Suppose 40 mL of an iodine solution contains 10 mL of (solute) pure iodine. Express the strength of this solution as a ratio, a fraction, and a percentage.

The strength of a solution may be expressed as the ratio of the *amount of pure drug in the solution to the total amount of the solution.* The amount of the solution is always expressed in milliliters, and because iodine is a liquid in pure form, the amount of iodine is also expressed in milliliters.

There are 10 mL of pure iodine in the 40 mL of the solution, so the strength of this solution, expressed as a ratio, is ten to forty. The ratio may also be written as *10:40, 10 to 40,* or in fractional form as $\frac{10}{40}$. This fraction could then be simplified to $\frac{1}{4}$, which is equal to 25%.

So, the strength of this iodine solution may be expressed as the ratio *1:4*, the fraction $\frac{1}{4}$ strength, and as the percentage 25%.

Dry Solutes

The ratio *1:20* means 1 part of the solute in 20 parts of solution, or 2 parts of the solute in 40 parts of solution, or 3 parts in 60, or 4 parts in 80, or 5 parts in 100, and so on. When a pure drug is in *dry* form, the ratio *1:20* means 1 g of pure drug in every 20 mL of solution. So 100 mL of a *1:20* potassium permanganate solution means 5 g of pure potassium permanganate dissolved in water to make a total of 100 mL of the solution. A *1:20* solution is the same as a 5% solution. If each tablet is 5 g, then you would prepare this solution by placing 1 tablet of the pure potassium permanganate in a graduated cylinder and adding some water to dissolve the tablet; then add more water until the level in the graduated cylinder reaches 100 mL.

Because a 5% potassium permanganate solution means 5 g of pure potassium permanganate in 100 mL of solution, the strength is also written as $\frac{5\,g}{100\,mL}$ or $\frac{1\,g}{20\,mL}$. • **Figure 8.7.**

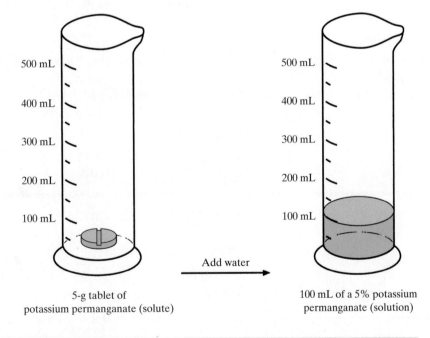

Add water

5-g tablet of potassium permanganate (solute)

100 mL of a 5% potassium permanganate (solution)

• **Figure 8.7**
Preparing a 5% solution from a pure, dry drug.

EXAMPLE 8.3

One liter of an isotonic normal saline solution contains 9,000 mg of sodium chloride. Express the strength of this solution both as a ratio and as a percentage.

The strength of a solution may be expressed as the ratio of the *amount of solute* in the solution to the *total amount of the solution.* Because sodium chloride (NaCl) is a *solid* in pure form, the amount of NaCl (9,000 mg) must be expressed in *grams* (9 g). The *amount of the solution* (1 L) must always be expressed in *milliliters* (1,000 mL).

Because there are 9 g of pure NaCl in 1,000 mL of the solution, the strength of this solution, expressed as a ratio, is *nine to one thousand*.

This ratio may also be written as *9 to 1,000*, *9:1,000*, or in fractional form as $\frac{9}{1,000}$. This fraction could be written in decimal form as 0.009, which is equal to 0.9%.

So, the strength of this isotonic normal saline solution may be expressed as the ratio *9:1,000* or as the percentage *0.9%*.

EXAMPLE 8.4

Read the label in • Figure 8.8 and verify that the two strengths stated on the label are equivalent.

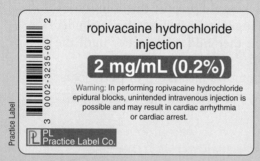

• **Figure 8.8**
Practice Label for ropivacaine HCl.
(For educational purposes only)

The two strengths stated on this label are *2 mg/mL and 0.2%*. To show that they are equivalent, take either one of these strengths and show how to change it to the other. For example, if you start with 0.2%, you must change this to 2 mg/mL.

A solution whose strength is 0.2% has 0.2 g of solute (ropivacaine HCl) in 100 mL of solution. As a fraction, this is $\frac{0.2\,g}{100\,mL}$.

You need to change this fraction to mg/mL. That is,

$$\frac{0.2\ g}{100\ mL} = \frac{?\ mg}{mL}$$

DIMENSIONAL ANALYSIS

To change the grams in the numerator to milligrams, use the equivalence 1 g = 1,000 mg

$$\frac{0.2\ \cancel{g}}{1\,0\,0\ mL} \times \frac{1,0\,0\,0\ mg}{1\ \cancel{g}} = \frac{2\ mg}{mL}$$

MOVING THE DECIMAL POINT

Another way to change $\frac{0.2\ g}{100\ mL}$ to $\frac{?\ mg}{mL}$ is to convert 0.2 g to *mg* by moving the decimal point three places to the right as follows:

$$0.2\ g = 0.200\ g = 0\,2\,0\,0.\ mg = 200\ mg$$

Therefore,

$$\frac{0.2\ g}{100\ mL} = \frac{200\ mg}{100\ mL} = \frac{200\ mg}{100\ mL} = \frac{2\ mg}{1\ mL}$$

So, the two strengths (0.2% and 2 *mg/mL*) on the label are equivalent.

Determining the Amount of Solute in a Given Amount of Solution

Either Dimensional Analysis or Ratio & Proportion can be used to determine the amount of solute in a given amount of a solution of known strength.

The units of measurement for the amount of solution (volume), strength of the solution, and amount of solute are listed as follows:

Amount of solution: Use *milliliters*.

Strength: Always write as a fraction for calculations.

For liquid solutes:

1:40 acetic acid solution is written as $\frac{1\,mL}{40\,mL}$

5% acetic acid solution is written as $\frac{5\,mL}{100\,mL}$

For dry or powder solutes:

1:20 potassium permanganate solution is written as $\frac{1\,g}{20\,mL}$

12% potassium permanganate solution is written as $\frac{12\,g}{100\,mL}$

Amount of solute: Use *milliliters* for liquids.

Use *grams* for tablets or powders.

To prepare a given amount of a solution of a given strength, you must first determine the amount of solute that will be in that solution. The following examples illustrate how this is done.

EXAMPLE 8.5

How would you prepare 500 mL of a 0.45% sodium chloride solution using 2.25 g sodium chloride tablets?

The 0.45% strength means that there is 0.45 g of sodium chloride in every 100 mL of this solution. You need to determine the number of grams of sodium chloride contained in 500 mL of this solution.

DIMENSIONAL ANALYSIS

Given: Amount of solution: 500 mL
        Strength: 0.45%
Find: Amount of pure drug: ? g

Convert the amount of solution (500 mL) to the amount of solute

$$500\ mL = ?\ g$$

Write the strength of the solution, 0.45%, as the unit fraction $\frac{0.45\ g}{100\ mL}$

$$500\ \cancel{mL} \times \frac{0.45\ g}{100\ \cancel{mL}} = 2.25\ g$$

RATIO & PROPORTION

Determine the number of grams of sodium chloride that are in 500 mL of this strength solution *(? g = 500 mL)*.

Think of the problem as:

$$0.45\,g = 100\,mL$$

$$x\,g = 500\,mL$$

Because the number of grams of solute is proportional to the number of milliliters of solution, a proportion could be used to solve the problem. The proportion could be set up as

$$\frac{g}{mL} = \frac{g'}{mL'}$$

Substituting, you get

$$\frac{0.45\,g}{100\,mL} = \frac{x\,g}{500\,mL}$$

Eliminate the units of measurement and cross multiply

$$\frac{0.45}{100} = \frac{x}{500}$$

$$(x)(100) = (0.45)(500)$$
$$100x = 225$$
$$x = 2.25$$

Because 500 mL of the solution must contain 2.25 g of sodium chloride, and each tablet contains 2.25 g, you would need 1 tablet.

So, you would place 1 tablet into a graduated cylinder, add some water to dissolve the tablet, and then add water until the 500 mL level is reached.

EXAMPLE 8.6

Read the label in • Figure 8.9. How many grams of dextrose are contained in 30 mL of this solution?

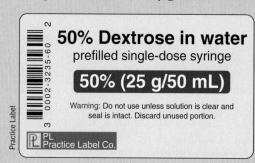

3 0002-3235-60 2

50% Dextrose in water
prefilled single-dose syringe

50% (25 g/50 mL)

Warning: Do not use unless solution is clear and seal is intact. Discard unused portion.

PL
Practice Label Co.

Practice Label

• **Figure 8.9**
Practice label for 50% Dextrose.
(For educational purposes only)

DIMENSIONAL ANALYSIS

Given: Amount of solution: 30 mL

Strength: 50% or $\dfrac{50\,g}{100\,mL}$

Find: Amount of solute: ? g

$$30\,mL = ?\,g$$

$$30\,mL \times \frac{50\,g}{100\,mL} = ?\,g$$

$$30\,mL \times \frac{50\,g}{100\,mL} = 15\,g$$

RATIO & PROPORTION

The 50% strength means that there are 50 g of dextrose in every 100 mL of this solution *(50g = 100mL)*. You need to determine the number of grams of dextrose that are in 30 mL of this strength solution *(?g = 30mL)*.

Think of the problem as:

$$50g = 100\,mL$$
$$xg = 30\,mL$$

The proportion could be set up as

$$\frac{g}{mL} = \frac{g'}{mL'}$$

Substituting, you get

$$\frac{50\,g}{100\,mL} = \frac{x\,g}{30\,mL}$$

Eliminate the units of measurement and cross multiply

$$\frac{50}{100} = \frac{x}{30}$$

$$100x = 1{,}500$$
$$x = 15$$

So, 15 g of dextrose are contained in 30 mL of a 50% dextrose solution.

EXAMPLE 8.7

How would you prepare 2,000 mL of a *1:10* Clorox solution?

DIMENSIONAL ANALYSIS

Given: Amount of solution: 2,000 mL

Strength: 1:10 or $\frac{1}{10}$

Find: Amount of solute: ? mL

Because Clorox is a liquid in its pure form, it is measured in milliliters. So, a *1:10* strength means that 1 mL of Clorox is in each 10 mL of the solution.

You want to convert the amount of the solution (2,000 mL) to the amount of the pure Clorox.

$$2{,}000 \text{ mL} = ? \text{ mL}$$

The preceding expression contains mL on both sides. This can be confusing! To make it clearer, note that on the left side "mL" refers to the volume of the solution, whereas on the right side "mL" refers to the volume of the full-strength Clorox.

So, you have the following:

2,000 mL (solution) = ? mL (Clorox)

The strength of the solution, *1:10*, gives the unit fraction

$$\frac{1 \text{ mL (Clorox)}}{10 \text{ mL (solution)}}$$

$$2{,}00\,\cancel{0 \text{ mL (solution)}} \times \frac{1 \text{ mL (Clorox)}}{1\,\cancel{0 \text{ mL (solution)}}}$$

$$= 200 \text{ mL (Clorox)}$$

RATIO & PROPORTION

Because Clorox is a liquid in its pure form, it is measured in milliliters. So, *1:10* strength means 1 mL of Clorox in each 10 mL of the solution *(1 mL of Clorox = 10 mL of solution)*. You need to determine the number of mL of Clorox that are in 2,000 mL of this solution *(? mL of Clorox = 2,000 mL of solution)*.

Think of the problem as:

1 mL (Clorox) = 10 mL (solution)

x mL (Clorox) = 2,000 mL (solution)

Because the number of milliliters of solute is proportional to the number of milliliters of solution, a proportion could be used to solve the problem. The proportion could be set up as

$$\frac{mL(Clorox)}{mL(solution)} = \frac{mL(Clorox)'}{mL(solution)'}$$

Substituting, you get

$$\frac{1\,mL(Clorox)}{10\,mL(solution)} = \frac{x\,mL(Clorox)}{2{,}000\,mL(solution)}$$

Eliminate the units of measurement and cross multiply

$$\frac{1}{10} = \frac{x}{2{,}000}$$

$$10x = 2{,}000$$
$$x = 200$$

So, you need 200 mL of Clorox to prepare 2,000 mL of a *1:10* solution. This means that 200 mL of Clorox is diluted with water to 2,000 mL of solution.

EXAMPLE 8.8

How would you prepare 250 mL of a $\frac{1}{2}$% Lysol solution?

DIMENSIONAL ANALYSIS

Given: Amount of solution: 250 mL

Strength: $\frac{1}{2}$%

Find: Amount of pure Lysol: ? mL

Because Lysol is a liquid in undiluted form, the amount of Lysol to be found is measured in milliliters.

$\frac{1}{2}$% can be written as 0.5% or as

$$\frac{0.5 \text{ mL (Lysol)}}{100 \text{ mL (solution)}}$$

Convert the amount of the solution (250 mL) to the amount of Lysol.

$$250 \text{ mL (solution)} = ? \text{ mL (Lysol)}$$

Use the strength of the solution
$\frac{0.5 \text{ mL (Lysol)}}{100 \text{ mL (solution)}}$ as the unit fraction.

$$250 \, \overline{\text{mL (solution)}} \times \frac{0.5 \text{ mL (Lysol)}}{100 \, \overline{\text{mL (solution)}}}$$

$$= 1.25 \text{ mL (Lysol)}$$

RATIO & PROPORTION

Because Lysol is a liquid in its pure form, it is measured in milliliters. So, $\frac{1}{2}$% (0.5%) strength means 0.5 mL of Lysol is contained in each 100 mL of the solution *(0.5 mL of Lysol = 100 mL of solution)*. You need to determine the number of mL of Lysol that are contained in 250 mL of this solution *(? mL of Lysol = 250 mL of solution)*.

Think of the problem as:

$$0.5 \text{ mL (Lysol)} = 100 \text{ mL (solution)}$$
$$x \text{ mL (Lysol)} = 250 \text{ mL (solution)}$$

The proportion could be set up as

$$\frac{mL(\text{Lysol})}{mL(\text{solution})} = \frac{mL(\text{Lysol})'}{mL(\text{solution})'}$$

Substituting, you get

$$\frac{0.5 \, mL(\text{Lysol})}{100 \, mL(\text{solution})} = \frac{x \, mL(\text{Lysol})}{250 \, mL(\text{solution})}$$

Eliminate the units of measurement and cross multiply

$$\frac{0.5}{100} \diagdown \frac{x}{250}$$

$$100x = 125$$
$$x = 1.25$$

So, you need 1.25 mL of Lysol to prepare 250 mL of a $\frac{1}{2}$% Lysol solution. This means that 1.25 mL of Lysol is diluted with water to 250 mL of solution.

EXAMPLE 8.9

Read the label in • Figure 8.10 and determine the number of milligrams of lidocaine that are contained in 5 mL of this lidocaine solution.

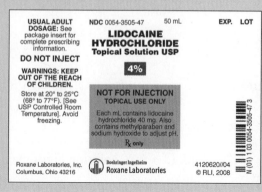

• **Figure 8.10**
Drug label for lidocaine.

DIMENSIONAL ANALYSIS

Given: Amount of solution: 5 mL

Strength: 4%

Find: Amount of solute: ? mg

You want to convert the amount of the solution (5 mL) to the amount of the solute (? mg).

$$5 \text{ mL} = ? \text{ mg}$$

Note that lidocaine is a powder in pure form, so the strength of the 4% solution is expressed in fraction form as $\dfrac{4 \text{ g}}{100 \text{ mL}}$.

This strength can be used to find the amount of lidocaine in grams.

$$5 \text{ mL} \times \frac{4 \text{ g}}{100 \text{ mL}} = ? \text{ mg}$$

But you want the answer in milligrams, so the equivalence 1 g = 1,000 mg must also be used. This can be written in one line as follows:

$$5 \text{ mL} \times \frac{4 \text{ g}}{100 \text{ mL}} \times \frac{1{,}000 \text{ mg}}{\text{g}} = 200 \text{ mg}$$

RATIO & PROPORTION

Because lidocaine is a solid in its pure form, it is measured in grams. So, 4% strength means 4 g of lidocaine in each 100 mL of the solution ($4\,g\,of\,lidocaine = 100\,mL\,of\,solution$). You need to determine the number of mg of lidocaine that are in 5 mL of this solution ($?\,mg\,of\,lidocaine = 5\,mL\,of\,solution$).

This problem expresses quantities of lidocaine in two different units of measure: grams *(4 g)* and milligrams *(? mg)*. To set up a proportion, you need to use a single unit of measurement for the lidocaine. To do this, change 4 g to 4,000 mg (by moving the decimal point three places). Now you can think of the problem as:

$$4{,}000 \text{ mg (lidocaine)} = 100 \text{ mL (solution)}$$
$$x \text{ mg (lidocaine)} = 5 \text{ mL (solution)}$$

The proportion could be set up as

$$\frac{mg}{mL} = \frac{mg'}{mL'}$$

Substituting, you get

$$\frac{4{,}000 \, mg}{100 \, mL} = \frac{x \, mg}{5 \, mL}$$

Eliminate the units of measurement and cross multiply

$$\frac{4{,}000}{100} = \frac{x}{5}$$

$$100x = 20{,}000$$
$$x = 200$$

So, 200 milligrams of lidocaine are contained in 5 milliliters of a 4% Lidocaine solution.

Determining the Amount of Solution That Contains a Given Amount of Solute

In the previous examples, you were given a volume of solution of known strength and had to find the amount of solute in that solution. Now, the process will be reversed. In the following examples, you will be given an amount of the solute in a solution of known strength and have to find the volume of that solution.

EXAMPLE 8.10

How many milliliters of a 20% magnesium sulfate solution will contain 40 g of magnesium sulfate?

DIMENSIONAL ANALYSIS

You need to determine the number of milliliters of this solution that contains 40 g of magnesium sulfate.

Given: Amount of solute: 40 g

           Strength: 20%

Find: Amount of solution: ? mL

You want to convert the 40 g of solute to milliliters of solution.

$$40 \text{ g} = ? \text{ mL}$$

You want to cancel the grams and obtain the equivalent amount in milliliters.

$$40 \text{ g} \times \frac{? \text{ mL}}{? \text{ g}} = ? \text{ mL}$$

In a 20% solution there are 20 g of magnesium sulfate per 100 mL of solution. So, the fraction is

$$\frac{100 \text{ mL}}{20 \text{ g}}$$

$$\overset{2}{40} \text{ g} \times \frac{100 \text{ mL}}{\underset{1}{20} \text{ g}} = 200 \text{ mL}$$

RATIO & PROPORTION

The 20% strength means that there is 20 g of magnesium sulfate in every 100 mL of this solution ($20g = 100mL$). You ne0o determine the number of milliliters of this solution that contain 40 g of the pure drug magnesium sulfate ($40g = ?mL$).

Think of the problem as:

$$20g = 100mL$$
$$40g = x\,mL$$

The proportion could be set up as

$$\frac{g}{mL} = \frac{g'}{mL'}$$

Substituting, you get

$$\frac{20g}{100mL} = \frac{40g}{x\,mL}$$

Eliminate the units of measurement and cross multiply

$$\frac{20}{100} = \frac{40}{x}$$

$$4,000 = 20x$$
$$200 = x$$

So, 200 mL of a 20% magnesium sulfate solution contains 40 g of magnesium sulfate.

EXAMPLE 8.11

How many milliliters of a *1:40* acetic acid solution will contain 25 mL of acetic acid?

DIMENSIONAL ANALYSIS

You need to determine the number of milliliters of this solution that contain 25 mL of acetic acid.

Given: Amount of solute: 25 mL (acid)

           Strength: *1:40*

Find: Amount of solution: ? mL (solution)

You want to convert the 25 mL of full-strength acetic acid to milliliters of solution.

$$25 \text{ mL (acid)} = ? \text{ mL (solution)}$$

RATIO & PROPORTION

The *1:40* strength means that there is 1 mL of acetic acid in every 40 mL of this solution *(1 mL of acetic acid = 40 mL of solution)*. You need to determine the number of milliliters of this solution that contain 25 mL of the pure acetic acid *(25 mL of acetic acid = x mL of solution)*.

Think of the problem as:

$$1\,mL\,(\text{acetic acid}) = 40\,mL\,(\text{solution})$$
$$25\,mL\,(\text{acetic acid}) = x\,mL\,(\text{solution})$$

There may be some confusion in the meaning of the previous line because there are milliliters on both sides of the equal sign. To aid your understanding, the parentheses are included to indicate whether "mL" refers to the amount of solute or to the amount of solution.

You want to cancel the milliliters of acid and obtain the equivalent amount in milliliters of solution.

$$25 \text{ mL (acid)} \times \frac{? \text{ mL (solution)}}{? \text{ mL (acid)}}$$

$$= ? \text{ mL(solution)}$$

In a *1:40* acetic acid solution there is 1 mL of pure acetic acid in 40 mL of solution. So, the fraction is

$$\frac{40 \text{ mL (solution)}}{1 \text{ mL (acid)}}$$

$$25 \; \overline{\text{mL (acid)}} \times \frac{40 \text{ mL (solution)}}{1 \; \overline{\text{mL (acid)}}}$$

$$= 1{,}000 \text{ mL (solution)}$$

The proportion could be set up as

$$\frac{mL\,(acetic\,acid)}{mL\,(solution)} = \frac{mL\,(acetic\,acid)'}{mL\,(solution)'}$$

Substituting you get

$$\frac{1\,mL}{40\,mL} = \frac{25\,mL}{x\,mL}$$

Eliminate the units of measurement and cross multiply

$$\frac{1}{40} = \frac{25}{x}$$

$$1{,}000 = 1x$$
$$1{,}000 = x$$

So, 1,000 mL of a *1:40* acetic acid solution contain 25 mL of acetic acid.

EXAMPLE 8.12

How many milliliters of ondansetron solution (• Figure 8.11) contain 10 mg of the drug?

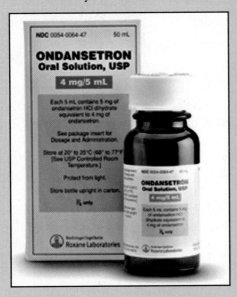

• **Figure 8.11**
Drug label for ondansetron.

NOTE

Because the strength (*4 mg/5 mL*) stated on the ondansetron label in Figure 8.11 uses mg/mL instead of g/mL, it is not a *4:5* solution.

DIMENSIONAL ANALYSIS

You need to determine the number of milliliters of the solution that contains 10 mg of the solute.

Given: Amount of solute: 10 mg
          Strength: 4 mg/5 mL
Find: Amount of solution: ? mL

You want to convert the amount of the solute (10 mg) to the amount of the solution (? mL).

$$10 \text{ mg} = ? \text{ mL}$$

Use the strength of the solution $\dfrac{4 \text{ mg}}{5 \text{ mL}}$ as the unit fraction. In this case, the milligrams need to cancel. So, the fraction must be inverted to have mg in the denominator

$$10 \text{ mg} \times \frac{5 \text{ mL}}{4 \text{ mg}} = 12.5 \text{ mL}$$

RATIO & PROPORTION

The *4 mg/5 mL* strength means that there is 4 mg of the pure drug (zoledronic acid) in every 5 mL of this solution. You need to determine the number of milliliters of this solution that contain 10 mg of the pure drug.

Think of the problem as:

$$4 \text{ mg (drug)} = 5 \text{ mL (solution)}$$
$$10 \text{ mg (drug)} = x \text{ mL (solution)}$$

The proportion could be set up as

$$\frac{mg}{mL} = \frac{mg'}{mL'}$$

Substituting, you get

$$\frac{4 \text{ mg}}{5 \text{ mL}} = \frac{10 \text{ mg}}{x \text{ mL}}$$

Eliminate the units of measurement and cross multiply

$$\frac{4}{5} = \frac{10}{x}$$

$$50 = 4x$$
$$\frac{50}{4} = x$$
$$12.5 = x$$

So, 12.5 mL of the ondansetron solution contain 10 mg of ondansetron.

Irrigating Solutions, Soaks, and Oral Feedings

Sometimes healthcare professionals are required to prepare irrigating solutions, soaks, and nutritional feedings. These may be supplied in ready-to-use form, or they can be prepared from dry powders or from liquid concentrates.

Irrigating solutions and soaks are used for sterile irrigation of body cavities, wounds, indwelling catheters; washing and rinsing purposes; or for soaking of surgical dressings, instruments, and laboratory specimens.

Enteral feedings are nutritional solutions which can be supplied in ready-to-use form, or they may be reconstituted from powders or from liquid concentrates. The nutritional solutions may be administered either orally or parenterally.

EXAMPLE 8.13

ALERT

Full-strength (ready-to-use) hydrogen peroxide is generally supplied as a 3% solution. This stock solution may be diluted to form weaker solutions depending on the application. These dilutions must be performed using aseptic techniques.

Using a full-strength hydrogen peroxide solution, how would you prepare 300 mL of $\frac{2}{3}$ strength hydrogen peroxide solution for a wound irrigation, using normal saline as the diluent?

The $\frac{2}{3}$ strength means that there are 2 mL of full-strength hydrogen peroxide in every 3 mL of the $\frac{2}{3}$ strength solution *(2 mL of full-strength hydrogen peroxide = 3 mL of $\frac{2}{3}$ strength solution)*. You need to determine the number of milliliters of full-strength hydrogen peroxide that are contained in 300 mL of the $\frac{2}{3}$ strength solution.

DIMENSIONAL ANALYSIS

Hint: *Think of the full-strength solution as the solute.*

Given: 300 mL $\left(\frac{2}{3}\ strength\right)$

Equivalence: *2 mL (full-strength) / 3 mL $\left(\frac{2}{3}\ strength\right)$*

Find: Amount of solute ? mL *(full-strength)*

300 mL $\left(\frac{2}{3}\ strength\right)$ = ? mL *(full-strength)*

$$\frac{300\ \cancel{mL}\left(\frac{2}{3}str\right)}{1} \times \frac{2\ mL\ (full\text{-}str)}{3\ \cancel{mL}\left(\frac{2}{3}str\right)}$$

= 200 mL *(full-strength)*

RATIO & PROPORTION

(? mL of full-strength hydrogen peroxide = 300 mL of 2/3 strength solution).

Think of the problem as:

2 mL (full-strength hydrogen peroxide) = 3 mL (2/3 strength solution)

x mL (full-strength hydrogen peroxide) = 300 mL (2/3 strength solution)

The proportion could be set up as

$$\frac{mL\ (full\text{-}strength)}{mL\ (2/3\ strength\ solution)}$$
$$= \frac{mL\ (full\text{-}strength)'}{mL\ (2/3\ strength\ solution)'}$$

Substituting, you get

$$\frac{2\ mL\ (full\text{-}strength)}{3\ mL\ (2/3\ strength\ solution)}$$
$$= \frac{x\ mL\ (full\text{-}strength)}{300\ mL\ (2/3\ strength\ solution)}$$

Eliminate the units of measurement and cross multiply

$$\frac{2}{3} = \frac{x}{300}$$

$$3x = 600$$
$$x = 200$$

So, 200 mL of full-strength hydrogen peroxide would be diluted with 100 mL of normal saline to make 300 mL of a $\frac{2}{3}$ strength solution.

EXAMPLE 8.14

How many ounces of $\frac{1}{4}$ strength Sustacal can be made from a 12-ounce can of full-strength Sustacal?

The $\frac{1}{4}$ strength means that there is 1 ounce of full-strength Sustacal in every 4 ounces of this solution *(1 oz of full-strength Sustacal = 4 oz of $\frac{1}{4}$ strength solution)*. You need to determine the number of ounces of $\frac{1}{4}$ strength Sustacal that can be made from 12 oz of full-strength Sustacal *(12 oz of full-strength Sustacal = ? oz of $\frac{1}{4}$ strength solution)*.

DIMENSIONAL ANALYSIS

Hint: *Think of the full-strength solution as the solute.*

Given: 12 oz *(full-strength)*

Equivalence: 1 oz *(full-strength)* / 4 oz *($\frac{1}{4}$ strength)*

Find: ? oz *($\frac{1}{4}$ strength)*

$$12 \text{ oz } (full\text{-}strength) = ? \text{ oz } \left(\tfrac{1}{4} strength\right)$$

$$\frac{12 \; \overline{oz\,(full\text{-}str)}}{1} \times \frac{4 \text{ oz } (\tfrac{1}{4}\text{-}str)}{1 \; \overline{oz\,(full\text{-}str)}}$$

$$= 48 \text{ oz } \left(\frac{1}{4} \; strength\right)$$

RATIO & PROPORTION

Think of the problem as:

$$1 \text{ oz (full-strength Sustacal)} = 4 \text{ oz } (\tfrac{1}{4} \text{ strength soltuion})$$

$$12 \text{ oz (full-strength Sustacal)} = x \text{ oz } (\tfrac{1}{4} \text{ strength soltuion})$$

The proportion could be set up as

$$\frac{oz\,(full\text{-}strength)}{oz\,(1/4\,strength\,solution)}$$
$$= \frac{oz\,(full\text{-}strength)'}{oz\,(1/4\,strength\,solution)'}$$

Substituting, you get

$$\frac{1\,oz\,(full\text{-}strength)}{4\,oz\,(1/4\,strength\,solution)}$$
$$= \frac{12\,oz\,(full\text{-}strength)}{x\,oz\,(1/4\,strength\,solution)}$$

Eliminate the units of measurement and cross multiply

$$\frac{1}{4} = \frac{12}{x}$$

$$48 = 1x$$

$$x = 48 \text{ ounces}$$

So, 48 ounces of $\frac{1}{4}$ strength Sustacal can be made from a 12-ounce can of full-strength Sustacal by adding the 12-ounce can of Sustacal to 36 ounces of water.

EXAMPLE 8.15

How would you prepare 240 mL of $\frac{1}{2}$ strength Ensure from full-strength Ensure? Which size can(s) of Ensure would you use to minimize the amount of discarded Ensure if the supply consists of 8- and 12-oz cans?

The $\frac{1}{2}$ strength means that there is 1 ounce of full-strength Ensure in every 2 ounces of this solution. You need to determine the number of ounces of full-strength Ensure that are contained in 240 mL of the $\frac{1}{2}$ strength solution.

DIMENSIONAL ANALYSIS

You need to work with a single unit of measurement; either *ounces* or *milliliters*. If you decide to work in *ounces*, one way to do this is to use the equivalence *30 mL = 1 oz* to change *240 mL* to *8 oz*.

Given: 8 oz (half-strength)

Equivalence: 1 oz (full-strength)/2 oz (half-strength)

Find: ? oz (full-strength)

8 oz (half-strength) = ? oz (full-strength)

$$\frac{8 \; \overline{oz \; (half\text{-}str)}}{1} \times \frac{1 \; oz \; (full\text{-}str)}{2 \; \overline{oz \; (half\text{-}str)}}$$

$$= 4 \; oz \; (full\text{-}strength)$$

RATIO & PROPORTION

This problem expresses the quantities of $\frac{1}{2}$ strength Ensure in two different units of measure: ounces *(2 oz)* and milliliters *(240 mL)*. To set up a proportion, you need to use a single unit of measurement for the $\frac{1}{2}$ strength Ensure; either ounces or milliliters. One way to do this is to use the equivalence 30 mL = 1 oz to change 240 milliliters to 8 ounces.

Now think of the problem as:

1 oz (full-strength Ensure) = 2 oz ($\frac{1}{2}$ strength solution)

x oz (full-strength Ensure) = 8 oz ($\frac{1}{2}$ strength solution)

Now, a proportion could be set up as

$$\frac{1 \; oz \, (full\text{-}strength)}{2 \; oz \, (1/2 \, strength \, solution)}$$

$$= \frac{x \; oz \, (full\text{-}strength)}{8 \; oz \, (1/2 \, stength \, solution)}$$

Eliminate the units of measurement and cross multiply

$$\frac{1}{2} = \frac{x}{8}$$

$$2x = 8$$

$$x = 4 \; ounces$$

So, 4 oz of full-strength Ensure are contained in 240 mL of $\frac{1}{2}$ strength Ensure. To prepare the solution, add 4 ounces of water to 4 ounces of full-strength Ensure to make 8 ounces of the $\frac{1}{2}$-strength solution. Because 4 ounces of full-strength Ensure are needed, using a 8-oz can would result in discarding 4 oz of Ensure, whereas using a 12-oz can would result in discarding 8 oz of Ensure. Therefore, use one 8-oz can to minimize waste.

Summary

In this chapter, you learned that there are three important quantities associated with a solution: the *strength* of the solution, the *amount of solute* dissolved in the solution, and the total *volume of the solution*. If any two of these three quantities are known, the remaining quantity can be found.

- The *strength* of a solution is the ratio of the *amount of solute* dissolved in the solution to the total *volume of the solution*.
- The strength of a solution may be expressed in the form of a *ratio, fraction,* or *percentage*.
- A $\frac{1}{2}$ *strength* solution is a *1:2* or a *50%* solution and should not be confused with a $\frac{1}{2}$% solution.
- The amount of solute dissolved in the solution should be expressed in *milliliters* if the solute is a *liquid*.
- The amount of solute dissolved in the solution should be expressed in *grams* if the solute is a *solid* or *powder*.
- The *volume of a solution* should be expressed in *milliliters*.

- $$\boxed{\text{Strength} = \frac{\text{Solute}}{\text{Solution}}}$$

- To determine the amount of solute contained in a given amount of a solution of known strength, use the strength as the known equivalence.
- To determine amount of a solution of known strength containing a given amount of solute, use the strength as the known equivalence.
- Use aseptic technique when diluting stock solutions for irrigations, soak, and nutritional liquids.
- The strength of a particular solution may be written in many different forms. The following strengths are all equivalent:

With stated Units of Measurement

$$\text{Rates} \begin{cases} 500 \text{ mg/mL} \\ 500 \text{ mg per mL} \\ \dfrac{500 \ mg}{1 \ mL} \end{cases}$$

Equivalence   500 mg = 1 mL

Without stated Units of Measurement

Fraction	$\frac{1}{2}$ strength
Ratio	1:2
Precentage	50%

Case Study 8.1

Read the Case Study and answer the questions. Answers can be found in Appendix A.

A 75-year-old female is admitted to a long-term care facility status post-mitral valve replacement. She has a past medical history of osteoarthritis; hypertension; atrial fibrillation; and insulin-dependent diabetes mellitus. Skin assessment reveals a 3-cm wound on the right heel. She is alert and oriented to person, place, time, and recent memory and she rates her pain level as 6 on a scale of 0–10. Vital signs are: T 98.7 °F; P 68; R 18; B/P 124/76.

Her orders are as follows:

- Persantine (dipyridamole) 75 mg PO, q.i.d.
- Cordarone (amiodarone hydrochloride) 400 mg PO daily; notify MD if P less than 60
- Cardizem SR(diltiazem) 180 mg PO daily

- Relafen (nabumetone) 1,000 mg PO daily
- KCl oral solution 20 mEq PO b.i.d.
- Multivitamin 1 tab PO daily
- Tylenol 650 mg PO q4h prn T above 101
- Humulin R insulin 10 units and Humulin N insulin 38 units subcutaneous 30 minutes ac breakfast
- Humulin R insulin 10 units and Humulin N insulin 30 units 30 minutes ac dinner
- Pneumovax 0.5 mL IM stat for 1 dose
- Cleanse right heel with NS solution (0.9% NaCl) and apply a DSD daily
- 1,800 calorie ADA 2 g sodium diet

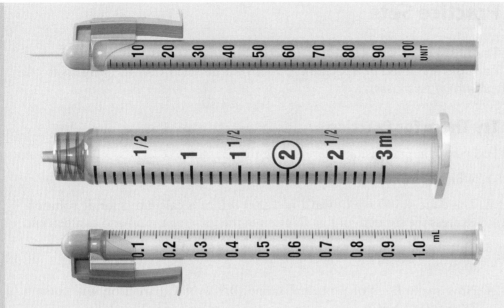

1. The Pneumovax vial contains 2.5 mL. Choose the appropriate syringe from those given and place an arrow at the dose.

2. Cardizem SR is available in 60 mg and 120 mg tablets. Which strength will you use and how many tablets for the daily dose?

3. The KCl solution label reads 40 mEq/15 mL. How many milliliters will you administer?

4. The dipyridamole is available in 25-, 50-, and 75-mg tablets. Which strength tablets will you administer and how many?

5. The strength of the nabumetone tablets is 500 mg. How many tablets will you administer?

6. Describe how you will measure the morning insulin. Select the appropriate syringe from those given and mark the dose of Humulin R and Humulin N.

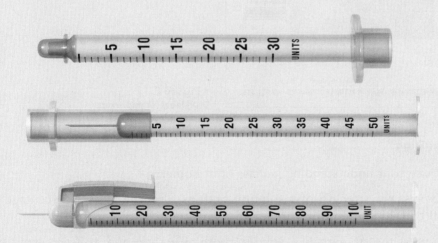

7. How many grams of sodium chloride (NaCl) are in 1 liter of the normal saline (NS) solution?

Workspace

Practice Sets

The answers to *Try These for Practice*, *Exercises*, and *Cumulative Review Exercises* are found in Appendix A. Ask your instructor for the answers to the *Additional Exercises*.

Try These for Practice

Test your comprehension after reading the chapter.

1. Which is stronger: a half-strength solution or a $\frac{1}{2}$% solution?

2. There are 4,500 *mg* of CaCl in 1,000 *mL* of a calcium chloride solution. Express the strength of this solution in the form of a ratio and as a percent.

3. Calculate the number of *grams* of dextrose in 500 *mL* of a 5% dextrose solution.

4. How many *liters* of a normal saline (0.9% NaCl) solution will contain 18 *grams* of NaCl?

5. How many milliliters of the naproxen solution (• **Figure 8.12**) contain 100 mg of the pure drug?

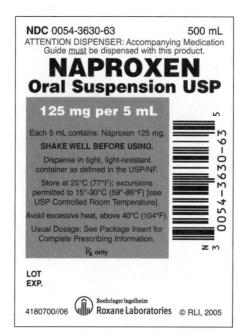

• **Figure 8.12**
Drug label for naproxen.

Exercises

Reinforce your understanding in class or at home.

1. Express the strength of a solution both as a ratio and as a percentage if 500 mL of the solution contain 25 mL of solute.

2. Express the strength of a solution both as a ratio and as a percentage if 200 mL of the solution contain 40 g of solute.

3. Express the strength of a solution both as a ratio and as a percentage if 2 L of the solution contain 400 mg of solute.

4. Betadine solution is a 10% povidone-iodine solution. Express this strength both as a fraction and as a ratio.

5. Thorazine is available in a strength of 25 mg/mL. Express this strength as a percent.

6. Which of the following could be solution strengths?

1:10,000; 0.5%; 25 mL; $\frac{1}{3}$; 2 mg/mL; 100 g

7. Fill in the following chart of equivalent strengths.

Ratio	Fraction	Percent
1:5		
	$\frac{1}{4}$	
		10%
1:200		
	$\frac{9}{1,000}$	

8. How many mL of a 10% magnesium sulfate solution will contain 14 grams of magnesium sulfate?

9. A pharmaceutical company sells ropivacaine HCl in various strengths as listed in the chart. Find the error in the "strength" column of the table by trying to verify that each of the four "concentrations" listed are equivalent to each of the corresponding "strengths."

Concentration	Strength	Vial Size
2 mg/mL	0.2%	100 mL
5 mg/mL	0.4%	30 mL
7.5 mg/mL	0.75%	20 mL
10 mg/mL	1%	20 mL

10. How many mL of the lidocaine viscous solution shown in • Figure 8.13 will contain 10 mg of lidocaine?

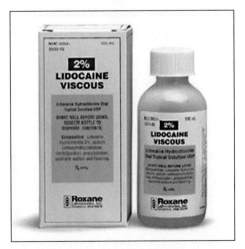

• Figure 8.13
Drug packaging for 2% Lidocaine Viscous.

11. How many mg of fluconazole are contained in 200 mL of a 0.2% solution?

12. Express as a percent the strength of the pneumococcal vaccine whose label is in • **Figure 8.14**.

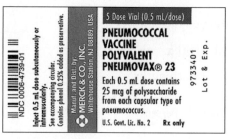

• **Figure 8.14**
Drug label for pneumococcal vaccine.

13. The nutritional formula Sustacal is supplied in 10-ounce cans. How would you prepare 40 ounces of a half-strength Sustacal solution?

14. How would you prepare 1 liter of a 25% boric acid solution from boric acid crystals?

15. How would 400 mL of a 20% solution be prepared using tablets that each contain 10 grams of the drug?

16. How many mg of NaCl are contained in 250 mL of a 0.45% NaCl solution?

17. The label on the vial of metoprolol tartrate indicates a strength of 5 mg/5 mL. How many mg of metoprolol tartrate are contained in 87 mL of this solution?

18. Are the following two strengths equivalent? 2% and 20 mg/mL.

19. The label on a 20 mL aminophylline vial indicates a strength of 500 mg/20 mL.
    (a) How many mL of aminophylline would contain 200 mg of this drug?
    (b) How many mg of aminophylline would be contained in 1 mL of this solution?

20. How many milliliters are in one spray of the ipratropium bromide solution shown in • **Figure 8.15**?

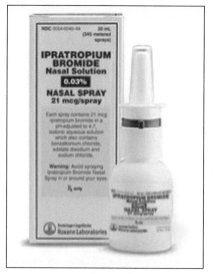

• **Figure 8.15**
Container and packaging for ipratropium bromide.

Additional Exercises

Now, test yourself!

1. 750 mL of a solution contain 15 mL of a pure drug. Express the strength of this solution both as a ratio and as a percentage.

2. Two liters of a solution contain 60 g of a pure drug. Express the strength of this solution both as a ratio and as a percentage.

3. How would 300 mL of a 0.9% sodium chloride solution be prepared using sodium chloride crystals?

4. Read the label in • **Figure 8.16** and determine the number of milligrams of hydroxyzine pamoate that are contained in the vial of Vistaril.

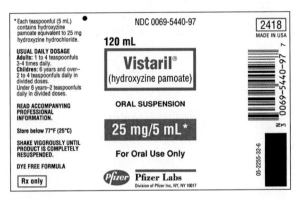

• **Figure 8.16**
Drug label for Vistaril.
(Reg. trademark of Pfizer Inc. Reproduced with permission.)

5. How many milliliters of Vistaril (Figure 8.16) contain 20 mg of hydroxyzine pamoate?

6. How would 400 mL of a 50% solution be prepared from a drug that in its pure form is a liquid?

7. How many milliliters of a 6% solution contain 18 g of the pure drug?

8. Read the label in • **Figure 8.17**. How many milliliters of the lidocaine hydrochloride solution contain 300 mg of lidocaine hydrochloride?

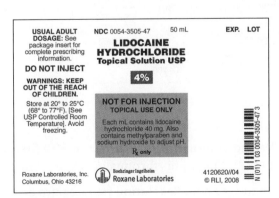

• **Figure 8.17**
Drug label for lidocaine HCl.

9. Read the packaging information shown in • **Figure 8.18** to determine the number of milligrams of acetylcysteine that are contained in 5 milliliters of the solution.

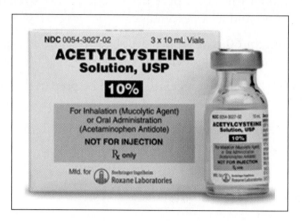

• **Figure 8.18**
Packaging and Drug Guide information for acetylcysteine.

10. A drug has a strength of 125 mg/mL. Write this strength in the form of a ratio, a fraction, and a percentage.

11. The nutritional formula Sustacal is supplied in 10-ounce cans. How would you prepare 1,600 mL of a 3/4 strength Sustacal solution?

12. If 600 mL of a solution contain 120 mL of a pure drug, express the strength of this solution both as a ratio and as a percentage.

13. If 1 L of a solution contains 2,000 mg of a pure drug, express the strength of this solution both as a ratio and as a percentage.

14. How would 800 mL of a 10% solution be prepared using tablets each containing 20 g?

15. Read the label in • **Figure 8.19** and determine the number of milligrams of erythromycin ethylsuccinate that are contained in 2 mL of the solution.

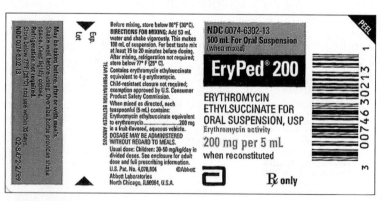

• **Figure 8.19**
Drug label for EryPed 200.

16. Read the label in Figure 8.19 and determine the number of milliliters of the solution that would contain 250 mg of erythromycin ethylsuccinate.

17. How would you prepare 1,200 mL of a 25% solution from a pure drug in solid form?

18. A drug label states the strength of the solution is 10 mg/mL or 1%. Verify that the two stated strengths are equivalent.

19. A drug has a strength of 25 mg/mL. Write this strength in the form of a ratio, a fraction, and a percentage.

20. The nutritional formula Isomil is supplied in 4-, 8-, and 12-ounce cans. How would you prepare 6 oz of a 2/3 strength Isomil solution. What size can(s) would you use in order to minimize the amount of discarded Isomil?

Cumulative Review Exercises

Review your mastery of previous chapters.

1. 0.4 *g* = _____ *mg*

2. 3 *oz* = _____ *T*

3. 88 *lb* = _____ *kg*

4. 3.4 *mm* = _____ *cm*

5. 15 *mL* = _____ *oz*

6. 50 *mg/day* = _____ *mg/week*

7. Each serving of the nutritional supplement *BoostPlus* provides 360 calories and 14 g of protein.
   (a) How many servings of BoostPlus contain 1,440 calories?
   (b) How many grams of protein are contained in 10 servings?

8. *Order: Accupril (quinapril HCl) 80 mg po daily.* How many *grams* of this ACE inhibitor will the patient receive in a week?

9. A therapy starts at 9:15 PM on Monday. It continues for 6 hours and 45 minutes. At what time and on what day will it finish (use military time)?

10. Geodon (ziprasidone) is available in the concentration of 20 mg/mL. The order is *Geodon 10 mg IM q2h for 4 doses.* How many *mL* of this antipsychotic drug will be administered in 8 hours?

11. A patient weighs 220 *lb*. Find the patient's weight in *kilograms*.

12. Order: *Provera (medroxprogesterone acetate) 5 mg po daily for 5 days.* The tablets are supplied in 10 *mg* scored tablets. How many tablets of this hormone will you administer each day?

13. Order: *Zithromax (azithromycin) 500 mg po daily for 3 days.* It is supplied as an oral suspension with strength of 100 *mg/5 mL*. How many *mL* of this macrolide antibiotic will you administer?

14. How many *mg* of NaCl are contained in 200 *mL* of a 0.9% NaCl solution?

15. What is the weight in *grams* of an infant who weighs 6 *pounds*.

nursing.pearsonhighered.com
Prepare for success with animated examples, practice questions, challenge tests, and interactive assignments.

Chapter

9

Parenteral Medications

Learning Outcomes

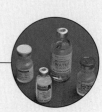

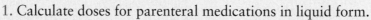

After completing this chapter, you will be able to

1. Calculate doses for parenteral medications in liquid form.
2. Interpret the directions on drug labels and package inserts for reconstituting medications supplied in powdered form.
3. Label reconstituted multidose medication containers with the necessary information.
4. Choose the most appropriate diluent volume when reconstituting a multiple-strength medication.
5. Calculate doses of parenteral medications measured in units.

This chapter introduces the calculations you will use to prepare and administer parenteral medications safely. Chapter 2 discussed the most common parenteral sites: intramuscular (IM), subcutaneous (subcut), intravenous (IV), intradermal (ID), intracardiac (IC), intrathecal, and epidural. This chapter will focus on calculations for administering medications via the subcutaneous and intramuscular routes.

Parenteral Medications

Parenteral medications are those that are injected into the body by various routes. Drugs for parenteral medications may be packaged in a variety of forms, including ampules, vials, and prefilled cartridges or syringes. Prefilled cartridges and syringes were discussed in Chapter 7.

An *ampule* is a glass container that holds a single dose of medication. It has a narrowed neck that is designed to snap open. The medication is aspirated into a syringe by gently pulling back on the plunger, which creates a negative pressure and allows the liquid to be pulled into the syringe (• **Figure 9.1**).

A *vial* is a glass or plastic container that has a rubber membrane on the top. This membrane is covered with a lid that maintains the sterility of the membrane until the vial is used for the first time. Multidose vials contain more than one dose of a medication. Single-dose vials contain one dose of medication, and many drugs are now prepared in single-dose format to reduce the chance of error. The medication in a vial may be supplied in liquid or powdered form (• **Figure 9.2**).

NOTE

Be sure to use a plastic ampule opener to safely break the ampule and a filter needle to withdraw the contents from the ampule. *Do not* use the filter needle to administer the medication.

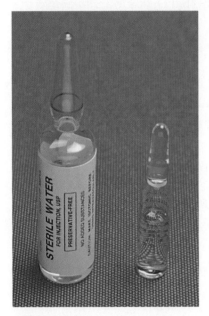

• **Figure 9.1**
Ampules.

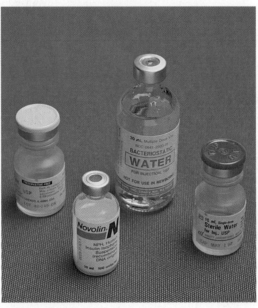

• **Figure 9.2**
Vials.

Parenteral Medications Supplied as Liquids

When parenteral medications are in liquid form, you must calculate the volume of the solution that contains the prescribed amount of the medication. To perform this calculation you also need to know the strength of the solution. You will use dimensional analysis to calculate the volume that will be administered.

The following rough guidelines for the volumes generally administered subcutaneously or intramuscularly can be used to test the reasonableness of your calculated dosages.

Subcut:	Infant:	less than 0.1 mL
	Child:	less than 0.5 mL
	Adult:	from 0.5 mL to 1 mL

NOTE

Single-dose ampules and vials may contain a little more drug than indicated on the label. Therefore, if the order is for the exact amount of medication stated on the label, it is very important to carefully measure the amount of medication to be withdrawn. Before a fluid can be extracted from a vial, that same volume of air must be injected into the vial.

IM:	Infant:	less than 1 mL
	Child:	less than 2 mL
	Adult:	less than 3 mL (in the deltoid less than 2 mL)

EXAMPLE 9.1

The prescriber ordered *nalbuphine 15 mg subcut q6h prn moderate-severe pain*. Read the label in • Figure 9.3(a) and determine how many milliliters of this analgesic drug you will prepare. The dose is indicated on the syringe shown in • Figure 9.3(b).

ALERT

In Example 9.1, the strength indicates that 20 mg = 1 mL. Because the order (15 mg) is less than 20 mg, you would administer less than 1 mL. Always check to see whether the amount of drug prescribed is smaller (or larger) than the amount of drug stated in the strength available.

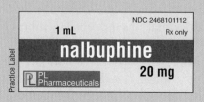

Practice Label

NDC 2468101112

1 mL   Rx only

nalbuphine

PL Pharmaceuticals   **20 mg**

• Figure 9.3(a)
Drug label for nalbuphine.
(For educational purposes only)

Begin by determining how many milliliters contain the prescribed quantity of the medication. That is, you want to convert mg to an equivalent in milliliters.

$$15 \text{ mg} = ? \text{ mL}$$

DIMENSIONAL ANALYSIS

You cancel the milligrams and obtain the equivalent quantity in milliliters.

$$15 \text{ mg} \times \frac{? \, mL}{? \, mg} = ? \, mL$$

The label reads 20 milligrams per 1 milliliter. So, the unit fraction is $\frac{1 \, mL}{20 \, mg}$

$$15 \text{ mg} \times \frac{1 \, mL}{20 \, mg} = 0.75 \text{ mL}$$

FORMULA METHOD

D (desired dose) = 15 mg
H (dose on hand) = 20 mg
Q (dosage unit) = 1 mL
X (unknown) = ? mL

Fill in the formula $\dfrac{D}{H} \times Q = X$

$$\frac{15 \, mg}{20 \, mg} \times 1 \, mL = ? \, mL$$

Cancel $\dfrac{\overset{3}{\cancel{15} \, mg}}{\underset{4}{\cancel{20} \, mg}} \times 1 \, ml = ? \, mL$

Multiply $\dfrac{3}{4} \times 1 \, mL = \dfrac{3}{4} \text{ mL}$

So, you would administer 0.75 mL using a 1 mL syringe.

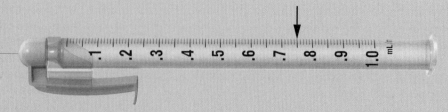

• Figure 9.3(b)
Syringe with 15 mg of nalbuphine.

EXAMPLE 9.2

The prescriber ordered *quinidine gluconate 600 mg IM stat and 400 mg IM q4h prn*. Read the label in •Figure 9.4 and calculate the number of milliliters of this antiarrhythmic drug you will administer to the patient as needed.

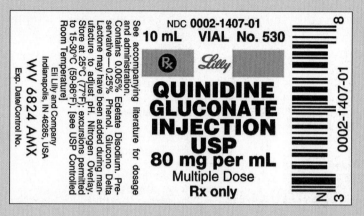

•**Figure 9.4**
Drug label for quinidine gluconate.
(Copyright Eli Lilly and Company. Used with permission.)

Begin by determining how many milliliters of the liquid in the vial contain the prescribed quantity of the medication (400 mg of quinidine gluconate—the question asks for the as needed dose). That is, you want to convert 400 mg to an equivalent in milliliters.

DIMENSIONAL ANALYSIS

$$400 \text{ mg} = ? \text{ mL}$$

You cancel the milligrams and obtain the equivalent quantity in milliliters.

$$400 \text{ mg} \times \frac{? \text{ mL}}{? \text{ mg}} = ? \text{ mL}$$

The label reads 80 mg per milliliter, which means the solution strength is 80 mg/1 mL.

So, the unit fraction is $\dfrac{1 \text{ mL}}{80 \text{ mg}}$

$$400 \text{ mg} \times \frac{1 \text{ mL}}{80 \text{ mg}} = 5 \text{ mL}$$

RATIO & PROPORTION

Think of the problem as:

$$400 \text{ mg (quinidine)} = x \text{ mL (solution)} \quad \text{(dose)}$$
$$80 \text{ mg (quinidine)} = 1 \text{ mL (solution)} \quad \text{(strength)}$$

The proportion could be set up as

$$\frac{mg}{mL} = \frac{mg'}{mL'}$$

Substituting, you get

$$\frac{400 \, mg}{x \, mL} = \frac{80 \, mg}{1 \, mL}$$

Eliminate the units of measurement and cross multiply

$$\frac{400}{x} = \frac{80}{1}$$

$$80x = 400$$

Divide both sides by the coefficient of x

$$x = \frac{400}{80}$$

$$x = 5$$

So, you would administer 5 mL to the patient. Because of the large volume, the dosage would be **divided** in two syringes.

EXAMPLE 9.3

The prescriber ordered *amikacin sulfate IM loading dose* for an adult patient who weighs 110 pounds and has a severe infection. Read the label and the Drug Guide information in • Figure 9.5.

(a) How many mg/kg will the prescriber order for the maximum dose?

(b) Calculate the number of milliliters of this aminoglycoside antibiotic you would administer.

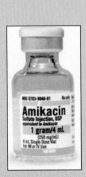

	ROUTE & DOSAGE
AMIKACIN SULFATE (am-i-kay'sin) Amikin **Classification:** AMINOGLYCOSIDE ANTIBIOTIC Therapeutic: ANTIBIOTIC **Prototype:** Gentamicin **Pregnancy Category:** C	**Moderate to Severe Infections** *Adult:* **IV/IM** 5–7.5 mg/kg loading dose, then 7.5 mg/kg q12h (max: 15 mg/kg/day) for 7–10 days *Child:* **IV/IM** 5–7.5 mg/kg loading dose, then 5 mg/kg q8h or 7.5 mg/kg q12h for 7–10 days (max: 1.5 g/day) *Neonate:* **IV/IM** 10 mg/kg loading dose, then 7.5 mg/kg q12h for 7–10 days

• **Figure 9.5**
Drug vial and information for amikacin sulfate.

(a) First read the information in the Drug Guide, and you will see that the maximum loading dose should be 7.5 mg/kg.

DIMENSIONAL ANALYSIS

(b) You must first convert the patient's weight to kilograms using the unit fraction $\dfrac{1\,kg}{2.2\,lb}$

$$110\,lb \times \frac{1\,kg}{2.2\,lb}$$

Then, multiply the patient's weight (in kg) by the order to obtain the dose in milligrams.

$$110\,lb \times \frac{1\,kg}{2.2\,lb} \times \frac{7.5\,mg}{kg} = ?\,mL$$

Finally, use the strength to obtain the unit fraction $\dfrac{1\,mL}{250\,mg}$ to change the mg to mL.

$$110\,lb \times \frac{1\,kg}{2.2\,lb} \times \frac{7.5\,mg}{kg} \times \frac{1\,mL}{250\,mg} = 1.5\,mL$$

FORMULA METHOD

(b) You must first convert the patient's weight from pounds to kilograms. This can be done by dividing the weight in kilograms by 2.2.

$$\frac{110}{2.2} = 50\,kg$$

Determine the dose in milligrams by using the formula:

Size of the Patient × Order = Dose

$$50\,kg \times \frac{7.5\,mg}{kg} = 375\,mg$$

Now, think of the problem as:

D (desired dose) = 375 mg
H (dose on hand) = 250 mg
Q (dosage unit)   = 1 mL
X (unknown)   = ? mL

Fill in the formula $\dfrac{D}{H} \times Q = X$

$$\frac{375\,mg}{250\,mg} \times 1\,mL = ?\,mL$$

Cancel	$\dfrac{\overset{3}{\cancel{375}}\ \cancel{mg}}{\underset{2}{\cancel{250}}\ \cancel{mg}} \times 1\,ml = ?\,mL$
Multiply	$\dfrac{3}{2} \times 1\,mL = 1.5\,mL$

So, you would administer 1.5 mL IM to the patient.

EXAMPLE 9.4

The prescriber ordered *haloperidol 3 mg IM q4h prn*. Read the label in • Figure 9.6(a) and determine how many milliliters of this antipsychotic drug you will prepare. Indicate the dose on the syringe in • Figure 9.6(b).

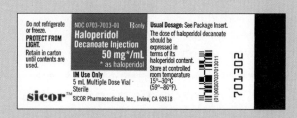

• **Figure 9.6(a)**
Drug label for haloperidol.

You have a 5 mL multiple dose vial, and the label indicates the strength is 50 mg/mL. Begin by determining how many milliliters of the solution in the vial contain the prescribed quantity of the medication. That is, you want to convert 3 mg to an equivalent in milliliters.

FORMULA METHOD

D (desired dose) = 3 mg
H (dose on hand) = 50 mg
Q (dosage unit) = 1 mL
X (unknown) = ? mL

Fill in the formula $\dfrac{D}{H} \times Q = X$

$$\dfrac{3\,\overset{\frown}{mg}}{50\,\overset{\frown}{mg}} \times 1\,mL = ?\,mL$$

Cancel $\dfrac{3\,\overset{\frown}{g}}{50\,\overset{\frown}{mg}} \times 1\,ml = ?\,mL$

Multiply $\dfrac{3}{50} \times 1\,mL = 0.06\,mL$

RATIO & PROPORTION

$3\,mg = x\,mL$ [ordered dose]
$50\,mg = 1\,mL$ [strength]

$$\dfrac{3\,mg}{x\,mL} = \dfrac{50\,mg}{1\,mL}$$

$$50x = 3$$

$$x = \dfrac{3}{50}$$

$$x = 0.06$$

So, you would use a 1 mL syringe and give the patient 0.06 mL.

0.06 mL

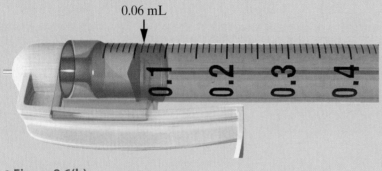

• **Figure 9.6(b)**
Syringe with 3 mg of haloperidol (0.06 mL).

EXAMPLE 9.5

The prescriber ordered *Tigan (trimethobenzamide hydrochloride) 200 mg IM stat*. You have a 20 mL multidose vial, and the label indicates that the strength is 100 mg/mL. How many milliliters of this antiemetic drug will you prepare?

Begin by determining how many milliliters of the solution in the vial contain the prescribed quantity of the medication. That is, you want to convert 200 mg to an equivalent in milliliters.

DIMENSIONAL ANALYSIS

$$200 \text{ mg} = ? \text{ mL}$$

You cancel the milligrams and obtain the equivalent quantity in milliliters.

$$200 \text{ mg} \times \frac{? \text{ mL}}{? \text{ mg}} = ? \text{ mL}$$

The label indicates that there are 100 mg per milliliter.

So, the unit fraction is $\dfrac{1 \text{ mL}}{100 \text{ mg}}$

$$200 \text{ mg} \times \frac{1 \text{ mL}}{100 \text{ mg}} = 2 \text{ mL}$$

RATIO & PROPORTION

$$200 \text{ mg} = x \text{ mL} \quad \text{(dose)}$$
$$100 \text{ mg} = 1 \text{ mL} \quad \text{(strength)}$$

$$\frac{200 \text{ mg}}{x \text{ mL}} = \frac{100 \text{ mg}}{1 \text{ mL}}$$

$$100x = 200$$

$$x = \frac{200}{100}$$

$$x = 2$$

So, you would give the patient 2 mL.

EXAMPLE 9.6

The order for an adult who has adrenal insufficiency is *dexamethasone sodium phosphate 5 mg IM q12h*. The patient weighs 100 kg, and the strength in the vial is 4 mg/mL.

(a) If the recommended daily dosage is 0.03–0.15 mg/kg, is the prescribed dosage safe?

(b) How many milliliters will you administer?

DIMENSIONAL ANALYSIS

(a) Using the recommended daily dosage, calculate the minimum and maximum number of milligrams the patient should receive each day.

Minimum Daily Dosage

Because the *minimum* recommended daily dosage (0.03 mg/kg) is based on the size of the patient (100 kg), multiply these as follows:

$$100\,\cancel{kg} \times \frac{0.03\,mg}{\cancel{kg}} = 3\,mg$$

Maximum Daily Dosage

Because the *maximum* recommended daily dosage (0.15 mg/kg) is based on the size of the patient (100 kg), multiply these as follows:

$$100\,\cancel{kg} \times \frac{0.15\,mg}{\cancel{kg}} = 15\,mg$$

So, the safe dose range for this patient is 3–15 mg daily.

The prescribed dosage is safe because the prescribed dosage of 5 mg q12h means the patient would receive 10 mg per day, which is in the safe dose range of 3–15 mg per day.

(b) Begin by determining how many milliliters of liquid in the vial contain the prescribed quantity of the medication. That is, you want to convert 5 mg to an equivalent in milliliters.

$$5\ mg = ?\ mL$$

You cancel the milligrams and obtain the equivalent quantity in milliliters.

$$5\ mg \times \frac{?\ mL}{?\ mg} = ?\ mL$$

The label reads 4 milligrams per milliliter, therefore, the unit fraction is $\dfrac{1\ mL}{4\ mg}$

$$5\,\cancel{mg} \times \frac{1\ mL}{4\,\cancel{mg}} = 1.25\ mL$$

RATIO & PROPORTION

(a) Using the recommended daily dosage, calculate the minimum and maximum number of milligrams the patient should receive each day.

Minimum Daily Dosage

Because the *minimum* recommended daily dosage (0.03 mg/kg) is based on the size of the patient (100 kg), multiply these as follows:

$$100\,\cancel{kg} \times \frac{0.03\,mg}{\cancel{kg}} = 3\,mg$$

Maximum Daily Dosage

Because the *maximum* recommended daily dosage (0.15 mg/kg) is based on the size of the patient (100 kg), multiply these as follows:

$$100\,\cancel{kg} \times \frac{0.15\,mg}{\cancel{kg}} = 15\,mg$$

So, the safe dose range for this patient is 3–15 mg daily.

The prescribed dosage is safe because the prescribed dosage of 5 mg q12h means the patient would receive 10 mg per day, which is in the safe dose range of 3–15 mg per day.

(b)
$$4\,mg = 1\,mL \quad \text{(strength)}$$
$$5\,mg = x\,mL \quad \text{(dose)}$$
$$\frac{4\,mg}{1\,mL} = \frac{5\,mg}{x\,mL}$$
$$5 = 4x$$
$$\frac{5}{4} = x$$
$$1.25 = x$$

So, you would administer 1.3 mL.

Parenteral Medications Supplied in Powdered Form

Some parenteral medications are unstable when stored in liquid form, so they are packaged in powdered form. Before they can be administered, the powder in the vial must be diluted with a liquid (*diluent* or *solvent*). This process is referred to as *reconstitution*.

NOTE

If there are no directions for reconstitution on the label or package insert, consult appropriate resources such as the *PDR*, the pharmacist, or the prescribing information on the manufacturer's Web site before reconstituting.

Sterile water for injection and 0.9% sodium chloride (normal saline) are the most commonly used *diluents*. Both the type and amount of diluent to be used must be determined when reconstituting parenteral medications. This information is found on the medication label or package insert. Because many reconstituted parenteral medications can be administered intramuscularly or intravenously, it is essential to verify the route ordered **before** reconstituting the medication, because different routes may require different strengths.

Drugs dissolve completely in the diluent. Some drugs do not add any volume to the amount of diluent added, whereas other drugs increase the amount of total volume. This increase in volume is called the *displacement factor*. For example, directions for a 1 g powdered medication may state to add 2 mL of diluent to provide an approximate volume of 2.5 mL. When the 2 mL of diluent is added, the 1 g of powdered drug displaces an additional 0.5 mL for a total volume of 2.5 mL. The available strength after reconstitution is 1 g in 2.5 mL or 400 mg/mL.

To reconstitute a powdered medication:

- Follow the directions on the label or package insert exactly as specified.
- Check the expiration dates of the drug and the diluent.
- Add the diluent to the vial.
- Shake, roll, or invert the vial as directed.
- Make sure that the powder is fully dissolved.

EXAMPLE 9.7

The prescriber ordered *ceftriaxone 250 mg IM stat* to treat a patient who has gonorrhea.

Read the label and the directions for reconstitution in • Figure 9.7 determine how to prepare and administer this cephalosporin antibiotic.

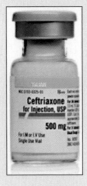

| | Amount of Diluent to be Added | |
Vial Dosage Size	250 mg/mL	350 mg/mL
250 mg	0.9 mL	—
500 mg	1.8 mL	1.0 mL
1 g	3.6 mL	2.1 mL
2 g	7.2 mL	4.2 mL

• **Figure 9.7**
Ceftriaxone vial and portion of reconstitution directions.

Directions for Use

Intramuscular Administration

Reconstitute ceftriaxone for injection powder with sterile water for injection. Inject diluent into vial, shake vial thoroughly to form solution.

After reconstitution, each 1 mL of solution contains approximately 250 mg or 350 mg equivalent of ceftriaxone, according to the amount of diluent indicated.

As with all intramuscular preparations, ceftriaxone for injection, USP, should be injected well within the body of a relatively large muscle; aspiration helps to avoid unintentional injection into a blood vessel.

To prepare the solution, inject 1.8 mL of air into the vial of sterile water for injection and withdraw 1.8 mL of sterile water. Then inject the 1.8 mL of sterile water into the 500 mg ceftriaxone vial and shake well to form a solution. • **Figure 9.8.**

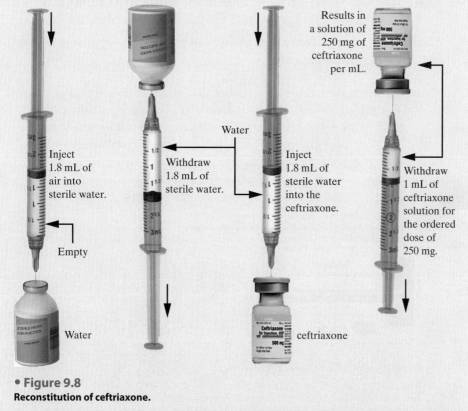

• **Figure 9.8**
Reconstitution of ceftriaxone.

Now the vial contains a reconstituted solution in which 1 mL = 250 mg.

So, you would withdraw 1 mL from the vial and administer it to the patient.

> **NOTE**
>
> The label in Example 9.7 states that when 1.8 mL of diluent is added, the resulting solution has a strength of 250 mg/ mL. There is an approximate volume of 2 mL due to the displacement factor of 0.2 mL, which adds 0.2 mL to the 1.8 mL of diluent, to yield a total solution of 2 mL.

When you reconstitute a multiple-dose vial of powdered medication, it is important that you clearly label the vial with the following:

1. date and time of preparation
2. strength of the solution
3. date and time that the reconstituted solution will expire
4. storage directions
5. your initials

ALERT

Proper labeling of reconstituted medication is critical for safe administration.

Suppose that at 6 P.M. on January 23, 2013, Marie Colon, R.N., reconstitutes a drug to a strength of 50 mg/mL, which will retain its potency for one week if kept refrigerated. Nurse Colon would write the following information on the label:

> *1/23/2013, 1800h, 50 mg/mL,*
> *Expires 1/30/2013, 1800h,*
> *Keep refrigerated, MC*

EXAMPLE 9.8

Order: *Unasyn (ampicillin sodium/sulbactam sodium) 1,700 mg IM q6h.* Read the drug label and portion of the package insert in • Figure 9.9. The package insert indicates that the solution must be used within one hour of preparation.

(a) How much diluent must be added to the vial?

(b) If Nurse Susan Green reconstitutes the Unasyn at 0600h on February 1, 2013, complete the label she will place on the vial.

(c) Determine how many milliliters of this antibiotic Nurse Green will give the patient.

(a) First, prepare the solution. Because the vial contains 3 g, inject 6.4 mL of air into a vial of Sterile Water for Injection and withdraw 6.4 mL of sterile water. Add the sterile water to the Unasyn 3 g vial and be sure the solution is completely mixed.

(b) Nurse Green would write the following on the label:

> *2/1/2013, 0600h, reconstituted strength 375 mg/mL.*
> *Expires 2/1/2013, 0700h, SG*

NOTE

If the vial label does not contain reconstitution directions, refer to the drug package insert or contact the pharmacist. If directions are given for both IM and IV reconstitution, be careful to use the directions appropriate for the route prescribed.

NOTE

When reconstituting a multiple-strength parenteral medication, select a solution strength that results in a volume appropriate for the route of administration, for example, a volume of no more than 3 mL per IM dose. Also, consider the patient's age and size.

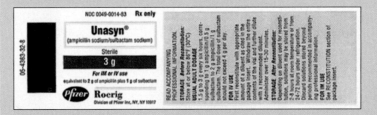

Preparation for Intramuscular Injection

1.5 g and 3.0 g Standard Vials:Vials for intramuscular use may be reconstituted with Sterile Water for Injection USP, 0.5% Lidocaine Hydrochloride Injection USP or 2% Lidocaine Hydrochloride Injection USP.Consult the following table for recommended volumes to be added to obtain solutions containing 375 mg UNASYN per mL (250 mg ampicillin/125 mg sulbactam per mL). Note:Use only freshly prepared solutions and administer within one hour after preparation.

UNASYN Vial Size	Volume of Diluent to be Added	Withdrawal Volume*
There is sufficient excess present to allow withdrawal and administration of the stated volumes.		
1.5 g	3.2 mL	4.0 mL
3.0 g	6.4 mL	8.0 mL

• **Figure 9.9**
Drug label and portion of package insert for Unasyn.

(c) To calculate the amount of this solution, you need to convert the milligrams to milliliters.

DIMENSIONAL ANALYSIS

$$1{,}700 \text{ mg} \times \frac{? \, mL}{? \, mg} = ? \text{ mL}$$

The vial contains 375 mg per 1 mL, so the unit fraction is $\dfrac{1 \, mL}{375 \, mg}$

$$1{,}700 \, \overline{mg} \times \frac{1 \, mL}{375 \, \overline{mg}} = 4.533 \text{ mL}$$

FORMULA METHOD

D (desired dose) = 1,700 mg

H (dose on hand) = 375 mg

Q (dosage unit)   = 1 mL

X (unknown)   = ? mL

Fill in the formula $\dfrac{D}{H} \times Q = X$

$$\frac{1700 \, mg}{375 \, mg} \times 1 \, mL = ? \, mL$$

Cancel $\dfrac{1700 \, \overline{mg}}{375 \, \overline{mg}} \times 1 \, ml = ? \, mL$

Multiply $4.533 \times 1 \, mL = 4.533 \, mL$

So, Nurse Green would withdraw 4.5 mL and administer it to the patient in two injections.

EXAMPLE 9.9

An order requires 80 mg of a drug to be administered IM stat. The vial has the following three choices of strength after reconstitution:

> 10 mg/mL
> 20 mg/mL
> 40 mg/mL

For each of the three strengths:

(a) Determine the required volume of the solution to be administered.

(b) Choose the most appropriate strength.

NOTE

In Example 9.9, the *stronger* the strength (concentration) of the reconstituted drug, the *smaller* the volume to be administered.

DIMENSIONAL ANALYSIS

(a) To calculate the amount of the 10 mg/mL solution (weakest strength), you need to convert the milligrams prescribed to milliliters.

$$80 \text{ mg} \times \frac{? \, mL}{? \, mg} = ? \text{ mL}$$

- The vial contains 10 mg per 1 mL, so, the unit fraction is $\dfrac{1 \, mL}{10 \, mg}$

$$80 \, \overline{mg} \times \frac{1 \, mL}{10 \, \overline{mg}} = 8 \text{ mL}$$

RATIO & PROPORTION

(a) Using 10 mg/mL (weakest strength)

Think:

$$10 \, mg = 1 \, mL \quad \text{(strength)}$$
$$80 \, mg = x \, mL \quad \text{(dose)}$$

One way to set up the proportion is

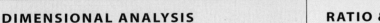

$$\frac{10 \, mg}{1 \, mL} = \frac{80 \, mg}{x \, mL}$$

$$80 = 10x$$

$$8 \, mL = x$$

- Using the 20 mg/mL solution (moderate strength), the unit fraction is $\dfrac{1\ mL}{20\ mg}$

$$80\ \cancel{mg} \times \frac{1\ mL}{20\ \cancel{mg}} = 4\ mL$$

- Using the 40 mg/mL solution (strongest strength), the unit fraction is $\dfrac{1\ mL}{40\ mg}$

$$80\ \cancel{mg} \times \frac{1\ mL}{40\ \cancel{mg}} = 2\ mL$$

Using 20 mg/mL (moderate strength)

Think:

$$20\,mg = 1\,mL \quad \text{(strength)}$$
$$80\,mg = x\,mL \quad \text{(dose)}$$

One way to set up the proportion is

$$\frac{20\,mg}{1\,mL} \diagdown\!\!\!= \frac{80\,mg}{x\,mL}$$

$$80 = 20x$$
$$4\,mL = x$$

Using 40 mg/mL (strongest strength)

Think:

$$40\,mg = 1\,mL \quad \text{(strength)}$$
$$80\,mg = x\,mL \quad \text{(dose)}$$

One way to set up the proportion is

$$\frac{40\,mg}{1\,mL} \diagdown\!\!\!= \frac{80\,mg}{x\,mL}$$

$$80 = 40x$$
$$2\,mL = x$$

In summary:

(Weakest)	10 mg/mL	requires 8 mL
(Moderate)	20 mg/mL	requires 4 mL
(Strongest)	40 mg/mL	requires 2 mL

(b) **Weakest: 10 mg/mL** requires 8 mL to be administered. However, IM volumes are generally less that 3 mL. Therefore, this strength *should not be selected.*

Moderate: 20 mg/mL requires 4 mL to be administered. However, IM volumes are generally less that 3 mL. Therefore, this strength is a *poor choice.* However, the 4 mL could be divided into two syringes and administered at two different sites.

Strongest: 40 mg/mL requires 2 mL to be administered. This is less than 3 mL and is the *best choice.*

EXAMPLE 9.10

NOTE

After you reconstitute the Pfizerpen, you would write the following information on the label: 7/27/13, 0600h, 1mL = 250,000 units.

A prescriber ordered *Pfizerpen (penicillin potassium) 200,000 units IM stat and q6h.* Read the label in ● Figure 9.10 and calculate how many milliliters of this penicillin antibiotic you will administer to the patient.

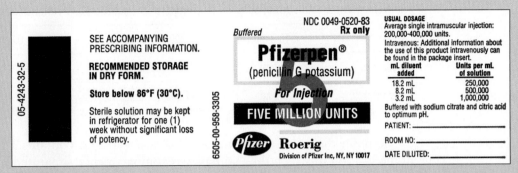

• Figure 9.10
Drug label for Pfizerpen.

(Reg. trademark of Pfizer Inc. Reproduced with permission.)

First, reconstitute the solution. The label lists three options: 250,000 units/mL, 500,000 units/mL, and 1,000,000 units/mL. If you choose the first option, 18.2 mL of diluent must be added to obtain a dosage strength of 250,000 units/mL.

Now, inject 18.2 mL of air into a vial of sterile water for injection and then withdraw 18.2 mL of sterile water. Add the sterile water to the Pfizerpen vial and shake well. Now the vial contains a solution in which 1 mL = 250,000 units.

To calculate the amount of this solution to be administered, you need to convert units to milliliters.

> **NOTE**
>
> Some medications must be reconstituted immediately before administering them because they lose potency rapidly. Ampicillin, for example, must be used within one hour of being reconstituted.

FORMULA METHOD

D (desired dose) = 200,000 units
H (dose on hand) = 250,000 units
Q (dosage unit)   = 1 mL
X (unknown)   = ? mL

Fill in the formula $\dfrac{D}{H} \times Q = X$

$$\dfrac{200,000\,units}{250,000\,units} \times 1\,mL = {?}\,mL$$

Cancel $\dfrac{\overset{4}{\cancel{200,000}}\ \cancel{units}}{\underset{5}{\cancel{250,000}}\ \cancel{units}} \times 1\,ml = {?}\,mL$

Multiply $\dfrac{4}{5} \times 1\,mL = 0.8\,mL$

RATIO & PROPORTION

250,000 units = 1 mL   (strength)
200,000 units = x mL   (dose)

$$\dfrac{250,000\,units}{1\,mL} = \dfrac{200,000\,units}{x\,mL}$$

$$200,000 = 250,000x$$

$$\dfrac{200,000}{250,000} = x$$

$$0.8 = x$$

So, you would withdraw 0.8 mL from the vial and administer it to the patient.

In Example 9.10, if a *stronger concentration* had been chosen for the reconstitution, then a *smaller volume* of the solution would be administered. The calculations would be similar to those just completed. The last two lines of the following table show the volumes for the other two options.

Concentration	Amount of diluent	Strength of the solution	Volume to administer
Weakest	18.2 mL	250,000 units/mL	0.8 mL
Moderate	8.2 mL	500,000 units/mL	0.4 mL
Strongest	3.2 mL	1,000,000 units/mL	0.2 mL

Some medications are manufactured in a vial that contains a single dose of medication in which the vial has two compartments, separated by a rubber stopper. The top portion contains a sterile liquid (diluent), and the bottom portion contains the medication in powder form. When pressure is applied to the top of the vial, the rubber stopper that separates the medication from the diluent is released. This allows the diluent and powder to mix. • Figure 9.11.

How to use a Mix-O Vial

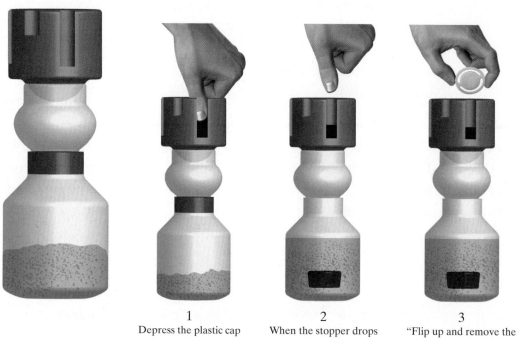

1
Depress the plastic cap so the diluent can mix into the bottom chamber

2
When the stopper drops into the bottom chamber, it allows the diluent to mix with the drug"

3
"Flip up and remove the protective cover, and insert needle squarely through the center to aspirate medication"

• **Figure 9.11**
How to prepare a Mix-O Vial.

EXAMPLE 9.11

The prescriber ordered *Cortef (hydrocortisone) 200 mg IM q6h.* You have a mix-o-vial of Cortef 500 mg. The directions on the label state: "Each mL when mixed contains 125 mg of Cortef." How many milliliters will you administer?

First, reconstitute the solution. Depress the plastic cover and allow the diluent into the bottom chamber of the vial and be sure that the powder is dissolved. See Figure 9.11.

Now the vial contains a solution in which 1 mL = 125 mg

To calculate the amount of this solution to be administered, you need to convert mg to milliliters.

DIMENSIONAL ANALYSIS

$$200 \text{ mg} \times \frac{? \text{ mL}}{? \text{ mg}} = ? \text{ mL}$$

The vial contains 125 mg per 1 mL, so the unit fraction is $\dfrac{1 \text{ mL}}{125 \text{ mg}}$

$$\overset{8}{200} \text{ mg} \times \frac{1 \text{ mL}}{\underset{5}{125} \text{ mg}} = 1.6 \text{ mL}$$

RATIO & PROPORTION

$$125 \text{ mg} = 1 \text{ mL} \quad [\text{Strength}]$$
$$200 \text{ mg} = x \text{ mL} \quad [\text{dose}]$$

$$\frac{125\,mg}{1\,mL} = \frac{200\,mg}{x\,mL}$$

$$200 = 125x$$

$$\frac{200}{125} = x$$

$$1.6 = x$$

So, you would administer 1.6 mL of Cortef.

Heparin

Heparin sodium is a potent anticoagulant that inhibits clot formation and blood coagulation. Heparin is a high-alert drug and can be administered subcutaneously or intravenously. It is *never given intramuscularly because of the danger of hematomas*. According to the ISMP, anticoagulant medications are more likely to cause harm due to complex dosing, insufficient monitoring, and inconsistent patient compliance. The Joint Commission now requires a National Patient Safety Goal to reduce the likelihood of patient harm associated with use of anticoagulant therapy.

Like insulin, penicillin, and some other medications, heparin is supplied and ordered in units. Heparin is available in single and multidose vials, as well as in commercially prepared IV solutions. It is available in a variety of strengths, ranging from 10 units/mL to 50,000 units/mL. See • Figure 9.12(a). Heparin is also available in prepackaged syringes. Lovenox (enoxaprin) and Fragmin (dalteparin sodium) are examples of low molecular weight heparin. They are used to prevent and treat deep vein thrombosis (DVT) following abdominal surgery, hip or knee replacement, unstable angina, and acute coronary syndromes.

ALERT

Fatal hemorrhages have occurred in pediatric patients due to medication errors in which 1 mL heparin sodium injection vials were confused with 1 mL "catheter lock flush" vials. Carefully examine all heparin sodium injection vials to confirm the correct vial choice prior to administration of the drug.

Practice Label

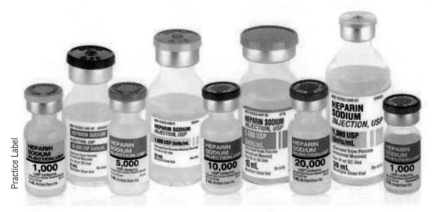

• **Figure 9.12(a)**
Heparin vials.

Heparin requires close monitoring of the patient's blood work because of the bleeding potential associated with anticoagulant drugs. To assure accuracy of dose measurement, a 1 mL syringe should be used to administer heparin subcutaneously. Healthcare providers should know and follow agency policies when administering heparin.

Heparin flush solutions (e.g., Hep-Flush, or Hep-Lock) are used for maintaining the patency of indwelling IV catheters. These solutions are available in strengths of 10 units/mL and 100 units/mL see • **Figure 9.12(b)**. Heparin sodium injection and heparin flush solutions are different and can not be used interchangeably. Note the large differences in dosage strength between heparin sodium (1,000 to 50,000 units/mL) and heparin flush solutions (10 to 100 units/mL). Thus, the healthcare provider must be careful when preparing heparin.

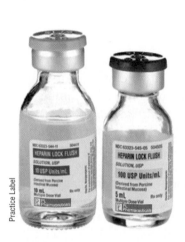

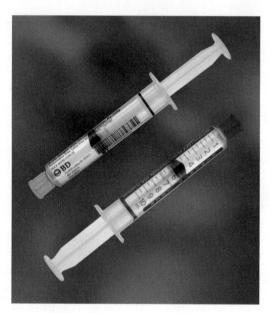

• **Figure 9.12(b)**
Heparin flush.
(For educational purposes only)

Heparin flush syringe.

EXAMPLE 9.12

The prescriber ordered *heparin 4,000 units subcut q12h*. Read the drug label in • Figure 9.13(a).

(a) Calculate the number of milliliters you will administer to the patient.

(b) Indicate the dose on the syringe in • Figure 9.13(b).

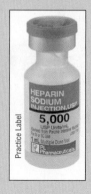

• **Figure 9.13(a)**
Vial of heparin.

(**a**) You want to convert units to milliliters.

$$4,000 \text{ units} = ? \text{ mL}$$

DIMENSIONAL ANALYSIS

(a) You want to convert units to milliliters.

$$4,000 \text{ units} = ? \text{ mL}$$

You cancel the units and obtain the equivalent amount in milliliters.

$$4,000 \text{ units} \times \frac{? \text{ mL}}{? \text{ units}} = ? \text{ mL}$$

The strength on the vial is 5,000 units per milliliter, so the unit fraction is

$$\frac{1 \text{ mL}}{5,000 \text{ units}}$$

$$4,000 \text{ units} \times \frac{1 \text{ mL}}{5,000 \text{ units}} = \frac{4 \text{ mL}}{5} = 0.8 \text{ mL}$$

RATIO & PROPORTION

$$5,000 \text{ units} = 1 \text{ mL} \quad [\text{strength}]$$
$$4,000 \text{ units} = x \text{ mL} \quad [\text{order}]$$

One way to set up the proportion is

$$\frac{5,000 \text{ units}}{1 \text{ mL}} = \frac{4,000 \text{ units}}{x \text{ mL}}$$

$$4,000 = 5,000x$$

$$\frac{4,000}{5,000} = x$$

$$0.8 = x$$

So, you would use a 1 mL syringe and administer 0.8 mL of heparin.

(b)

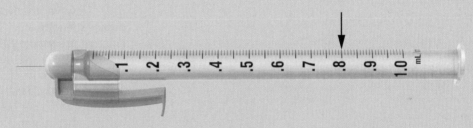

• **Figure 9.13(b)**
Syringe containing 4,000 units of heparin in 0.8 mL.

EXAMPLE 9.13

The prescriber ordered *heparin 4,000 units subcut q12h*. Read the drug label in • Figure 9.14(a).

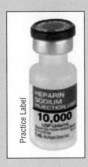

• **Figure 9.14(a)**
Vial of heparin.

(a) Calculate the number of milliliters you will administer to the patient.

(b) Indicate the dose on the syringe shown in • Figure 9.14(b).

FORMULA METHOD

D (desired dose) = 4,000 units

H (dose on hand) = 10,000 units

Q (dosage unit)   = 1 mL

X (unknown)   = ? mL

Fill in the formula $\dfrac{D}{H} \times Q = X$

$$\frac{4,000\,units}{10,000\,units} \times 1\,mL = ?\,mL$$

Cancel $\dfrac{4,\cancel{000}\,\overset{2}{\cancel{units}}}{\cancel{10,000}\,\underset{5}{\cancel{units}}} \times 1\,ml = ?\,mL$

Multiply $\dfrac{2}{5} \times 1\,mL = 0.4\,mL$

RATIO & PROPORTION

$$10,000\,units = 1\,mL \quad [\text{strength}]$$
$$4,000\,units = x\,mL \quad [\text{ordered dose}]$$

One way to set up the proportion is

$$\frac{10,000\,units}{1\,mL} = \frac{4,000\,units}{x\,mL}$$

$$4,000 = 10,000x$$

$$\frac{4,000}{10,000} = x$$

$$0.4 = x$$

ALERT

Observe that, in examples 9.12 and 9.13, the order for heparin is exactly the same (4,000 units subcutaneously q12h). However, the available dosage strengths are different. In example 9.13, the strength (10,000 units/mL) is twice the strength of that in example 9.12 (5,000 units/mL). Therefore, only half the amount of the stronger solution is needed.

So, you would use a 1 mL syringe and administer 0.4 mL of heparin.

(b)

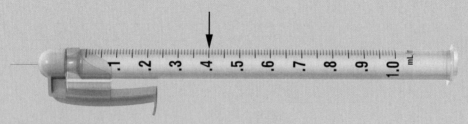

• **Figure 9.14(b)**
Syringe containing 4,000 units of heparin in 0.4 mL.

EXAMPLE 9.14

The prescriber ordered *Fragmin (dalteparin sodium) 120 units/kg subcutaneously q12h* for a patient who weighs 138 pounds. See •Figure 9.15 and determine how many milliliters of this low molecular weight heparin you will need to administer the dose.

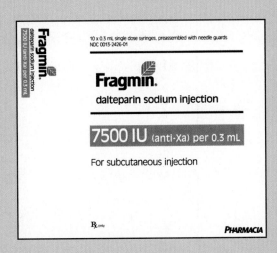

•**Figure 9.15**
Box label for Fragmin single-dose syringes.

Because this example contains a lot of information, it is useful to summarize it as follows:

Given: 138 lb (single unit of measurement)

Known equivalences: 1 kg = 2.2 lb (needed to convert lb to kg)

                          120 units/kg (order)

                          7,500 units/0.3 mL (strength on the drug label)

Volume you want to find: ? mL

DIMENSIONAL ANALYSIS

You want to convert a single unit of measurement (138 lb) to another single unit of measurement (mL).

$$138 \text{ lb} = ? \text{ mL}$$

You want to cancel lb. To do this you must use a unit fraction containing lb in the denominator. Using the equivalence 1 kg = 2.2 lb, this fraction will be $\dfrac{1 \text{ kg}}{2.2 \text{ lb}}$

$$138 \cancel{\text{ lb}} \times \frac{1 \text{ kg}}{2.2 \cancel{\text{ lb}}} = ? \text{ mL}$$

Now, on the left side kg is in the numerator. To cancel the kg will require a unit fraction with kg in the denominator, namely, $\dfrac{120 \text{ units}}{\text{kg}}$

$$138 \cancel{\text{ lb}} \times \frac{1 \text{ kg}}{2.2 \cancel{\text{ lb}}} \times \frac{120 \text{ units}}{\text{kg}} = ? \text{ mL}$$

FORMULA METHOD

First change the weight of 138 pounds to kilograms by dividing by 2.2.

$$\frac{132}{2.2} \approx 62.7$$

So, the patient weighs 62.7 kg.
Because the order is based on the size of the patient, use the formula:

size of the patient × *the order* = *dose*

$$62.7 \, kg \times \frac{120 \, units}{kg} = 7{,}524 \; units$$

Now, you need to convert 7,524 units to milliliters.

D (desired dose) = 7,524 units

H (dose on hand) = 7,500 units

Q (dosage unit)   = 0.3 mL

X (unknown)   = ? mL

Now, on the left side units is in the numerator. To cancel the units will require a fraction with units in the denominator, namely, $\dfrac{0.3\ \text{mL}}{7,500\ \text{units}}$

$$138\ \cancel{\text{lb}} \times \frac{1\ \text{kg}}{2.2\ \cancel{\text{lb}}} \times \frac{120\ \cancel{\text{units}}}{\text{kg}}$$

$$\times \frac{0.3\ \boxed{\text{mL}}}{7500\ \cancel{\text{units}}} = ?\ \text{mL}$$

after cancelation, only mL remains on the left side. This is what you want. Now multiply the numbers

$$138\ \cancel{\text{lb}} \times \frac{\cancel{\text{kg}}}{2.2\ \cancel{\text{lb}}} \times \frac{120\ \cancel{\text{units}}}{\cancel{\text{kg}}}$$

$$\times \frac{0.3\ \text{mL}}{7,500\ \cancel{\text{units}}} = 0.301\ \text{mL}$$

Fill in the formula $\dfrac{D}{H} \times Q = X$

$$\frac{7,524\ units}{7,500\ units} \times 0.3\ mL = ?\ mL$$

Cancel

$$\frac{7,524\ \cancel{units}}{7,500\ \cancel{units}} \times 0.3\ ml = ?\ mL$$

Multiply

$$1.003 \times 0.3\ mL = 0.3009\ mL$$

Therefore, you would need to administer 0.3 mL.

Summary

In this chapter, you learned how to calculate doses for administering parenteral medications in liquid form, the procedure for reconstituting medications in powdered form, and how to calculate dosages for medications supplied in units.

- Medications supplied in powdered form must be reconstituted following the manufacturer's directions.
- You must determine the best dosage strength when there are several options for reconstituting the medication.
- After reconstituting a multiple-dose vial, label the medication vial with the dates and times of both preparation and expiration, storage directions, your initials, and strength.

- When directions on the label are provided for both IM and IV reconstitution, be sure to read the order and the label carefully to determine the necessary amount of diluent to use.
- Heparin is measured in USP units.
- It is especially important that heparin orders be carefully checked with the available dosage strength before calculating the amount to be administered.
- A tuberculin (1 mL) or a 0.5-mL syringe should be used when administering heparin.
- Heparin sodium and heparin flush solutions are different and should never be used interchangeably.

Case Study 9.1

Read the Case Study and answer the questions. Answers can be found in Appendix A.

A 69-year-old male is admitted to the ambulatory surgery unit for a laproscopic repair of a torn meniscus. He reports a past medical history of hypertension, hypercholesterolemia, osteoarthritis, and atrial fibrillation. Past surgical history of bilateral repair of rotator cuffs and right total hip replacement. He is 6 feet tall and weighs 175 pounds. He denies any allergies to food or drugs. His vital signs are: T 98.9 °F; B/P 138/90; P 96; R 18.

Pre-op orders:

- NPO
- IV RL @ 125 mL/h
- ondansetron hydrochloride 4 mg IM stat before anesthesia induction
- fentanyl 75 mcg IVP stat
- Transfer to OR

Post-op orders:

- NPO, progress to clear liquids as tolerated
- IV D5NS @ 125 mL/h until tolerating liquids
- Nexium (esomeprazole magnesium) 20 mg IVP stat
- Morphine sulfate 5 mg IM once if needed for pain
- V/S q15 min × 4, then q30 min × 2h, then q1h × 2h
- Cold compresses to right leg q1h × 20 minutes
- Discharge when stable

Discharge Orders

- losartan potassium-hydrochlorathiazide 100/12.5 mg PO daily
- lovastatin 20 mg PO daily
- escitalopram oxalate 15 mg PO daily
- warfarin 3.75 mg PO daily
- Nexium (esomeprazole magnesium) 20 mg PO 1h ac meals
- hydrocodone 5 mg PO q6h prn pain
- Cold compresses to right leg q1h × 20 minutes
- Make appointment for follow-up in one week

Refer to the labels in • **Figure 9.16** when necessary to answer the following questions.

1. The ondansetron hydrochloride is supplied in vials labeled 32 mg/5 mL

   (a) How many milliliters are needed for the prescribed dose?
   (b) What type of syringe is needed to administer the dose?

2. The fentanyl is supplied in vials labeled 0.05 mg/mL.

   (a) How many milliliters are needed for the prescribed dose?
   (b) What type of syringe is needed to administer the dose?

3. The anesthetist will be administering propofol 2 mg/kg IV q 10 seconds until induction onset.

   (a) How many milliliters will the anesthetist prepare?
   (b) What type of syringe will be used to draw up the propofol?

4. The esomeprazole magnesium is supplied in 40-mg vials, and the label states to reconstitute the powder with 5 mL of Normal Saline. Calculate how many milliliters the patient will receive.

5. During your discharge teaching, you are reviewing the patient's medication vials and dosages.

   (a) Select the correct label for the losartan potassium-hydrochlorathiazide order.
   (b) How many tablets should you instruct the patient to take?

6. (a) Select the correct label for the lovastatin dose.
   (b) How many tablets should you instruct the patient to take?

7. (a) Select the correct label for the escitalopram oxalate dose.
   (b) How many milliliters should you instruct the patient to take?

8. (a) Select the correct label for the hydrocodone dose.
   (b) How many tablets may the patient take in a 24h period?

9. How many tablets of warfarin should you instruct the patient to take each day?

10. How many milligrams of esomeprazole magnesium may the patient take each day?

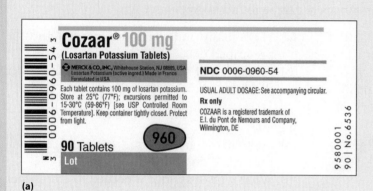

(a)

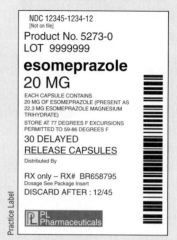

NDC 12345-1234-12
[Not on file]
Product No. 5273-0
LOT 9999999

esomeprazole
20 MG

EACH CAPSULE CONTAINS
20 MG OF ESOMEPRAZOLE (PRESENT AS
22.3 MG ESOMEPRAZOLE MAGNESIUM
TRIHYDRATE)
STORE AT 77 DEGREES F EXCURSIONS
PERMITTED TO 59-86 DEGREES F
30 DELAYED
RELEASE CAPSULES
Distributed By

RX only – RX# BR658795
Dosage See Package Insert
DISCARD AFTER : 12/45

PL Pharmaceuticals

(b) (For educational purposes only)

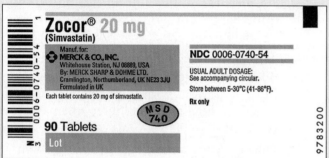

(c)

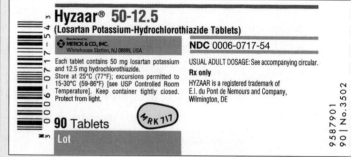

(d)

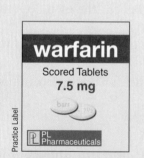

(e) (For educational purposes only)

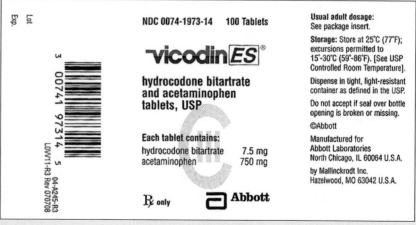

(f)

• **Figure 9.16**
Drug labels for Case Study.

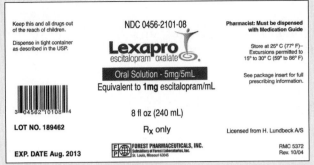

(g)

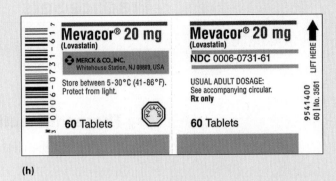

(h)

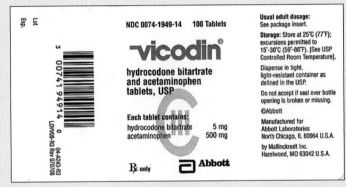

(i)

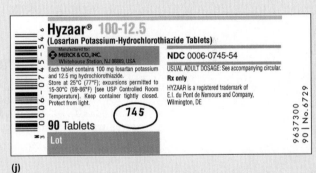

(j)

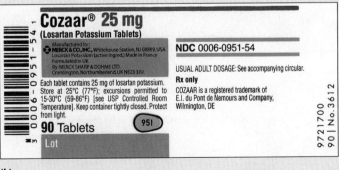

(k)

• **Figure 9.16**
(Continued)

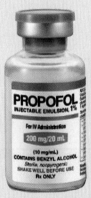

(l) (For educational purposes only)

Workspace

Practice Sets

The answers to *Try These for Practice*, *Exercises*, and *Cumulative Review Exercises* are found in Appendix A. Ask your instructor for the answers to the *Additional Exercises*.

Try These for Practice

Test your comprehension after reading the chapter.

1. Order:

   penicillin G procaine 250,000 units IM q6h

   Read the label in • **Figure 9.17**.
   (a) Calculate the number of milliliters of this antibiotic you would administer to the patient if you use the 8 mL of diluent to reconstitute the drug.
   (b) Indicate the dose by placing an arrow at the most appropriate syringe given.

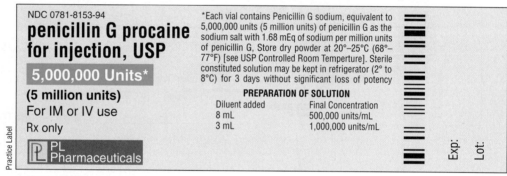

NDC 0781-8153-94	*Each vial contains Penicillin G sodium, equivalent to 5,000,000 units (5 million units) of penicillin G as the sodium salt with 1.68 mEq of sodium per million units of penicillin G, Store dry powder at 20°–25°C (68°–77°F) [see USP Controlled Room Temperture]. Sterile constituted solution may be kept in refrigerator (2° to 8°C) for 3 days without significant loss of potency

penicillin G procaine for injection, USP

5,000,000 Units*

(5 million units)
For IM or IV use
Rx only

PL Pharmaceuticals

PREPARATION OF SOLUTION

Diluent added	Final Concentration
8 mL	500,000 units/mL
3 mL	1,000,000 units/mL

Exp: Lot:

Practice Label

• **Figure 9.17**
Drug label for Penicillin G Procaine.
(For educational purposes only)

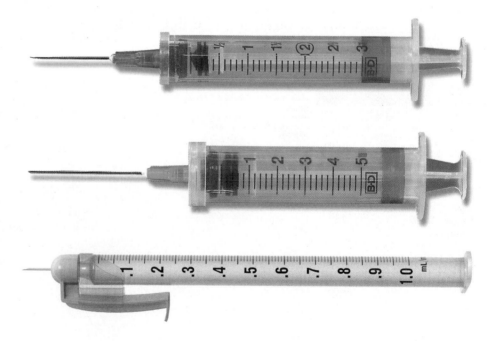

2. Order:

ticarcillin disodium 1 g IM q6h

The label reads, "reconstitute each 1 g of ticarcillin with 2 mL of Sterile Water for Injection or NS and use promptly. The resulting concentration is 1g/2.6 mL."
(a) Calculate the number of milliliters of this antibiotic you would administer to the patient.
(b) Indicate which size syringe you would use and place arrow at the dosage.

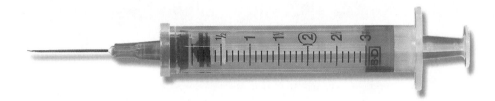

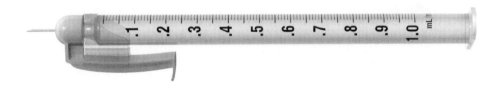

3. Order:

Relistor (methylnaltrexone bromide) 8 mg subcut every other day

The label reads "12 mg/0.6 mL."
(a) Calculate the number of milliliters of this narcotic antagonist you would administer to the patient.
(b) Indicate what size syringe you would use and place arrow at the dosage.

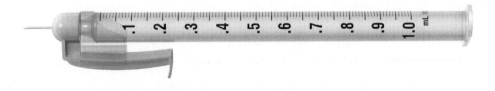

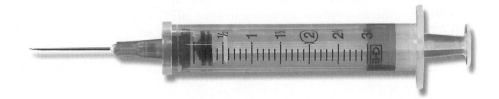

Workspace

4. Order:

Ativan (lorazepam) 0.05 mg/kg IM 20 min before surgery

Read the information in • **Figure 9.18**.
(a) Calculate the number of milliliters of this sedative-hypnotic you would administer to a patient who weighs 85 pounds.
(b) Indicate what size syringe you would use and place an arrow at the dosage.

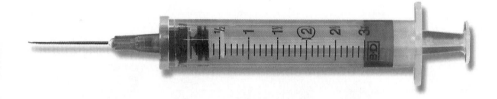

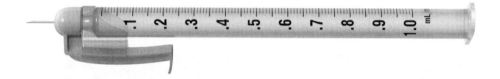

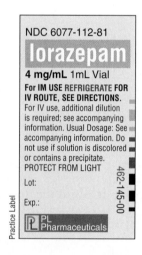

• **Figure 9.18**
Drug label for lorazepam.
(For educational purposes only)

5. Order:

Cefobid (cefoperazone sodium) 1.5g IM q12h

Use the portion of the package insert in • **Figure 9.19**.
(a) What vial would you use for reconstitution?
(b) How much diluent must be added to the vial?
(c) What is the reconstituted volume in the vial?
(d) What is the strength of the reconstituted solution?
(e) How many milliliters would you administer?
(f) How many full doses are in the vial?

Cefotaxime for injection for IM or IV administration should be reconstituted as follows:

Strength	Diluent (mL)	Withdrawable Volume (mL)	Approximate Concentration (mg/mL)
(*) in conventional vials			
500 mg vial* (IM)	2	2.2	230
1 g vial* (IM)	3	3.4	300
2 g vial* (IM)	5	6	330
500 mg vial* (IV)	10	10.2	50
1 g vial* (IV)	10	10.4	95
2 g vial* (IV)	10	11	180

● **Figure 9.19**
A portion of package insert instructions for cefotaxime.

Exercises

Reinforce your understanding in class or at home.

1. The prescriber ordered *Navane (thiothixene hydrochloride) 4 mg IM B.I.D.* The label on the vial reads 5 mg/mL. Calculate how many milliliters of this antipsychotic drug you would administer.

2. The prescriber ordered *Amevive (alefacept) 15 mg IM once per week for 12 weeks.*
   The instructions on the 15-mg vial states "reconstitute with 0.4 mL of the supplied diluent to yield 15 mg/0.5 mL". How many milliliters of this biologic response modifier would you administer?

3. The prescriber ordered *heparin 8,000 units subcut q8h.* Read the label in
   ● **Figure 9.20.**
   (a) How many milliliters of this anticoagulant will you administer?
   (b) What size syringe will you use?

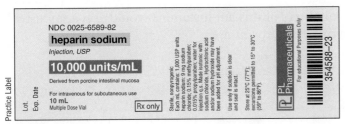

● **Figure 9.20**
Drug label for heparin.
(For educational purposes only)

4. The prescriber ordered *Unasyn (ampicillin sodium/sublactam sodium) 2g IM q6h.* Use the information from the package insert in ● **Figure 9.21.**
   (a) How much diluent must be added to the vial?
   (b) What is the reconstituted volume in the vial?
   (c) What is the strength of the reconstituted solution?
   (d) How many milliliters of this antibiotic will you administer?

Workspace

Workspace

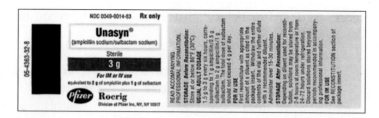

Unasyn Vial Size	Volume of Diluent to Be Added	Withdrawal Volume
1.5 g	3.2 mL	4 mL
3 g	6.4 mL	8 mL

• **Figure 9.21**
Drug label for and portion of package insert for Unasyn.

5. The prescriber ordered *lincomycin hydrochloride 600 mg IM q12h*. Read the label in • **Figure 9.22**. Calculate how many milliliters of this lincosamide antibiotic you would administer.

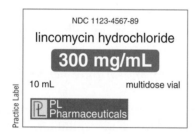

• **Figure 9.22**
Drug label for lincomycin.
(For educational purposes only)

6. The prescriber ordered *Benadryl (diphenhydramine hydrochloride) 45 mg IM q4h*. Read the label in • **Figure 9.23**. The manufacturer states not to exceed 400 mg/day.
   (a) Is this a safe dose?
   (b) How many milliliters of this antihistamine would you administer?
   (c) What size syringe would you use?

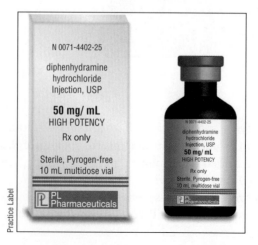

• **Figure 9.23**
Drug box and vial for diphenhydramine hydrochloride.
(For educational purposes only)

7. The prescriber ordered *fentanyl citrate 55 mcg IM prn pain*. Read the label in • **Figure 9.24.**
   (a) How many milliliters of this narcotic analgesic would you administer?
   (b) Which size syringe would you use?

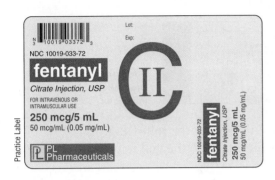

• **Figure 9.24**
Drug label for fentanyl citrate.
(For educational purposes only)

8. The prescriber ordered *ceftriaxone sodium 1,200 mg IM q12h for 4 days*. The instructions in the package insert state to reconstitute the 1g or 2g vial by adding 2.1 mL or 4.2 mL, respectively, of sterile water for injection, yields 350 mg/mL.
   (a) What vial would you use?
   (b) How many milliliters of this cephalosporin antibiotic would you administer?
   (c) What size syringe would you use?

9. The prescriber ordered *morphine sulfate 0.2 mg/kg IM q4h prn moderate-severe pain*. Read the label in • **Figure 9.25**.
   (a) How many milliliters of this narcotic analgesic would you administer to a patient who weighs 154 pounds?
   (b) What size syringe would you use?
   (c) The package insert states that the maximum dose is 10 mg/24h. Is the patient receiving a safe dose?

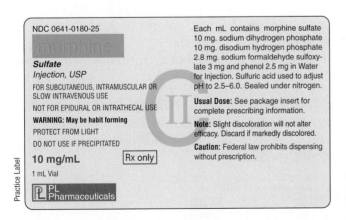

• **Figure 9.25**
Drug label for morphine sulfate.
(For educational purposes only)

10. The prescriber ordered *Kenalog (triamcinolone) 15 mg into the knee joint stat*. The medication is available in a 5 mL multi-dose vial with a strength of 10 mg/mL.
    (a) How many milliliters of this synthetic glucocorticoid will the patient receive?
    (b) How many doses of 15 mg are contained in the vial?

Workspace

Workspace

11. The prescriber ordered *leuprolide acetate injection 1 mg subcut now*. Read the information in • **Figure 9.26**.
    (a) How many milliliters of this hormone would you prepare?
    (b) What size syringe would you use?
    (c) How many doses are in the vial?

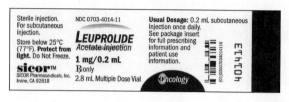

• **Figure 9.26**
Drug label for leuprolide acetate injection.

12. Use the label in • **Figure 9.27** to answer the following:
    (a) How much diluent must be added to the vial to prepare 500,000 units/mL strength?
    (b) What strength would be available if you added 18.2 mL of diluent?
    (c) What is the total dose of penicillin G potassium in the vial?
    (d) The prescriber ordered *penicillin G potassium 2 million units IM q4h*. Which dosage strength would you use?
    (e) How many milliliters of this antibiotic would you administer?

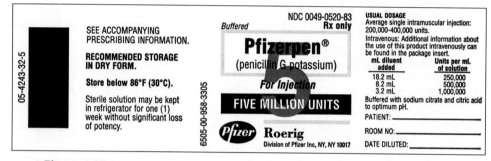

• **Figure 9.27**
Drug label for Pfizerpen.

13. The prescriber ordered *Ancef (cefazolin sodium) 250 mg IM q8h*. The directions for the 1g vial state "for IM administration add 2.5 mL of Sterile Water for Injection. Provides an approximate volume of 3 mL."
    (a) What is the total amount of Ancef in the vial?
    (b) How many milliliters of this cephalosporin antibiotic would you administer?

14. The prescriber ordered *furosemide 30 mg IM B.I.D.* Read the label in • **Figure 9.28**.
    (a) How many milliliters of this loop diuretic would you administer?
    (b) What size syringe would you use?

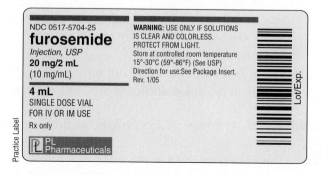

• **Figure 9.28**
Drug label for furosemide.
(For educational purposes only)

15. The prescriber ordered *streptomycin 15 mg/kg IM stat.* Use the label in • **Figure 9.29** to calculate the number of milliliters you would administer to a patient who weighs 150 pounds.)

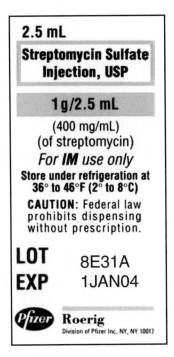

• **Figure 9.29**
Drug label for streptomycin.

16. The prescriber ordered *oxacillin 500* mg *IM q6h.* The instructions on the 2 g vial states to reconstitute the powder with 11.5 mL of Sterile Water for Injection, yielding 250 mg/1.5 mL.
    (a) What is the strength of the reconstituted solution?
    (b) How many milliliters would you administer?

17. The prescriber ordered *Humalog Mix 75/25 15 units subcut ac breakfast.* Use the label in • **Figure 9.30** to determine the following:
    (a) How many units will you administer?
    (b) How many units are contained in the pen?

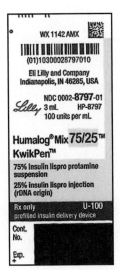

• **Figure 9.30**
Drug label for Humalog Mix 75/25.

Workspace

Workspace

18. Use the insulin "sliding scale" below to determine how much insulin you would give to a patient whose blood glucose is 244.

The prescriber ordered *Humulin R Unit 100 insulin subcutaneously for blood glucose levels as follows:*

Glucose less than 160	no insulin
Glucose 160–220	give 2 units
Glucose 221–280	give 4 units
Glucose 281–340	give 6 units
Glucose 341–400	give 8 units
Glucose more than 400	hold insulin and call MD stat

19. A patient weighs 110 pounds. The daily recommended safe dose range for a certain drug is 0.03–0.04 mg/kg.
    (a) What is the minimum number of milligrams of this drug that this patient should receive each day?
    (b) What is the maximum number of milligrams of this drug that this patient should receive each day?

20. The prescriber ordered *terbutaline 0.25 mg subcut q15 to 30 minutes, no more than 0.5 mg in 4 h*. Read the label in • **Figure 9.31** to answer the following:
    (a) How many milliliters would you administer?
    (b) What size syringe would you use?
    (c) How many milliliters of this bronchodilator may the patient receive in 30 minutes?

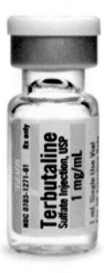

• **Figure 9.31**
Drug label for terbutaline.

Additional Exercises

Now, test yourself!

1. The prescriber ordered *ampicillin 750 mg IM q6h*.
   The directions for the 1 g ampicillin vial state, "reconstitute with 3.5 mL of diluent to yield 250 mg/mL." How many milliliters will contain the prescribed dose?

2. The prescriber ordered *Unasyn 1.5 g IM q6h.*
   The package insert for the label in •**Figure 9.32** states: Add 3.2 mL of sterile water for injection to yield 375 mg/mL (250 mg ampicillin and 125 mg sulbactam/mL). Calculate how many milliliters you will administer.

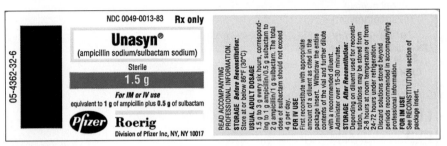

•**Figure 9.32**
Drug label for Unasyn.
(Reg. Trademark of Pfizer Inc. Reproduced with permission.)

3. The prescriber ordered *methylprednisolone 80 mg IM every other day for 1 month.* Read the label in •**Figure 9.33**.
   (a) Calculate how many milliliters of this adrenal corticosteroid you will administer.
   (b) What size syringe will you use to administer the dose?

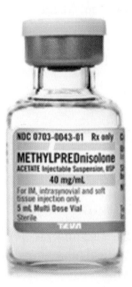

•**Figure 9.33**
Drug label for methylprednisolone.

4. The prescriber ordered *Claforan (cefotaxime) 1,200 mg IM q12h.* The directions for the 1 g vial state: "Add 3.2 mL of diluent to yield an approximate concentration of 300 mg/mL. The directions for the 2 g vial state: Add 5 mL of diluent to yield an approximate concentration of 330 mg/mL."
   (a) Which vial will you use?
   (b) How many milliliters will you administer?

5. The prescriber ordered *streptomycin 500 mg IM q12h for 7 days.* Read the label in •**Figure 9.34** and calculate how many milliliters of this antibiotic you will administer.

Workspace

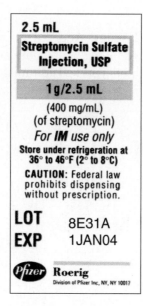

2.5 mL

Streptomycin Sulfate
Injection, USP

1 g/2.5 mL

(400 mg/mL)
(of streptomycin)
For IM use only
Store under refrigeration at
36° to 46°F (2° to 8°C)
CAUTION: Federal law
prohibits dispensing
without prescription.

LOT   8E31A
EXP   1JAN04

Pfizer Roerig
Division of Pfizer Inc, NY, NY 10017

• **Figure 9.34**
Drug label for Streptomycin.

(Reg. Trademark of Pfizer Inc. Reproduced with permission.)

6. The prescriber ordered *Stelazine (trifluoperazine hydrochloride) 1.4 mg IM (give deep IM) q6h prn.* The label on the 10 mL multidose vial reads 2 mg/mL injection.
   (a) Calculate the number of milliliters of this antipsychotic drug that contain this dose.
   (b) What size syringe will you use?

7. The prescriber ordered 1 dose of the pneumovax vaccine IM for a patient. Read the label in • **Figure 9.35**.
   (a) How many milliliters will you administer?
   (b) What size syringe will you use to administer the dose?
   (c) How many doses are in the vial?

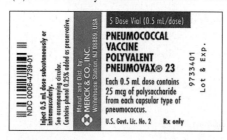

5 Dose Vial (0.5 mL/dose)

**PNEUMOCOCCAL
VACCINE
POLYVALENT
PNEUMOVAX® 23**

Each 0.5 mL dose contains
25 mcg of polysaccharide
from each capsular type of
pneumococcus.

U.S. Govt. Lic. No. 2   Rx only

Inject 0.5 mL dose subcutaneously or intramuscularly.
See accompanying circular.
Contains phenol 0.25% added as preservative.

Manuf. and Dist. by
MERCK & CO., INC.
Whitehouse Station, NJ 08889, USA

NDC 0006-4739-01

9733401   Lot & Exp.

• **Figure 9.35**
Drug label for Pneumovax.

8. The prescriber ordered *promethazine hydrochloride 12.5 mg IM q4h prn nausea/vomiting.* Read the label in • **Figure 9.36** and calculate how many milliliters of this antiemetic drug you will administer.

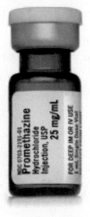

• **Figure 9.36**
Drug label for promethazine hydrochloride.

9. The prescriber ordered *gentamicin 60 mg IM q12h*. The drug is supplied in a 20 mL multidose vial. The label reads 40 mg/mL. How many milliliters will you administer?

10. The prescriber ordered *morphine sulfate 5 mg subcutaneously q4h prn*. The drug is supplied in a 1 mL vial that is labeled 15 mg/mL.
    (a) How many milliliters will you administer?
    (b) What size syringe will you use?

11. The prescriber ordered *Lasix (furosemide) 30 mg IM stat*. The drug is supplied in a vial labeled 40 mg/mL. How many milliliters will you administer?

12. A patient is to receive *Ativan (lorazepam) 3 mg IM, 2 hours before surgery*. The drug is supplied in a vial labeled 4 mg/mL. How many milliliters of this sedative hypenotic will you administer?

13. Use the insulin "sliding scale" below to determine how much insulin you will give to a patient whose blood glucose is 320.

    Order: Give Humulin R Unit-100 insulin subcutaneously for blood glucose levels as follows:

    Glucose less than 160-no insulin
    Glucose 160–220-2 units
    Glucose 221–280-4 units
    Glucose 281–340-6 units
    Glucose 341–400-8 units
    Glucose more than 400-hold insulin and call MD stat

14. The prescriber ordered *heparin 3,500 units subcutaneously q12h*. The label on the vial states 5,000 units/mL.
    (a) How many milliliters will you administer?
    (b) What size syringe will you use?

15. The prescriber ordered *Humulin N insulin pen 15 units subcut ac breakfast*. Read the label in • **Figure 9.37** and determine how many doses are contained in the Pen.

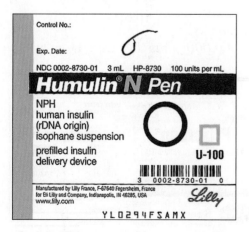

• **Figure 9.37**
Drug label for Humulin N insulin pen.

16. Read the information in • **Figure 9.38** and use the highest concentration to determine how many milliliters contain 650,000 units.

Workspace

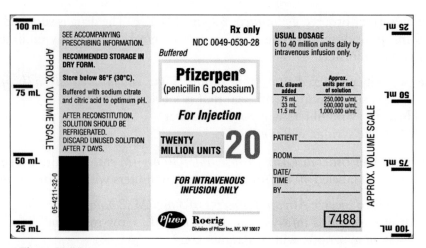

17. A patient is to receive *atropine sulfate 0.2 mg IM 30 minutes before surgery*. The vial is labeled 0.4 mg/mL.
    (a) How many milliliters of this anticholenergic drug will you administer?
    (b) What size syringe will you use?

18. The order is *Phenergan (promethazine hydrochloride) 12.5 mg IM q4h prn nausea*. The vial is labeled 50 mg/mL.
    (a) How many milliliters of this antiemetic drug will you administer?
    (b) What size syringe will you use?

19. The order is *Thorazine (chlorpromazine hydrochloride) 40 mg IM q6h prn for agitation*. The vial is labeled 25 mg/mL.
    (a) How many milliliters of this antipsychotic drug will you administer?
    (b) What size syringe will you use?

20. Use the information in • **Figure 9.39** and answer the following:
    (a) How much diluent must be added to the vial to prepare a 250,000 units/mL strength?
    (b) How much diluent must be added to the vial to prepare a 500,000 units/mL strength?
    (c) What is the total dose of this vial?
    (d) The order is *penicillin G 2,000,000 units IM stat*. How will you prepare this dose?

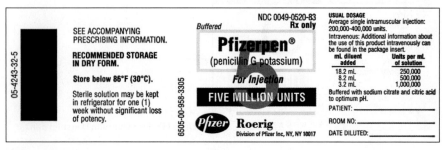

Cumulative Review Exercises

Review your mastery of previous chapters.

Read the label in • **Figure 9.40** to answer questions 1 through 4.

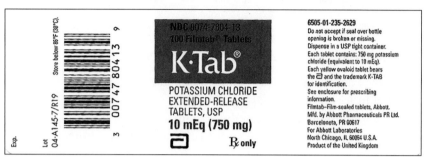

• **Figure 9.40**
Drug label for K-Tab.

1. What is the generic name of this drug?

2. What is the route of administration?

3. What is the name of the manufacturer?

4. A patient is to receive 750 mg twice a day. How many milliequivalents will you prepare?

5. The prescriber ordered *Biaxin (clarithromycin) 500 mg PO q12h*. Read the label in • **Figure 9.41(a)**.
   (a) How many milliliters will the container have when reconstituted?
   (b) What is the dosage strength when reconstituted?
   (c) Calculate the number of milliliters you will administer.
   (d) Indicate the dose on the medication cup in • **Figure 9.41(b)**.

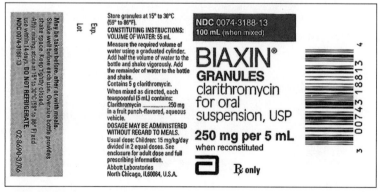

• **Figure 9.41(a)**
Drug label for Biaxin.

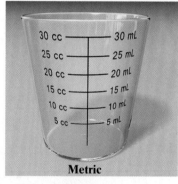

• **Figure 9.41(b)**
Medication Cup.

Read the label in • **Figure 9.42** to answer questions 6 through 9.

6. What is the generic name of this drug?

7. What is the route of administration?

8. How many milliliters must be added to result in a 5 mg/mL strength?

Workspace

Workspace

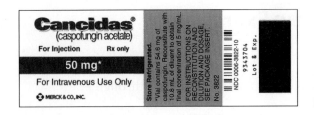

• Figure 9.42
Drug label for Cancidas.

9. A patient is to receive 70 mg. How many vials are needed?

10. The prescriber ordered *Zostavax 1 vial subcut stat.*
    Read the label in • **Figure 9.43.**
    (a) Determine how many milliliters the patient will receive.
    (b) Draw a line on the appropriate syringe to indicate the dosage.

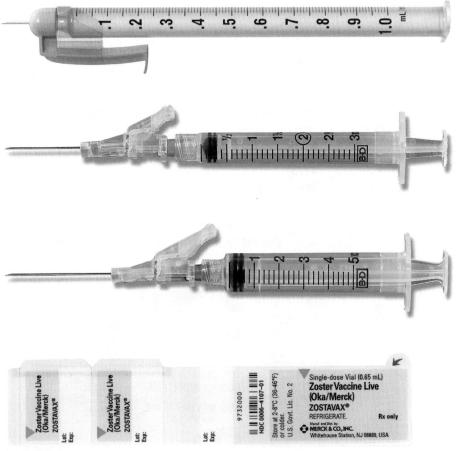

• Figure 9.43
Drug label for Zostavax.

11. How many grams of dextrose are contained in 2,000 mL of a 10% dextrose solution?

12. The prescriber ordered *Suprax (cefixime) 400 mg PO daily.* The label on the 75 mL bottle reads 100 mg/5 mL. How many milliliters of this cephalosporin antibiotic would the patient receive?

13. The prescriber ordered *Crixivan (indinavir sulfate) 800 mg PO q8h, 1 h before meals or 2 h after meals.* Read the label in •**Figure 9.44** and calculate how many capsules of this protease inhibitor drug you would administer.

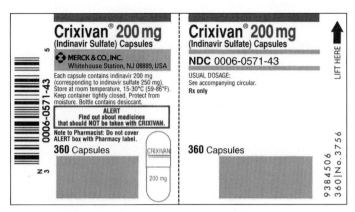

• **Figure 9.44**
Drug label for Crixivan.

14. The prescriber ordered 240 mL of *2/3 strength Sustacal PO B.I.D.* How will you prepare this solution using a 240 mL can of Sustacal?

15. The prescriber ordered *Demerol (meperidine hydrochloride) 75 mg IM stat.* The label on the 20 mL multi-dose vial reads 100 mg/mL.
    (a) How many milliliters of this narcotic analgesic drug would you administer?
    (b) What size syringe would you use?

Unit

4

Infusions and Pediatric Dosages

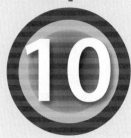

Flow Rates and Durations of Enteral and Intravenous Infusions

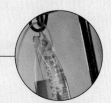

Learning Outcomes

After completing this chapter, you will be able to

1. Describe the basic concepts and standard equipment used in administering enteral and intravenous (IV) infusions.
2. Quickly convert flow rates between gtt/min and mL/h.
3. Calculate the flow rates of enteral and IV infusions.
4. Calculate the durations of enteral and IV infusions.
5. Determine fluid replacement volumes.

T his chapter introduces the basic concepts and standard equipment used in enteral and intravenous therapy. You will also learn how to calculate flow rates for these infusions and to determine how long it will take for a given amount of solution to infuse (its duration).

Introduction to Enteral and Intravenous Solutions

Fluids can be given to a patient slowly over a period of time through a vein (*intravenous*) or through a tube inserted into the alimentary tract (*enteral*). The rate at which these fluids flow into the patient is very important and must be controlled precisely.

Enteral Feedings

When a patient cannot ingest food or if the upper gastrointestinal tract is not functioning properly, the prescriber may write an order for an *enteral* feeding (*"tube feeding"*). Enteral feedings provide nutrients and other fluids by way of a tube inserted directly into the gastrointestinal system (alimentary tract).

There are various types of tube feedings. A gastric tube may be inserted into the stomach through the nares (**nasogastric**, as shown in •**Figure 10.1**) or through the mouth (**orogastric**). A longer tube may be similarly inserted, but would extend beyond the stomach into the upper small intestine, jejunum (**nasojejunum** or **orojejunum**).

For long-term feedings, tubes can be inserted surgically or laproscopically through the wall of the abdomen and directly into either the stomach (gastrostomy) or through the stomach and on to the jejunum (jejunostomy). These tubes are sutured in place and are referred to as *percutaneous endoscopic gastrostomy (PEG)* tubes and *percutaneous endoscopic jejunostomy (PEJ) tubes,* respectively (•**Figure 10.2**).

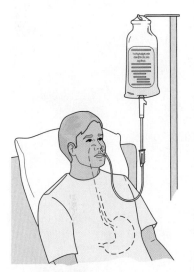

• **Figure 10.1**
A patient with a nasogastric tube.

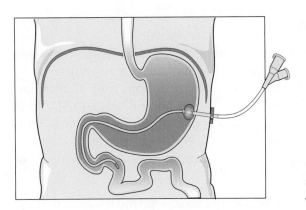

• **Figure 10.2**
A percutaneous endoscopic jejunostomy (PEJ) tube.

Enteral feedings may be given *continuously* (over a 24-hour period) or *intermittently* (over shorter periods, perhaps several times a day). There are many enteral feeding solutions, including Boost, Compleat, Ensure, Isocal, Resource, and Sustacal. Enteral feedings are generally administered via pump. •**Figure 10.3.**

Orders for enteral solutions always indicate a volume of fluid to be infused over a period of time; that is, a flow rate. For example, a tube feeding order might read *Isocal 50 mL/h via nasogastric tube for 6 hours beginning 6 A.M.* This order is for an intermittent feeding in which the name of the solution is Isocal, the rate of flow is 50 mL/h, the route of administration is via nasogastric tube, and the duration is 6 hours.

Intravenous Infusions

Intravenous (IV) means *through the vein.* Fluids are administered intravenously to provide a variety of fluids, including blood, water containing nutrients, electrolytes, minerals, and specific medications to the patient. IV fluids can replace lost fluids, maintain fluid and electrolyte balance, or serve as a medium to introduce medications directly into the bloodstream.

Replacement fluids are ordered for a patient who has lost fluids through hemorrhage, vomiting, or diarrhea. *Maintenance fluids* help sustain normal levels of fluids and electrolytes. They are ordered for patients who are at risk of becoming depleted; for example, patients who are NPO (nothing by mouth).

Intravenous infusions may be *continuous* or *intermittent.* Continuous IV infusions are used to replace or maintain fluids or electrolytes. Intermittent IV infusions—for example, IV piggyback (IVPB) and IV push (IVP)—are used to administer drugs and supplemental fluids. *Intermittent peripheral infusion devices* (saline locks or heparin locks) are used to maintain venous access without continuous fluid infusion. Intermittent IV infusions are discussed in Chapter 11.

A healthcare professional must be able to perform the calculations to determine the correct rate at which an enteral or intravenous solution will enter the body (*flow rate*). Infusion flow rates are usually measured in drops per minute (gtt/min) or milliliters per hour (mL/h). It is important to be able to convert each of these rates to the other and to determine how long a given amount of solution will take to infuse.

For example, a continuous IV order might read *IV fluids: D5W 125 mL/h for 8h.* In this case, the order is for an IV infusion in which the name of the solution is 5% dextrose in water, the rate of flow is 125 mL/h, the route of administration is intravenous, and the duration is 8 hours.

Intravenous Solutions

A **saline solution**, which is a solution of *sodium chloride (NaCl)* in sterile water, is commonly used for intravenous infusion. Sodium chloride is ordinary table salt. Saline solutions are available in various concentrations for different purposes. A 0.9% NaCl solution is also referred to as **normal saline (NS)**. Other saline solutions commonly used include **half-normal saline** (0.45% NaCl), written as $\frac{1}{2}$ NS; and **quarter-normal saline** (0.225% NaCl), written as $\frac{1}{4}$ NS.

Intravenous fluids generally contain dextrose, sodium chloride, or electrolytes:

- D5W, D5/W, or 5% D/W is a 5% dextrose solution, which means that 5 g of dextrose are dissolved in water to make each 100 mL of this solution. •**Figures 10.4a** and **10.4b**.

- NS or 0.9% NaCl is a solution in which each 100 mL contain 0.9 g of sodium chloride. •**Figures 10.4c** and **10.4d**.

- 5% D/0.45% NaCl is a solution containing 5 g of dextrose and 0.45 g of NaCl in each 100 mL of solution •**Figure 10.5b**.

- Ringer's Lactate (RL), also called Lactated Ringer's solution (LRS), is a solution containing electrolytes, including potassium chloride and calcium chloride. •**Figure 10.5c**.

Additional information on the many other IV fluids can be found in nursing and pharmacology textbooks.

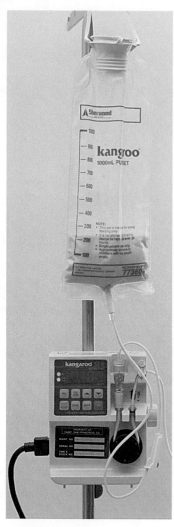

• **Figure 10.3**
Enteral feeding via pump.

(Photographer; Elena Dorfman)

NOTE

Pay close attention to the abbreviations of the names of the IV solutions. *Letters* indicate the solution compounds, whereas *numbers* indicate the solution strength (e.g., D5W).

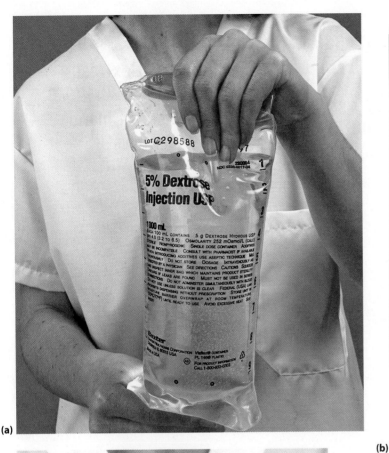

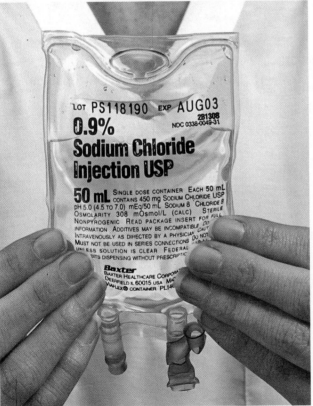

• **Figure 10.4**

Examples of IV bags and labels.

(10-04a Al Dodge/Al Dodge.   10-04b Courtesy of Baxter Healthcare Corporation. All rights reserved.   10-04c Al Dodge/Al Dodge.   10-04d Reproduced with permission of Abbott Laboratories)

(b)

LOT   EXP

NDC 0338-0017-04   280084

1
2
3

5% Dextrose Injection USP

1000 mL
EACH 100 mL CONTAINS   5 g DEXTROSE HYDROUS USP
pH 4.0 (3.2 TO 6.5)   OSMOLARITY 252 mOsmol/L (CALC)
STERILE   NONPYROGENIC   SINGLE DOSE CONTAINER   ADDITIVES
MAY BE INCOMPATIBLE   CONSULT WITH PHARMACIST IF AVAILABLE
WHEN INTRODUCING ADDITIVES USE ASEPTIC TECHNIQUE   MIX
THOROUGHLY   DO NOT STORE   DOSAGE   INTRAVENOUSLY AS
DIRECTED BY A PHYSICIAN   SEE DIRECTIONS   CAUTIONS   SQUEEZE
AND INSPECT INNER BAG WHICH MAINTAINS PRODUCT STERILITY
DISCARD IF LEAKS ARE FOUND   MUST NOT BE USED IN SERIES
CONNECTIONS   DO NOT ADMINISTER SIMULTANEOUSLY WITH BLOOD
DO NOT USE UNLESS SOLUTION IS CLEAR   FEDERAL (USA) LAW
PROHIBITS DISPENSING WITHOUT PRESCRIPTION   STORE UNIT IN
MOISTURE BARRIER OVERWRAP AT ROOM TEMPERATURE
(25°C/77°F) UNTIL READY TO USE   AVOID EXCESSIVE HEAT   SEE
INSERT

4
5
6
7

Baxter
BAXTER HEALTHCARE CORPORATION   VIAFLEX® CONTAINER
DEERFIELD IL 60015 USA   PL 146® PLASTIC
MADE IN USA   FOR PRODUCT INFORMATION
                                 CALL 1-800-933-0303

8
9

(d)

▱ **1000 mL** NDC 0074-7983-09

0.9% Sodium Chloride
Injection, USP

EACH 100 mL CONTAINS SODIUM CHLORIDE
900 mg IN WATER FOR INJECTION.
ELECTROLYTES PER 1000 mL: SODIUM 154 mEq;
CHLORIDE 154 mEq.
308 mOsm/LITER (CALC).   pH 5.6 (4.5–7.0)
ADDITIVES MAY BE INCOMPATIBLE. CONSULT
WITH PHARMACIST, IF AVAILABLE. WHEN
INTRODUCING ADDITIVES, USE ASEPTIC
TECHNIQUE, MIX THOROUGHLY AND DO NOT
STORE. SINGLE-DOSE CONTAINER. FOR
INTRAVENOUS USE. USUAL DOSE: SEE INSERT.
STERILE, NONPYROGENIC. CAUTION: FEDERAL
(USA) LAW PROHIBITS DISPENSING WITHOUT
PRESCRIPTION. USE ONLY IF SOLUTION IS CLEAR
AND CONTAINER IS UNDAMAGED. MUST NOT
BE USED IN SERIES CONNECTIONS.
                              PATENT PENDING

©ABBOTT 1988   PRINTED IN USA
ABBOTT LABORATORIES, NORTH CHICAGO, IL 60064, USA

0-1-2-3-4-5-6-7-8-9 0-1-2-3-4-5-6-7-8-9

• Figure 10.5
Examples of intravenous fluids.

(Reproduced with permission of Abbott Laboratories.)

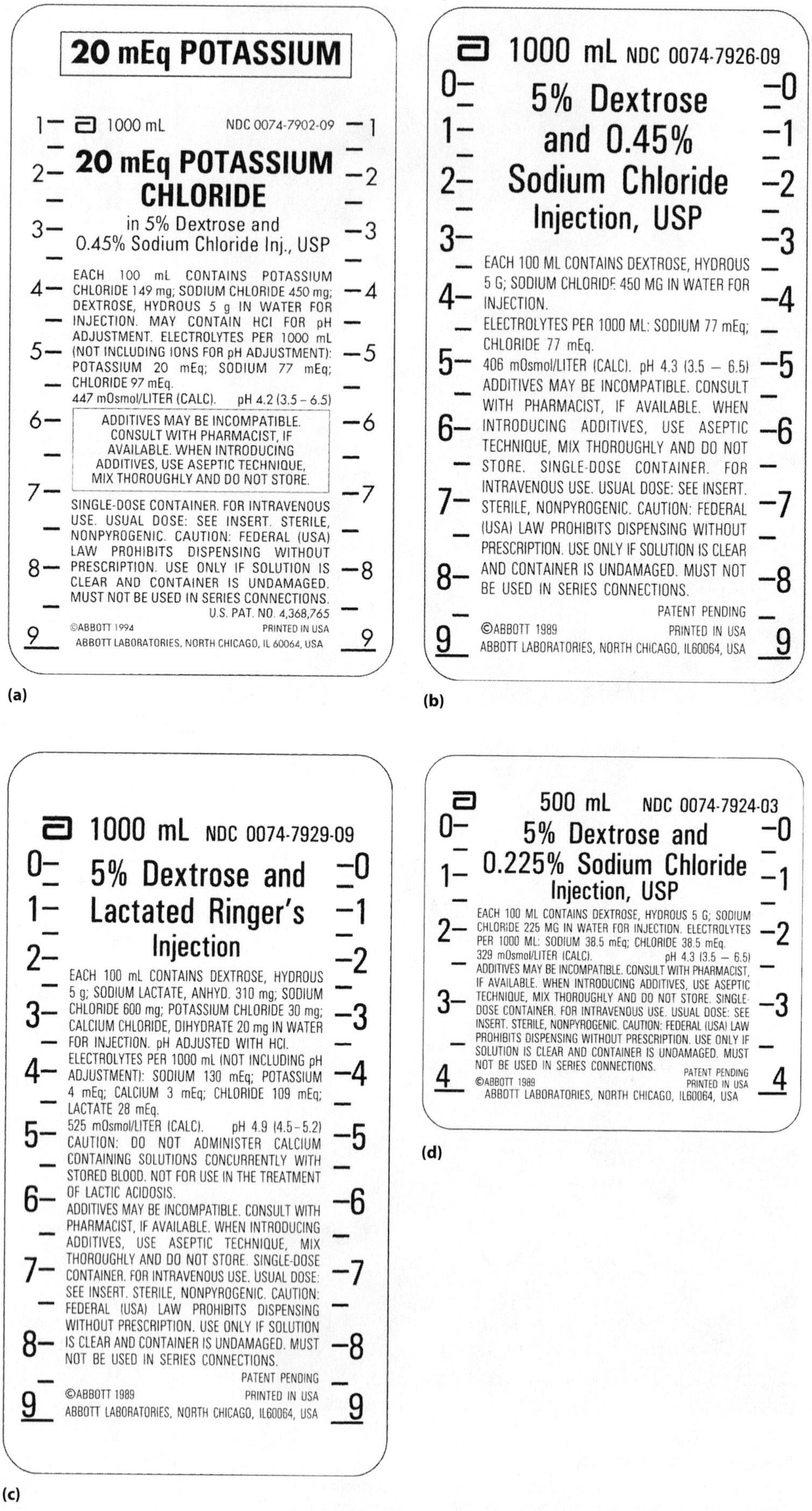

ALERT

In Figure 10.5, solutions (a) and (b) both contain 5% dextrose and $\frac{1}{2}$ NS. However, solution (a) also contains 20 mEq of potassium chloride, which is a high-alert medication. Do not confuse these two solutions.

20 mEq POTASSIUM

1 — 1000 mL   NDC 0074-7902-09 — 1

20 mEq POTASSIUM CHLORIDE

in 5% Dextrose and
0.45% Sodium Chloride Inj., USP

EACH 100 mL CONTAINS POTASSIUM CHLORIDE 149 mg; SODIUM CHLORIDE 450 mg; DEXTROSE, HYDROUS 5 g IN WATER FOR INJECTION. MAY CONTAIN HCl FOR pH ADJUSTMENT. ELECTROLYTES PER 1000 mL (NOT INCLUDING IONS FOR pH ADJUSTMENT): POTASSIUM 20 mEq; SODIUM 77 mEq; CHLORIDE 97 mEq.
447 mOsmol/LITER (CALC).   pH 4.2 (3.5 – 6.5)

ADDITIVES MAY BE INCOMPATIBLE. CONSULT WITH PHARMACIST, IF AVAILABLE. WHEN INTRODUCING ADDITIVES, USE ASEPTIC TECHNIQUE, MIX THOROUGHLY AND DO NOT STORE.

SINGLE-DOSE CONTAINER. FOR INTRAVENOUS USE. USUAL DOSE: SEE INSERT. STERILE, NONPYROGENIC. CAUTION: FEDERAL (USA) LAW PROHIBITS DISPENSING WITHOUT PRESCRIPTION. USE ONLY IF SOLUTION IS CLEAR AND CONTAINER IS UNDAMAGED. MUST NOT BE USED IN SERIES CONNECTIONS.
U.S. PAT. NO. 4,368,765
©ABBOTT 1994   PRINTED IN USA
ABBOTT LABORATORIES, NORTH CHICAGO, IL 60064, USA

(a)

1000 mL   NDC 0074-7926-09

5% Dextrose and 0.45% Sodium Chloride Injection, USP

EACH 100 ML CONTAINS DEXTROSE, HYDROUS 5 G; SODIUM CHLORIDE 450 MG IN WATER FOR INJECTION.
ELECTROLYTES PER 1000 ML: SODIUM 77 mEq; CHLORIDE 77 mEq.
406 mOsmol/LITER (CALC). pH 4.3 (3.5 – 6.5)
ADDITIVES MAY BE INCOMPATIBLE. CONSULT WITH PHARMACIST, IF AVAILABLE. WHEN INTRODUCING ADDITIVES, USE ASEPTIC TECHNIQUE, MIX THOROUGHLY AND DO NOT STORE. SINGLE-DOSE CONTAINER. FOR INTRAVENOUS USE. USUAL DOSE: SEE INSERT. STERILE, NONPYROGENIC. CAUTION: FEDERAL (USA) LAW PROHIBITS DISPENSING WITHOUT PRESCRIPTION. USE ONLY IF SOLUTION IS CLEAR AND CONTAINER IS UNDAMAGED. MUST NOT BE USED IN SERIES CONNECTIONS.
PATENT PENDING
©ABBOTT 1989   PRINTED IN USA
ABBOTT LABORATORIES, NORTH CHICAGO, IL60064, USA

(b)

1000 mL   NDC 0074-7929-09

5% Dextrose and Lactated Ringer's Injection

EACH 100 mL CONTAINS DEXTROSE, HYDROUS 5 g; SODIUM LACTATE, ANHYD. 310 mg; SODIUM CHLORIDE 600 mg; POTASSIUM CHLORIDE 30 mg; CALCIUM CHLORIDE, DIHYDRATE 20 mg IN WATER FOR INJECTION. pH ADJUSTED WITH HCl.
ELECTROLYTES PER 1000 mL (NOT INCLUDING pH ADJUSTMENT): SODIUM 130 mEq; POTASSIUM 4 mEq; CALCIUM 3 mEq; CHLORIDE 109 mEq; LACTATE 28 mEq.
525 mOsmol/LITER (CALC).   pH 4.9 (4.5 – 5.2)
CAUTION: DO NOT ADMINISTER CALCIUM CONTAINING SOLUTIONS CONCURRENTLY WITH STORED BLOOD. NOT FOR USE IN THE TREATMENT OF LACTIC ACIDOSIS.
ADDITIVES MAY BE INCOMPATIBLE. CONSULT WITH PHARMACIST, IF AVAILABLE. WHEN INTRODUCING ADDITIVES, USE ASEPTIC TECHNIQUE, MIX THOROUGHLY AND DO NOT STORE. SINGLE-DOSE CONTAINER. FOR INTRAVENOUS USE. USUAL DOSE: SEE INSERT. STERILE, NONPYROGENIC. CAUTION: FEDERAL (USA) LAW PROHIBITS DISPENSING WITHOUT PRESCRIPTION. USE ONLY IF SOLUTION IS CLEAR AND CONTAINER IS UNDAMAGED. MUST NOT BE USED IN SERIES CONNECTIONS.
PATENT PENDING
©ABBOTT 1989   PRINTED IN USA
ABBOTT LABORATORIES, NORTH CHICAGO, IL60064, USA

(c)

500 mL   NDC 0074-7924-03

5% Dextrose and 0.225% Sodium Chloride Injection, USP

EACH 100 ML CONTAINS DEXTROSE, HYDROUS 5 G; SODIUM CHLORIDE 225 MG IN WATER FOR INJECTION. ELECTROLYTES PER 1000 ML: SODIUM 38.5 mEq; CHLORIDE 38.5 mEq.
329 mOsmol/LITER (CALC).   pH 4.3 (3.5 – 6.5)
ADDITIVES MAY BE INCOMPATIBLE. CONSULT WITH PHARMACIST, IF AVAILABLE. WHEN INTRODUCING ADDITIVES, USE ASEPTIC TECHNIQUE, MIX THOROUGHLY AND DO NOT STORE. SINGLE-DOSE CONTAINER. FOR INTRAVENOUS USE. USUAL DOSE: SEE INSERT. STERILE, NONPYROGENIC. CAUTION: FEDERAL (USA) LAW PROHIBITS DISPENSING WITHOUT PRESCRIPTION. USE ONLY IF SOLUTION IS CLEAR AND CONTAINER IS UNDAMAGED. MUST NOT BE USED IN SERIES CONNECTIONS.
PATENT PENDING
©ABBOTT 1989   PRINTED IN USA
ABBOTT LABORATORIES, NORTH CHICAGO, IL60064, USA

(d)

Gravity Systems and Pumps

Equipment used for the administration of continuous IV infusions includes the IV solution and IV tubing, a drip chamber, at least one injection port, and a roller clamp. The tubing connects the IV solution to the hub of an IV catheter at the infusion site. The rate of flow of the infusion is regulated by an electronic infusion device (pump or controller) or by gravity. •**Figures 10.6** and **10.9.**

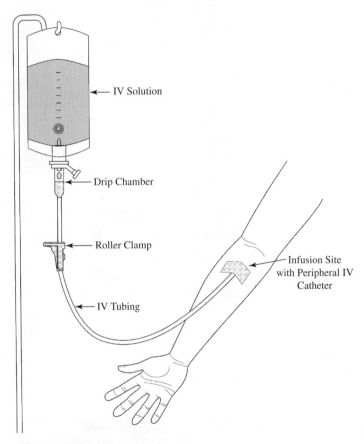

• **Figure 10.6**
Primary intravenous line (gravity flow).

IV Solution

Drip Chamber

Roller Clamp

IV Tubing

Infusion Site with Peripheral IV Catheter

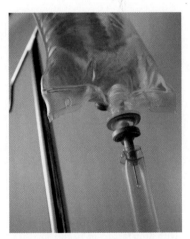

• **Figure 10.7**
Tubing with drip chamber.

(Photodisc/Getty Images)

The drip chamber (Figure 10.6) is located at the site of the entrance of the tubing into the container of intravenous solution. It allows you to count the number of drops per minute that the client is receiving (flow rate).

A roll valve clamp or clip is connected to the tubing and can be manipulated to increase or decrease the flow rate.

The size of the drop that IV tubing delivers is not standard; it depends on the way the tubing is designed. •**Figure 10.7.** Manufacturers specify the number of drops that equal 1 mL for their particular tubing. This equivalent is called the tubing's drop factor (•**Figure 10.8** and Table 10.1). You must know the tubing's **drop factor** when calculating the flow rate of solutions in drops per minute (gtt/min) or microdrops per minute (mcgtt/min).

It is difficult to visually make an accurate count of the drops falling per minute when setting the flow rate on a gravity system infusion. In addition,

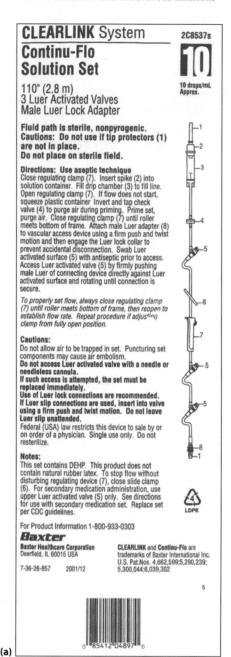

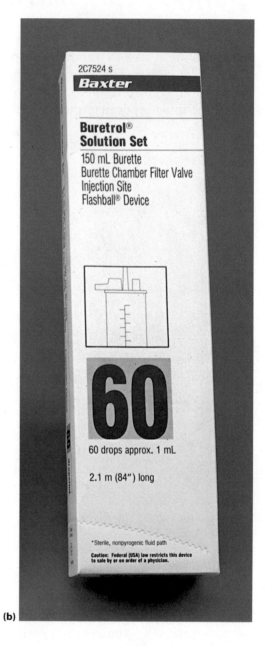

• **Figure 10.8**

Samples of IV tubing containers with drop factors of 10 and 60.

(10-8a Courtesy of Baxter Healthcare Corporation. All rights reserved. 10-8b Al Dodge/Al Dodge)

(a)

(b)

the flow rate of a gravity system infusion depends on the *relative heights* of the IV bag and the infusion site; changes in the relative position of either may cause flow rate changes. Electric IV pumps and controllers now make up the majority of infusion systems in use in health facilities.

NOTE

60 microdrops = 1 mL is a universal equivalent for IV tubing calibrated in microdrops.

Table 10.1 **Common Drop Factors**		
10 gtt = 1 mL		
15 gtt = 1 mL	}	macrodrops
20 gtt = 1 mL		
60 mcgtt = 1 mL	}	microdrops

An intravenous infusion can flow solely by the force of gravity or by an electronic infusion pump. There are many different types of electronic infusion pumps. •Figure 10.9.

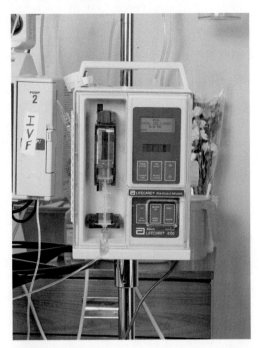

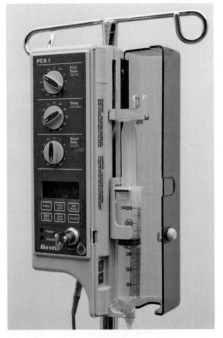

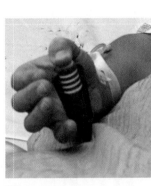

• **Figure 10.9**
Volumetric infusion pump.

(a)   **(b)**

• **Figure 10.10**
Patient-controlled analgesia (PCA) (a) pump (b) control button.

These electrically operated devices allow the rate of flow (usually specified in mL/h) to be simply keyed into the device by the user. The pumps can more precisely regulate the flow rate than can the gravity systems. For example, pumps detect an interruption in the flow (constriction) and sound an alarm to alert the nursing staff and the patient, sound an alarm when the infusion finishes, indicate the volume of fluid already infused, and indicate the time remaining for the infusion to finish. "Smart" pumps may contain libraries of safe dosage ranges that will help prevent the user from keying in an unsafe dosage.

A *patient-controlled analgesia (PCA) pump* (see •**Figure 10.10**) allows a patient to self-administer pain-relieving drugs. The dose is predetermined by the physician, and the pump is programmed accordingly. To receive the drug when pain relief is needed, the patient presses the button on the handset, which is connected to the PCA pump. A lockout device in the pump prevents patient overdose.

> **ALERT**
>
> A facility might use many different types of infusion pumps. The healthcare provider must learn how to program all of them. Be sure to use the specific tubing supplied by the manufacturer for each pump.

Calculations for Infusions

Most intravenous or enteral solutions are administered by using a pump that measures flow rates in *milliliters per hour*. Examples 10.1 through 10.6 illustrate problems where pumps are used.

The **flow rate** of an infusion is the *volume of fluid* that enters the patient over a *period of time*. For example, *25 mL/h* and *15 gtt/min* are flow rates. The following formula may be used to determine a flow rate.

$$Flow\,Rate = \frac{Volume}{Time}$$

EXAMPLE 10.1

Order: *NS 2,000 mL continuous IV for 24 h.* Find the pump setting in *milliliters per hour.*

Volume to be infused:	*2,000 mL*
Time:	*24 h*
Flow rate you want to find:	*? mL/h*

The flow rate $\dfrac{volume}{time}$ can be determined by placing the volume [*2,000 mL*] over the time [*24 h*].

$$\frac{2{,}000\ mL}{24\ h}$$

Reduce the fraction to obtain

$$\frac{250\ mL}{3\ h} = 88.33\ mL/h$$

So, the pump would be set for a flow rate of 83 *mL/h.*

EXAMPLE 10.2

A patient must receive a tube-feeding of *Ensure 120 milliliters in 90 minutes.* Calculate the flow rate in *milliliters per hour.*

Volume to be infused:	*120 mL*
Time:	*90 min*
Flow rate you want to find:	*? mL/h*

The flow rate $\dfrac{volume}{time}$ can be determined by placing the volume [*120 mL*] over the time [*90 min*].

$$\frac{120\ mL}{90\ min} = ?\ \frac{mL}{h}$$

DIMENSIONAL ANALYSIS

You want to change one flow rate [*mL/min*] to another flow rate [*mL/h*]. Each flow rate has *mL* in the numerator, which is what you want. You want to cancel *min*, which is in the denominator. To do this, you must use a unit fraction containing *min* in the numerator. Because 1 *h* = 60 *min*, this fraction will be $\dfrac{60\ min}{1\ h}$

$$\frac{120\ mL}{90\ \cancel{min}} \times \frac{60\ \cancel{min}}{1\ h} = \frac{80\ mL}{1\ h}$$

RATIO & PROPORTION

Because 1 hour = 60 minutes, the problem becomes

$$\frac{120\ mL}{90\ min} = ?\ \frac{mL}{60\ min}$$

$$\frac{120\ mL}{90\ min} = \frac{x\ mL}{60\ min}$$

$$90x = 7{,}200$$

$$x = 80$$

So, the flow rate is *80 milliliters per hour.*

EXAMPLE 10.3

Order: *Lactated Ringer's at 167 mL/h IV for 6 h*. How many milliliters will the patient receive in 6 hours?

DIMENSIONAL ANALYSIS

Time: 6 h   [single unit of measurement]

Flow rate: 167 mL/h   [equivalence]

Volume to be
infused: ? mL   [single unit of measurement]

In this example, you want to change the single unit of measurement [6 h] to another single unit of measurement [mL].

$$6 \, h = ? \, mL$$

The flow rate provides the equivalence [167 mL = 1 h] for the unit fraction.

$$6 \, \cancel{h} \times \frac{167 \, mL}{\cancel{h}} = 1{,}002 \, mL$$

RATIO & PROPORTION

This problem involves milliliters and hours. If you double the hours (time), you double the milliliters (volume) infused. Milliliters and hours in this problem are in proportion.

Think of the problem as:

$$167 \, mL = 1 \, h$$
$$x \, mL = 6 \, h$$

The proportion could be set up as

$$\frac{167 \, mL}{1 \, h} = \frac{x \, mL}{6 \, h}$$

$$x = 1{,}002$$

So, the patient will receive *1,002 milliliters* of Lactated Ringer's.

EXAMPLE 10.4

Order: *0.9% NaCl 500 mL IV at 125 mL/h*. How long will this infusion take?

DIMENSIONAL ANALYSIS

Volume to be
infused: 500 mL   [single unit of measurement]

Flow rate: 125 mL/h   [equivalence]

Time: ? h   [single unit of measurement]

In this example, you want to change the single unit of measurement [500 mL] to another single unit of measurement [h].

$$500 \, mL = ? \, h$$

The flow rate will provide the equivalence [125 mL = 1 h] for the unit fraction. In this case, you need to put mL in the denominator in order to cancel.

$$500 \, \cancel{mL} \times \frac{1 \, h}{125 \, \cancel{mL}} = 4 \, h$$

RATIO & PROPORTION

This problem involves milliliters and hours. If you double the hours (time), you double the milliliters (volume) infused. Milliliters and hours in this problem are in proportion.

Think of the problem as:

$$125 \, mL = 1 \, h$$
$$500 \, mL = x \, h$$

The proportion could be set up as

$$\frac{125 \, mL}{1 \, h} = \frac{500 \, mL}{x \, h}$$

$$500 = 125 \, x$$
$$4 = x$$

So, the infusion will take *4 hours*.

EXAMPLE 10.5

Order: $\frac{1}{2}$ NS 1,000 mL IV at 50 mL/h. If the IV starts at 1200h on Monday, at what time will it finish?

DIMENSIONAL ANALYSIS

Volume to be infused:	1,000 mL	[single unit of measurement]
Flow rate:	50 mL/h	[equivalence]
Time:	? h	[single unit of measurement]

In this example, you want to change the single unit of measurement [1,000 mL] to another single unit of measurement [h].

$$1,000 \ mL = ? \ h$$

The flow rate will provide the equivalence [50 mL = 1 h] for the unit fraction. In this case, you need to put mL in the denominator in order to cancel.

$$1,000 \ \cancel{mL} \times \frac{1 \ h}{50 \ \cancel{mL}} = 20 \ h$$

RATIO & PROPORTION

Think of the problem as:

$$50 \ mL = 1 \ h$$
$$1,000 \ mL = x \ h$$

The proportion could be set up as

$$\frac{50 \ mL}{1 \ h} = \frac{1,000 \ mL}{x \ h}$$

$$1,000 = 50 \ x$$
$$20 = x$$

So, the infusion will take 20 hours.

One way to continue is to add

$$\begin{array}{r} 1200h \\ + \ 2000h \\ \hline 3200h \end{array}$$

Because military time has a 24 clock, you must now subtract 2400h.

$$\begin{array}{r} 3200h \\ - \ 2400h \\ \hline 0800h \end{array}$$

So, the infusion will finish at 0800h on Tuesday.

EXAMPLE 10.6

Order: *Sustacal 240 mL infuse over 2 hours via a feeding tube stat.*

(a) Calculate the flow rate in *mL/h*.

(b) If after *1 hour and 30 minutes*, there is 50 mL left in the bag, how would the flow rate be adjusted so that the infusion would finish on time?

(c) If the facility has a policy that flow rate adjustments must not exceed 20% of the original rate, would the adjustment in part (b) be permitted?

(a) Volume to be infused:	240 mL
Time:	2 h
Flow rate you want to find:	? mL/h

The flow rate $\dfrac{volume}{time}$ can be determined by placing the volume [240 mL] over the time [2 h].

$$\frac{240\ mL}{2\ h} = \frac{120\ mL}{1\ h}$$

So, the pump would be set for a flow rate of 120 mL/h.

(b) The remaining volume [50 mL] must infuse in the remaining time [30 min].

The flow rate $\dfrac{volume}{time}$ can be determined by placing the volume over the time.

$$\frac{50\ mL}{30\ min} = ?\ \frac{mL}{h}$$

DIMENSIONAL ANALYSIS

You want to change one flow rate [mL/min] to another flow rate [mL/h]. Each flow rate has mL in the numerator, which is what you want. You want to cancel min, which is in the denominator. To do this, you must use a unit fraction containing min in the numerator. Because 1 h = 60 min, this fraction will be $\dfrac{60\ min}{1\ h}$

$$\frac{50\ mL}{30\ \cancel{min}} \times \frac{60\ \cancel{min}}{1\ h} = \frac{100\ mL}{1\ h}$$

RATIO & PROPORTION

Because 30 minutes = $\frac{1}{2}$ *hour*, the problem becomes

$$\frac{50\ mL}{\frac{1}{2}\ h} = \frac{x\ mL}{1\ h}$$

$$\frac{50\ mL}{\frac{1}{2}\ h} = \frac{x\ mL}{1\ h}$$

$$\frac{1}{2}x = 50$$

$$x = 100$$

So, the flow rate would be reset to 100 milliliters per hour.

(c) The guidelines indicate that an adjustment may not be more than 20% of the original rate [120 mL/h]. Therefore, the maximum allowable change in flow rate is

$$20\%\ of\ 120\ mL/h = 0.20 \times 120\ \frac{mL}{h} = 24\ mL/h$$

The flow rate in part (b) changed from 120 mL/h to 100 mL/h. This is a change of 20 mL/h. Because 20 ml/h is less than 24 mL/h, the flow rate adjustment would be permitted.

Flow Rate Conversion Number (FC)

Flow rates for gravity systems are measured in *drops/minute (gtt/min)*. A quick way to convert flow rates from *mL/h* to *gtt/min*, and vice versa, is to use the flow rate conversion number method.

The **flow rate conversion number**, abbreviated as **FC** (think: Flow Converter), is equal to the quotient of 60 and the drop factor (DF). That is,

$$FC = \frac{60}{DF}$$

For example, if the drop factor (DF) is 15 gtt/mL, then the flow rate conversion number is obtained as follows:

$$FC = \frac{60}{15} = 4$$

Table 10.2 shows the common drop factors and their corresponding flow rate conversion numbers.

Table 10.2	**Common Drop Factors and Corresponding Flow Rate Conversion Numbers**	
Drop Factor (DF)	**Flow Rate Conversion Number (FC)**	
10	$\dfrac{60}{10} = 6$	
15	$\dfrac{60}{15} = 4$	
20	$\dfrac{60}{20} = 3$	
60	$\dfrac{60}{60} = 1$	

To change flow rates between mL/h and gtt/min involves simply multiplying or dividing the given flow rate by the flow rate conversion number as follows:

To change from mL/h to gtt/min, divide the given rate by FC.
To change from gtt/min to mL/h, multiply the given rate by FC.

An easy way to remember the FC method is:

When you want <u>D</u>rops, <u>D</u>ivide.
When you want <u>M</u>illiliters, <u>M</u>ultiply.

Both dimensional analysis and FC methods will be illustrated in Examples 10.7 through 10.14.

EXAMPLE 10.7

The prescriber ordered $\frac{1}{4}$ *NS 850 mL IV in 8 hours.* The label on the box containing the intravenous set to be used for this infusion is shown in •Figure 10.11. Calculate the flow rate in drops per minute.

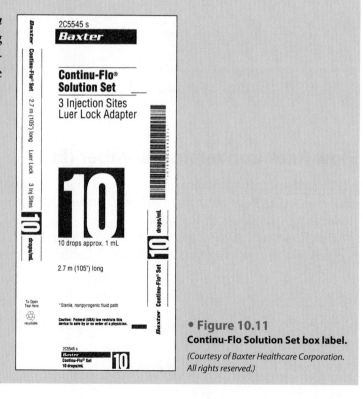

•**Figure 10.11**
Continu-Flo Solution Set box label.

(Courtesy of Baxter Healthcare Corporation. All rights reserved.)

DIMENSIONAL ANALYSIS

Given flow rate: 8.50 mL/8 h

Known equivalences: 10 gtt/mL (drop factor)

1 h = 60 min

Flow rate you want to find: ? gtt/min

You want to convert the flow rate from milliliters per hour to drops per minute.

$$\frac{850\ mL}{8\ h} = \frac{?\ gtt}{min}$$

You want to cancel mL. To do this you must use a unit fraction containing mL in the denominator. Using the drop factor, this fraction will be $\frac{10\ gtt}{1\ mL}$

$$\frac{850\ ml}{8\ h} \times \frac{10\ gtt}{1\ mL} = \frac{?\ gtt}{min}$$

Now, on the left side gtt is in the numerator, which is what you want. But h is in the denominator and it must be cancelled. This will require a unit fraction with h in the numerator, namely, $\frac{1\ h}{60\ min}$

Now cancel and multiply the numbers

$$\frac{850\ mL}{8\ h} \times \frac{10\ gtt}{1\ mL} \times \frac{1\ h}{60\ min} = 17.7\ \frac{gtt}{min}$$

FC METHOD

The problem is

$$\frac{850\ mL}{8\ h} = ?\ \frac{gtt}{min}$$

Because

$$\frac{850}{8} = 106.25$$

The problem becomes

$$106.25\ \frac{mL}{h} = ?\ \frac{gtt}{min}$$

DF = 10, therefore

$$FC = \frac{60}{10} = 6$$

Because you want Drops per minute, Divide the given flow rate by 6

$$\frac{106.25}{6} = 17.7$$

So, the flow rate is 18 drops per minute.

EXAMPLE 10.8

The prescriber orders D5/0.45% NaCl IV to infuse at 21 drops per minute. If the drop factor is 20 drops per milliliter, how many milliliters per hour will the patient receive?

Given flow rate: 21 gtt/min

Known equivalences: 20 gtt/mL (drop factor)

1 h = 60 min

Flow rate you want to find: ? mL/h

You want to convert a flow rate of 21 drops per minute to a flow rate in milliliters per hour.

$$\frac{21\ gtt}{min} = \frac{?\ mL}{h}$$

DIMENSIONAL ANALYSIS

You want to cancel gtt. To do this you must use a unit fraction containing *gtt* in the denominator.

Using the drop factor, this fraction is $\dfrac{1 \text{ mL}}{20 \text{ gtt}}$

$$\frac{21 \text{ gtt}}{\text{min}} \times \frac{1 \text{ mL}}{20 \text{ gtt}} = \frac{? \text{ mL}}{\text{h}}$$

Now, on the left side *mL* is in the numerator, which is what you want. But *min* is in the denominator and it must be cancelled. This will require a unit fraction with *min* in the numerator, namely, $\dfrac{60 \text{ min}}{1 \text{ h}}$

Now cancel and multiply the numbers

$$\frac{21 \text{ gtt}}{\text{min}} \times \frac{1 \text{ mL}}{20 \text{ gtt}} \times \frac{60 \text{ min}}{1 \text{ h}} = 63 \frac{\text{mL}}{\text{h}}$$

FC METHOD

The problem is

$$21 \frac{gtt}{min} = ? \frac{mL}{h}$$

DF = 20, therefore

$$FC = \frac{60}{20} = 3$$

Because you want <u>M</u>illiliters per hour, <u>M</u>ultiply the given flow rate by 3

$$21 \times 3 = 63$$

So, the flow rate is 63 mL per hour.

EXAMPLE 10.9

The order reads *125 mL 5% D/W IV in 1 hour.* **What is the flow rate in microdrops per minute?**

DIMENSIONAL ANALYSIS

Given flow rate:	125 mL/h
Known equivalences:	60 mcgtt/mL (drop factor for microdrops) 1 h = 60 min
Flow rate you want to find:	? mcgtt/min

NOTE

In Example 10.9, it is shown that 125 mL per hour is the same flow rate as 125 microdrops per minute because the 60s always cancel. The flow rates of *milliliters per hour* and *microdrops per minute* are equivalent. Therefore, calculations are not necessary to change mL/h to mcgtt/min.

FC METHOD

The problem is

$$\frac{125 \, mL}{1 \, h} = ? \frac{mcgtt}{min}$$

Because this is a conversion from *mL/h* to *gtt/min*, use the FC technique.

It is standard that *60 mcgtt = 1 mL*, therefore, use DF = 60 to calculate FC

$$FC = \frac{60}{DF}$$

$$FC = \frac{60}{60} = 1$$

Because you want <u>D</u>rops per minute, <u>D</u>ivide the given flow rate by FC

$$\frac{125}{1} = 125$$

You want to change the flow rate from 125 mL per hour to microdrops per minute.

$$\frac{125 \text{ mL}}{\text{h}} = \frac{? \text{ mcgtt}}{\text{min}}$$

You want to cancel mL. To do this you must use a unit fraction containing mL in the denominator. Using the drop factor, this fraction will be $\dfrac{60 \text{ mcgtt}}{1 \text{ mL}}$

$$\frac{125 \text{ mL}}{\text{h}} \times \frac{60 \text{ mcgtt}}{1 \text{ mL}} = \frac{? \text{ mcgtt}}{\text{min}}$$

Now, on the left side mcgtt is in the numerator, which is what you want. But h is in the denominator and it must be cancelled. This will require a unit fraction with h in the numerator, namely, $\dfrac{1 \text{ h}}{60 \text{ min}}$

Now cancel and multiply the numbers

$$\frac{125 \text{ mL}}{\text{h}} \times \frac{60 \text{ mcgtt}}{1 \text{ mL}} \times \frac{1 \text{ h}}{60 \text{ min}} = 125 \frac{\text{mcgtt}}{\text{min}}$$

So, 125 mL per hour is the same rate of flow as 125 microdrops per minute.

EXAMPLE 10.10

(a) The order is *500 mL of 5% D/W to infuse IV in 5 hours.* Calculate the flow rate in drops per minute if the drop factor is 15 drops per milliliter.

(b) When the nurse checks the infusion 2 hours after it started, 400 mL remain to be absorbed in the remaining 3 hours. Recalculate the flow rate in drops per minute for the remaining 400 mL.

DIMENSIONAL ANALYSIS

(a) Given flow rate: 500 mL/5 h
    Known equivalences: 15 gtt/mL
                         (drop factor)
                         1 h = 60 min

    Flow rate you want to find: ? gtt/min

You want to convert the flow rate from 500 mL in 5 hours to drops per minute.

$$\frac{500 \text{ mL}}{5 \text{ h}} = \frac{? \text{ gtt}}{\text{min}}$$

As in the previous examples, you can do this in one line as follows:

$$\frac{500 \text{ mL}}{5 \text{ h}} \times \frac{\overset{1}{15} \text{ gtt}}{1 \text{ mL}} \times \frac{1 \text{ h}}{\underset{4}{60} \text{ min}} = 25 \frac{\text{gtt}}{\text{min}}$$

FC METHOD

(a) The problem is

$$\frac{500 \text{ mL}}{5 \text{ h}} = ? \frac{\text{gtt}}{\text{min}}$$

Because

$$\frac{500}{5} = 100$$

The problem becomes

$$100 \frac{\text{mL}}{\text{h}} = ? \frac{\text{gtt}}{\text{min}}$$

DF = 15, therefore

$$FC = \frac{60}{15} = 4$$

Sometimes, for a variety of reasons the infusion flow rate can change. A change may affect the prescribed duration of time in which the solution will be administered. For example, with a gravity system, raising or lowering the infusion site or moving the patient's body or bed relative to the height of the bag may change the flow rate of the IV infusion. Therefore, the flow rate must be periodically assessed, and adjustments made if necessary. Example 10.10 illustrate the computations involved in this process.

So, the flow rate is 25 drops per minute.

(b) When the nurse checks the infusion, 400 mL need to be infused in 3 hours.

So, you now want to convert 400 mL in 3 hours to drops per minute.

$$\frac{400 \text{ mL}}{3 \text{ h}} = \frac{? \text{ gtt}}{\text{min}}$$

In a similar manner to part (a), you can do this in one line as follows:

$$\frac{400 \text{ mL}}{3 \text{ h}} \times \frac{\overset{1}{\cancel{15} \text{ gtt}}}{1 \text{ mL}} \times \frac{1 \text{ h}}{\underset{4}{\cancel{60} \text{ min}}} = 33.3 \frac{\text{gtt}}{\text{min}}$$

Because you want Drops per minute, Divide the given flow rate by 4

$$\frac{100}{4} = 25$$

So, the flow rate is 25 gtt/min.

(b) When the nurse checks the infusion, 400 mL need to be infused in 3 hours. So the problem is

$$\frac{400 \text{ mL}}{3 \text{ h}} = ? \frac{\text{gtt}}{\text{min}}$$

Because

$$\frac{400}{3} \approx 133.3$$

The problem becomes

$$133.3 \frac{\text{mL}}{\text{h}} = ? \frac{\text{gtt}}{\text{min}}$$

Because you want Drops per minute, Divide the given flow rate by FC, which is 4.

$$\frac{133.3}{4} = 33.3$$

So, in order for the infusion to be completed within the 5-hour period as ordered, the flow rate must be increased to 33 drops per minute.

EXAMPLE 10.11

A continuous IV of D5W has a drip rate of *20 gtt/min*. If the drop factor of the tubing is *15 gtt/mL*, how long will it take for 200 mL of D5W to infuse?

DIMENSIONAL ANALYSIS

| Volume to be infused: | 200 mL | [single unit of measurement] |
| Flow rate: | 20 gtt/min | [equivalence] |

FC METHOD AND PROPORTION

It is usually easier to work in *mL/h* rather than *gtt/min*. So, the first step is

$$20 \frac{\text{gtt}}{\text{min}} = ? \frac{\text{mL}}{\text{h}}$$

Drop factor:	15 gtt/mL	[equivalence]
Time:	? h	[single unit of measurement]

In this example, you want to change the single unit of measurement [*200 mL*] to another single unit of measurement [*h*].

$$500 \ mL = ? \ h$$

The problem becomes $500 \ ml \rightarrow ? \ gtt \rightarrow ? \ min$

To convert *mL to drops*, use the drop factor [*15 gtt/mL*]. To convert *gtt to min* use the flow rate [*20 gtt/min*].

$$200 \ \cancel{mL} \times \frac{15 \ \cancel{gtt}}{\cancel{mL}} \times \frac{min}{20 \ \cancel{gtt}} = 150 \ min$$

DF = 15, therefore

$$FC = \frac{60}{15} = 4$$

Because you want Milliliters per hour, Multiply the given flow rate by 4

$$20 \times 4 = 80$$

So, the flow rate is *80 mL/h*.

Now, you can set up a proportion:

$$\frac{80 \ mL}{1 \ h} = \frac{200 \ mL}{x \ h}$$

$$200 = 80 x$$

$$2.5 = x$$

So, the infusion will take *150 minutes* or *2½ hours*.

EXAMPLE 10.12

An infusion of 5% D/W is infusing at a rate of 20 drops per minute. If the drop factor is 15 drops per milliliter, how many hours will it take for the remaining solution in the bag (●Figure 10.12) to infuse?

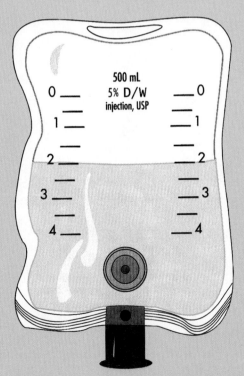

●**Figure 10.12**
5% D/W intravenous solution.

In Figure 10.12 you can see that 500 mL of solution were originally in the bag, and that the patient has received 200 mL. Therefore, 300 mL remain to be infused.

DIMENSIONAL ANALYSIS

Given:　300 mL (volume to be infused)

Known equivalences:　15 gtt/mL (drop factor)

　　20 gtts/min (flow rate)

　　1 h = 60 min

Find:　? h

You want to convert this single unit of measurement 300 mL to the single unit of measurement *hours*.

$$300 \text{ mL} = ? \text{ h}$$

You want to cancel mL. To do this you must use a unit fraction containing mL in the denominator. Using the drop factor, this fraction will be $\dfrac{15 \text{ gtt}}{1 \text{ mL}}$

$$300 \text{ mL} \times \frac{15 \text{ gtt}}{1 \text{ mL}} = ? \text{ h}$$

Now, on the left side gtt is in the numerator, but you don't want gtt. You need a unit fraction with gtt in the denominator to cancel. Using the flow rate, this fraction is $\dfrac{1 \text{ min}}{20 \text{ gtt}}$

$$300 \text{ mL} \times \frac{15 \text{ gtt}}{1 \text{ mL}} \times \frac{1 \text{ min}}{20 \text{ gtt}} = ? \text{ h}$$

Now, on the left side min is in the numerator, but you don't want min. You need a fraction with min in the denominator to cancel, namely, $\dfrac{1 \text{ h}}{60 \text{ min}}$

Now cancel and multiply the numbers.

$$300 \text{ mL} \times \frac{15 \text{ gtt}}{\text{mL}} \times \frac{\text{min}}{20 \text{ gtt}} \times \frac{1 \text{ h}}{60 \text{ min}} = 3.75 \text{ h}$$

FC METHOD AND PROPORTION

The first problem is to convert the flow rate to mL/h.

$$20 \frac{gtt}{min} = ? \frac{mL}{h}$$

DF = 15, therefore

$$FC = \frac{60}{15} = 4$$

Because you want <u>M</u>illiliters per hour, <u>M</u>ultiply the given flow rate by 4

$$20 \times 4 = 80$$

So, the flow rate is 80 mL/h.

Now use the proportion

$$\frac{80\,mL}{1\,h} = \frac{300\,mL}{x\,h}$$

$$300 = 80x$$
$$3.75 = x$$

So, it will take $3\frac{3}{4}$ hours for the remaining solution to infuse.

EXAMPLE 10.13

An IV of 1,000 mL of 5% D/0.9% NaCl is started at 8 P.M. The flow rate is 38 drops per minute, and the drop factor is 10 drops per milliliter. At what time will this infusion finish?

DIMENSIONAL ANALYSIS

Given: 1,000 mL (volume to be infused)

Known equivalences: 10 gtt/mL (drop factor)
38 gtt/min (flow rate)
1 h = 60 min

Find: ? h

You must first find how many hours the infusion will take to finish. You want to convert the single unit of measurement 1,000 mL to the single unit of measurement *hours*.

$$1,000 \text{ mL} = ? \text{ h}$$

You want to cancel mL. To do this you must use a unit fraction containing mL in the denominator. This fraction will be $\dfrac{10 \text{ gtt}}{1 \text{ mL}}$

$$1,000 \text{ mL} \times \frac{10 \text{ gtt}}{1 \text{ mL}} = ? \text{ h}$$

Now, on the left side gtt is in the numerator, but you don't want gtt. You need a fraction with gtt in the denominator. Using the flow rate, this fraction is $\dfrac{1 \text{ min}}{38 \text{ gtt}}$

$$1,000 \text{ mL} \times \frac{10 \text{ gtt}}{1 \text{ mL}} \times \frac{1 \text{ min}}{38 \text{ gtt}} = ? \text{ h}$$

Now, on the left side min is in the numerator, but you don't want min. You need a fraction with min in the denominator, namely, $\dfrac{1 \text{ h}}{60 \text{ min}}$ Now, cancel and multiply the numbers.

$$1,000 \text{ mL} \times \frac{\overset{1}{10} \text{ gtt}}{1 \text{ mL}} \times \frac{1 \text{ min}}{38 \text{ gtt}} \times \frac{1 \text{ h}}{\underset{6}{60} \text{ min}} = 4.4 \text{ h}$$

You then convert 0.4 h to min.

$$0.4 \text{ h} \times \frac{60 \text{ min}}{1 \text{ h}} = 24 \text{ min}$$

FC METHOD AND PROPORTION

For duration problems first convert the flow rate to *mL/h*.

$$38 \frac{gtt}{min} = ? \frac{mL}{h}$$

DF = 10, therefore

$$FC = \frac{60}{10} = 6$$

Because you want Milliliters per hour, Multiply the given flow rate by 6

$$38 \times 6 = 228$$

So, the flow rate is 228 mL/h.

Now use the proportion

$$\frac{228\,mL}{1\,h} = \frac{1,000\,mL}{x\,h}$$

$$1,000 = 228x$$
$$4.4 \approx x$$

So, it will take 4.4 hours for the remaining solution to infuse.

To convert 0.4 hours to minutes, use the proportion

$$\frac{1\,h}{60\,min} = \frac{0.4\,h}{x\,min}$$

$$24 = x$$

Therefore, 0.4 hours equals about 24 minutes.

So, the IV will infuse for 4 hours and 24 minutes. Because the infusion started at 8 P.M., it will finish at 12:24 A.M. on the following day.

EXAMPLE 10.14

The order reads: *1,000 mL D5W IV over 8 hours.* The drop factor is 10 gtt/mL.

(a) Calculate the initial flow rate in gtt/min for this infusion.

(b) After 5 hours 700 mL remain to be infused. How must the flow rate be adjusted so that the infusion will finish on time?

(c) If the facility has a policy that flow rate adjustments must not exceed 25% of the original rate, was the adjustment required within the guidelines?

DIMENSIONAL ANALYSIS

(a) First, convert the flow rate of 1,000 mL in 8 hours to gtt/min. You can do this in one line as follows:

$$\frac{1,000 \text{ mL}}{8 \text{ h}} \times \frac{1 \text{ h}}{60 \text{ min}} \times \frac{10 \text{ gtt}}{\text{mL}} = 20.8 \frac{\text{gtt}}{\text{min}}$$

So, the initial flow rate is 21 gtt/min.

(b) After 5 hours, 700 mL remain to be infused in the remaining 3 hours. Now, the new flow rate must be calculated. That is, you must convert the flow rate of 700 mL in 3 hours to gtt/min. You can do this in one line as follows:

$$\frac{700 \text{ mL}}{3 \text{ h}} \times \frac{1 \text{ h}}{60 \text{ min}} \times \frac{10 \text{ gtt}}{\text{mL}} = 38.9 \frac{\text{gtt}}{\text{min}}$$

So, the adjusted flow rate is 39 gtt/min.

FC METHOD AND PROPORTION

(a) The problem is

$$\frac{1,000 \text{ mL}}{8 h} = ? \frac{gtt}{min}$$

Because

$$\frac{1,000}{8} = 125$$

the problem becomes

$$125 \frac{mL}{h} = ? \frac{gtt}{min}$$

DF = 10, therefore

$$FC = \frac{60}{10} = 6$$

Because you want Drops per minute, Divide the given flow rate by 6

$$\frac{125}{6} \approx 20.8$$

So, the new flow rate is 21 *gtt/min*.

(b) After 5 hours, 700 mL remain to be infused in the remaining 3 hours.

The problem is

$$\frac{700 \text{ mL}}{3 h} = ? \frac{gtt}{min}$$

Because

$$\frac{700}{3} \approx 233.3$$

then the problem becomes

$$233.3 \frac{mL}{h} = ? \frac{gtt}{min}$$

As in part (a) FC = 6.

> Because you want <u>Drops</u> per minute, <u>Divide</u> the given flow rate by 6
>
> $$\frac{233.3}{6} \approx 38.9$$

(c) Since the facility has a policy that flow rate adjustments must not exceed 25% of the original rate, you must now calculate 25% of the original rate; that is, 25% of 21 gtt/min.

$$25\% \text{ of } 21 \text{ gtt/min} = (.25 \times 21) \text{ gtt/min}$$
$$= 5.25 \text{ gtt/min}$$

So, the flow rate may not be changed by more than about 5 gtt/min. Therefore, the initial flow rate of 21 gtt/min can be changed to no less than 16 (21 minus 5) gtt/min and no more than 26 (21 plus 5) gtt/min.

Since 39 gtt/min is outside the acceptable range of roughly 16–26 gtt/min, this change is not within the guidelines, and the adjustment may not be made. You must contact the prescriber.

Fluid Balance: Intake/Output

To work well, the various body systems need a stable environment in which their tissues and cells can function properly. For example, the body requires somewhat constant levels of temperature, salts, glucose, and in particular, adequate hydration to maintain homeostasis.

Part of hydration management involves the monitoring of a patient's fluid intake and output. This is especially important with pediatric, geriatric, and critical care patients.

Fluid intake is the amount of fluid that enters the body (oral and parenteral fluids), whereas **fluid output** is the amount of fluid that leaves the body (urine, sweat, liquid stool, emesis, and drainage).

Fluid replacement is sometimes necessary to avoid dehydration. If (as in Example 10.15) a physician provides an order with a specific ratio comparing the necessary replacement fluid with the patient's fluid output and if the patient's fluid output is known, then dimensional analysis could be used to determine the volume of replacement fluid to give the patient.

EXAMPLE 10.15

Order: *For every 100 mL of urine output, replace with 40 mL of water via PEG tube q4h.* The patient's urine output is 300 mL. What is the replacement volume?

DIMENSIONAL ANALYSIS

Think of the problem as:

Output:	300 mL (out)	[single unit of measurement]
Replacement:	100 mL (out)/ 40 mL (in)	[equivalence]
Input:	? mL (in)	[single unit of measurement]

In this example, you want to change the single unit of measurement [*300 mL(out)*] to another single unit of measurement [*mL(in)*].

$$300 \; mL(out) = ? \; mL(in)$$

The flow rate provides the equivalence [*100 mL(out)/40 mL(in)*] for the unit fraction.

$$300 \; \overline{mL(out)} \times \frac{40 \; mL(in)}{100 \; \overline{mL(out)}} = 120 \; mL(in)$$

So, the replacement volume is *120 mL*.

RATIO & PROPORTION

Think of the problem as:

$$100 \, mL \, (output) = 40 \, mL \, (input) \quad [order]$$
$$300 \, mL \, (output) = x \, mL \, (input) \quad [patient]$$

The proportion could be set up as

$$\frac{Out}{In} = \frac{Out'}{In'}$$

Substituting, you get

$$\frac{100 \, mL}{40 \, mL} = \frac{300 \, mL}{x \, mL}$$

$$12,000 = 100x$$
$$120 = x$$

So, the replacement volume is 120 mL.

Summary

In this chapter, the basic concepts and standard equipment used in enteral and intravenous therapy were introduced.

- Fluids can be given to a patient slowly over a period of time through a vein (*intravenous*) or through a tube inserted into the alimentary tract (*enteral*).
- Enteral and IV fluids can be administered continuously or intermittently.
- There is a wide variety of commercially prepared enteral and IV solutions.
- In IV solutions, *letters* indicate solution compounds, whereas *numbers* indicate solution concentration.
- Care must be taken to eliminate the air from, and maintain the sterility of, IV tubing.
- An IV infusion can flow solely by the force of gravity or by an electronic infusion pump.
- Use the following formula to determine flow rate:

$$Flow \; Rate = \frac{Volume}{Time}$$

- Flow rates are usually given as either mL/h or gtt/min.
- The drop factor of the IV administration set must be known in order to calculate flow rates.
- *Microdrops/minute* are equivalent to *milliliters/hour*.
- For microdrops, the drop factor is 60 microdrops per milliliter.
- For macrodrops, the usual drop factors are 10, 15, or 20 drops per milliliter.
- The *Flow Rate Conversion Number (FC)* is the quotient of 60 and the *Drop Factor (DF)*; *that is*, $FC = \frac{60}{DF}$.
- Use the FC technique to convert between the flow rates $\frac{mL}{h}$ and $\frac{gtt}{min}$:

    To get Drops, Divide by FC.
    To get Milliliters, Multiply by FC.

- To calculate the duration of an IV solution, first determine the flow rate in ml/h.
- Know the policy of the facility regarding readjustment of flow rates.

Case Study 10.1

Read the Case Study and answer the questions. Answers can be found in Appendix A.

An 86-year-old female is transferred from a nursing home and admitted to the hospital with a diagnosis of pneumonia. She has no known allergies to food or drugs and has a history of osteoarthritis, congestive heart failure, and hypertension. She is 5 feet tall, weighs 100 pounds, and has a PEG feeding tube. Her vital signs are: T 101° F; B/P 100/80; P 100; R 24, shallow.

Her orders include:

- Chest X-ray stat
- Blood culture stat
- Urine analysis, and C&S stat
- NPO
- IV: NS @83 mL/h
- Pulmocare 480 mg daily via PEG over 6 hours, followed by 50 mL sterile water flush

- Cleocin (clindamycin phosphate) 150 mg via PEG q6h
- Duragesic (fentanyl citrate) 25 mcg/h patch q3d
- heparin 5,000 units subcut q12h
- Zantac (ranitidine) 150 mg via PEG q6h

1. The label on the Cleocin reads 75 mg/5 ml oral suspension. How many milliliters will you administer?
2. The IV is infusing via gravity flow. Calculate the rate in mcgtt/min.
3. The strength on the heparin vial is 10,000 units/mL. How many milliliters will you administer?
4. Place an arrow at the correct measurement on the most appropriate syringe to indicate the amount of heparin to be administered.

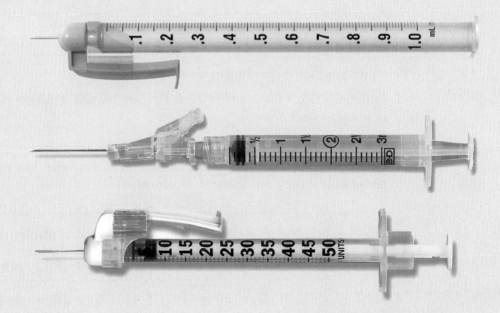

5. How many units of heparin is the patient receiving per day?
6. The strength of the ranitidine is 15 mg/mL. How many milliliters will you administer?
7. At what rate in mL/h will you set the feeding pump to administer the Pulmocare?

8. Calculate the total amount of enteral fluid the patient will receive in 24h.
9. How many milliliters of IV fluids is the patient receiving in 24h?
10. The fentanyl patch has been in place for 47 hours. How many milligrams has she received?

Practice Sets

Workspace

The answers to *Try These for Practice, Exercises,* and *Cumulative Review Exercises* are found in Appendix A. Ask your instructor for the answers to the *Additional Exercises.*

Try These for Practice

Test your comprehension after reading the chapter.

1. Order: *NS 1,000 mL IV infuse over 24 h.* Find the pump setting in *milliliters per hour.* _____

2. Order: *D_5W 1,000 mL IV infuse over 12 h.* Find the flow rate in *drops per minute if the drop factor is 20 gtt/mL.* _____

3. Order: *0.45% NaCl 500 mL IV infuse over 24 h.* Find the flow rate in *microdrops per minute.* _____

4. Order: $\frac{1}{2}$ *NS 400 mL IV at 25 mL/h.* If the IV starts at *1430h on Friday,* at what time will it finish? _____

5. Order: *For every 200 mL of urine output, replace with 50 mL of water via nasogastric tube q4h.* If the patient's urine output for the last four hours is 300 mL, what is the replacement volume of water needed?

_____

Exercises

Reinforce your understanding in class or at home.

1. Order: *5%D 0.45% NaCl 500 mL IV over 3 hours.* Find the pump setting in *milliliters per hour.*

_____

2. Order: *Ringer's Lactate 500 mL IV over 12 h.* Find the flow rate in *drops per minute if the drop factor is 15 gtt/mL.*

_____

3. D5/W is infusing at *90 mL/h* using an electronic controler. How much D5/W will infuse in 90 minutes?

_____

4. NS is infusing intravenously at *75 mL/h.* How long will it take for 500 mL to infuse?

_____

5. Order: 1,000 mL NS infuse at 75 mL/h. The infusion starts at 7 A.M. on Tuesday. When is the infusion scheduled to be completed?

_____

6. Order: *500 mL NS IV run 75 mL/h.* How many milliliters will infuse in 3 hours?

_____

7. *Order: NS 1,500 mL over 12 h.* After 3 hours *1,200 mL* remain in the bag. The facility policy indicates that flow rate adjustments may not exceed 25% of the original rate. Recalculate the flow rate so that the infusion will finish on time, and decide if the adjustment is within the guidelines.

8. Find the flow rate in *drops per minute* that is equivalent to a flow rate of *75 mL/h* when you are using *20 gtt/mL* macrodrip tubing.

9. A pump is set at *200 mL/h.* Find the flow rate in *gtt/min* if the drop factor is *10 gtt/mL.*

10. Find the flow rate in *microdrops per minute* that is equivalent to a rate of *35 mL/h.*

11. Order: *For every 100 mL of urine output, replace with 30 mL of H_2O through the persutaneous endoscopic gastrostomy (PEG) tube q4h.* If urine output for the last 4 hours is 500 mL, find the replacement fluid volume.

12. Determine the completion time of *200 mL* packed blood cells that ran at *50 mL/h.* The bag was hung at 3:15 P.M. on Monday.

13. Order: *RL 375 mL IV over 3 h.* The tubing has a drop factor of *10 gtt/mL.*
    (a) Calculate the initial flow rate in *gtt/min.*
    (b) After *1 hour, 175 mL* have infused. Determine the adjusted flow rate so that the infusion will finish on time.
    (c) If flow rate adjustments cannot exceed 25% of the original rate, is the adjustment in part (b) within the guidelines?

14. An infusion is running at *50 mL/h.* Find the equivalent flow rate in gtt/min when the drop factor is 15 gtt/mL.

15. Order: *NS 750 mL IV infuse at 75 mL/h.* If the IV started at 11 P.M. on Wednesday, at what time will it finish?

16. Order: *1,000 mL D5 $\frac{1}{2}$ NS to run at 90 mL/h.* Find the drip rate for 15 gtt/mL tubing.

17. Order: *NS 1,000 mL intravenous over 10 h.* At 0700h 400 mL has infused. At what time will the infusion finish?

18. Order: *RL 1,000 mL IV 8 A.M. – 8 P.M.* What is the pump setting in mL/h?

19. Order: *150 mL NS IV over 3 hours.* At how many mcgtt/min would you run this infusion?

_____

20. For every 200 mL of urine output, replace with 40 mL of H_2O through the jejunostomy (J-tube) tube q8h. If urine output for the last 8 hours is 700 mL, find the replacement fluid volume.

_____

Additional Exercises

Now, test yourself!

1. The physician ordered *750 mL of NS IV for 8 hours.* Calculate the flow rate in drops per minute. The drop factor is 10 gtt = 1 mL.

_____

2. The patient is to receive *375 mL of RL over 3 hours.* Set the rate on the infusion pump in milliliters per hour.

_____

3. Order: *For every 100 mL of urine output, replace with 30 mL of water via nasogastric tube q4h.* If the patient's urine output for the last four hours is 550 mL, what is the replacement volume of water needed?

_____

4. Order: *1,000 mL D_5W to infuse at 125 mL/h.* How long will this infusion take to finish?

_____

5. A patient is to receive 500 mL 5%D/0.45%NaCl IV in 3 hours. Calculate the flow rate in microdrops per minute.

_____

6. The order reads *1,500 mL D_5W IV over 12 hours.* The drop factor is 20 gtt/mL.
   (a) Find the flow rate in gtt/min for this infusion.
   (b) If after 3 hours 1,200 mL remain to be infused, how must the flow rate be adjusted so that the infusion will finish on time?
   (c) If the facility has a policy that flow rate adjustments must not exceed 25% of the original rate, is the adjustment required in part (b) within the guidelines?

_____

7. Order: *750 mL Ringer's Lactate IV in 8 hours.* Calculate the flow rate in drops per minute if the drop factor is 15 gtt/mL.

_____

8. An IV infusion of 750 mL Ringer's Lactate began at noon. It has been infusing at the rate of 125 mL/h. At what time is it scheduled to finish?

_____

9. A patient has an order for a total parenteral nutrition (TPN) solution 1,000 mL in 24 hours. At what rate in mL/h should the pump be set?

10. An IV is infusing at 90 mL/h. The IV tubing has a drop factor of 20 gtt/mL. Calculate the flow rate in gtt/min.

11. Order: *1,000 mL NS IV over 6 hours.* Calculate and set the flow rate in mL/h for the electronic controller.

12. Calculate the infusion time for an IV of 500 mL that is ordered to run at 40 mL/h.

13. The order reads *750 mL of NS IV. Infuse over a 24 h period.* Set the flow rate on the infusion pump in milliliters per hour.

14. An IV of 800 mL is to infuse over 8 hours at the rate of 20 gtt/min. After 4 hours and 45 minutes, only 300 mL had infused. Recalculate the flow rate in gtt/min. The set calibration is 15 gtt/mL.

15. The order reads *1,000 mL D$_5$W IV in 8 hours* start at 10 A.M. The IV was stopped at 4:30 P.M. for 45 minutes with 90 mL of fluid remaining. Determine the new flow rate setting for the infusion pump in mL/h so that the infusion finishes on time.

16. An IV bag has 350 mL remaining. It is infusing at 35 gtt/min, and a 15 gtt/mL set is being used. How long will it take to finish?

17. An IV solution is infusing at 32 microdrops per minute. How many milliliters of this solution will the patient receive in 6 hours?

18. A patient must have a tube feeding of 1,000 mL Ensure for 10 hours. The drop factor is 15 gtt/mL. After 5 hours, a total of 650 mL has infused. Recalculate the new gtt/min flow rate to complete the infusion on schedule.

19. An IV is infusing at a rate of 30 drops per minute. The drop factor is 15 gtt/mL. Calculate the flow rate in milliliters per hour.

20. A patient is to receive 1 unit (500 mL) of packed red blood cells over 4 hours. For the first 15 minutes, infuse at 50 mL/h. At what rate would you set the pump to complete the infusion?

Workspace

Cumulative Review Exercises

Workspace

Review your mastery of previous chapters.

1. 1 cm = ? inches

2. 35 mcgtt = ? mL

3. 200 lb = ? kg

4. 45 mm = ? cm

5. 60 mL = ? oz

6. How many milligrams of sodium chloride are contained in 1 L of 0.225% NaCl?

7. The order reads *Sustacal 240 mL via PEG over 8 h*. At how many mL/h will you set the pump?

8. An IV of 1,000 mL of 5% D/W is to infuse over 10 hours. After 5 hours, the patient had received 450 mL. The drop factor is 20 drops per milliliter. Recalculate the flow rate in gtt/min which will allow the infusion to finish on time.

9. Calculate the BSA of a patient who is 5 feet 2 inches and weighs 100 pounds.

10. The patient weighs 109 pounds. The order is for *oxymetholone 2 mg/kg po daily*. The drug is supplied in 50 mg tablets. How many tablets of this anabolic steroid will you prepare?

11. Order: *interferon beta-1a 0.25 mg subcut every other day*. The strength available is 0.25 mg/mL. How many mL will you administer?

12. Order: *Clarinex (desloratadine) 5 mg po daily*. How many 2.5-mg tablets of this antihistamine would you administer?

13. How many grams of a drug are contained in a bottle of 100 tablets if each tablet contains 50 mg of the drug?

14. How many mL of 2% lidocaine contain 3 grams of lidocaine?

15. If an IV starts at 2300h on Wednesday and lasts for 13 hours, when does it finish?

nursing.pearsonhighered.com
Prepare for success with animated examples, practice questions, challenge tests, and interactive assignments.

Flow Rates and Dosage Rates for Intravenous Medications

Chapter

11

Learning Outcomes

After completing this chapter, you will be able to

1. Describe intravenous (IV) medication administration.
2. Convert from dosage rates (drug/time) to IV rates (volume/time).
3. Convert from IV rates (volume/time) to dosage rates (drug/time).
4. Calculate infusion rates when medication must be added to the intravenous piggyback (IVPB) bag.
5. Calculate infusion rates based on the size (weight or body surface area [BSA]) of the patient.
6. Calculate flow rates for IV push medications.
7. Calculate the duration of an IVPB infusion.
8. Calculate flow rates for medication requiring titration.
9. Construct a titration table.

T his chapter extends the discussion of infusions to include the administration of intravenous *medications*.

In the previous chapter the focus was on **flow rates** (*volume of fluid per time, e.g., mL/h or gtt/min*). However, in this chapter, the infusing solutions will contain medication, so you will also calculate **dosage rates** (*amount of drug per time, e.g., mg/min or unit/hr*).

This chapter also introduces orders that indicate the dosage rate based on the size of the patient, namely, **compound rates** (*amount of drug per size of the patient per time, e.g., mg/kg/min or mcg/m²/min*).

The calculations involved in medication administered by *IV push* and *titration* are also introduced.

Intravenous Administration of Medications

Intravenous (IV) administration of medications provides rapid access to a patient's circulatory system, thereby presenting potential hazards. Errors in medications, dose, or dosage strength can prove fatal. Therefore, *caution must be taken in the calculation, preparation, and administration of IV medications.*

Typically, a **primary** IV line provides continuous fluid to the patient. **Secondary** lines can be attached to the primary line at injection ports, and these lines are often used to deliver *continuous or intermittent* medication intravenously. A secondary line is referred to as a **piggyback** or **intravenous piggyback** (**IVPB**). With intermittent IVPB infusions, the bags hold generally 50–250 mL of fluid containing dissolved medication and usually require 20–60 minutes to infuse. Like a primary line, an IVPB infusion may use a manually controlled gravity system or an electronic infusion device.

A **heplock**, or **saline lock**, is an infusion port attached to an indwelling needle or cannula in a peripheral vein. Intermittent IV infusions can be administered through these ports via IV lines connected to these ports. An **IV push** (**IVP**), or **bolus**, is a direct injection of medication either into the heplock/saline lock or directly into the vein.

Syringe pumps can also be used for intermittent infusions. A syringe with the medication is inserted into the pump. The medication is delivered at a set rate over a short period of time.

A **volume-control set** is a small container, called a burette, that is connected to the IV line. Burettes are often used in pediatric or geriatric care, where accurate volume control is critical. The danger of overdose is limited because of the small volume of solution in the burette. Burettes will be discussed in Chapter 12.

Intravenous Piggyback Infusions

Patients can receive a medication through a port in an existing IV line. This is called **intravenous piggyback (IVPB)**; •**Figure 11.1**. The medication is in a secondary bag. Notice in Figure 11.1 that the secondary bag is higher than the primary bag so that the pressure in the secondary line will be greater than the pressure in the primary line. Therefore, the secondary medication infuses first. Once the secondary infusion is completed, the primary line begins to flow. Be sure to keep both lines open. If you close the primary line, when the secondary IVPB is completed the primary line will not flow into the vein.

A typical IVPB order might read: *cimetidine 300 mg IVPB q6h in 50 mL NS infuse over 20 min.* This is an order for an IV piggyback infusion in which 300 mg of the drug cimetidine diluted in 50 mL of a normal saline solution must infuse in 20 minutes. So, the patient receives 300 mg of cimetidine in 20 minutes via a secondary line, and this dose is repeated every 6 hours.

In this chapter you will encounter both flow rates and dosage rate. The following formulas will apply:

$$Flow\,Rate = \frac{Volume}{Time}$$

$$Dosage\,Rate = \frac{Drug}{Time}$$

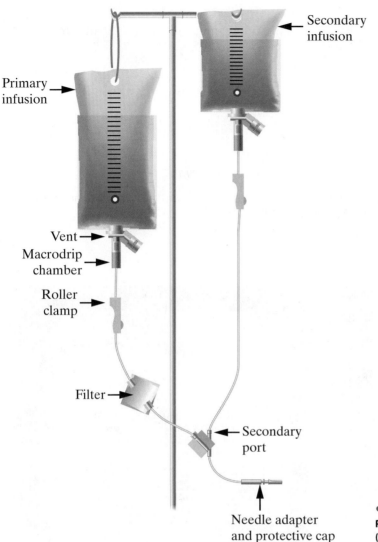

Primary infusion

Secondary infusion

Vent

Macrodrip chamber

Roller clamp

Filter

Secondary port

Needle adapter and protective cap

• Figure 11.1
Primary and secondary (IVPB) infusion setup.

EXAMPLE 11.1

Order: *cimetidine 300 mg IVPB q6h in 50 mL NS infuse in 20 min.* Find the

(a) IV flow rate measured in milliliters/min.

(b) Dosage rate measured in milligrams/min.

(a) Because 50 mL of solution must infuse in 20 minutes, the IV flow rate is

$$\frac{\text{volume}}{\text{time}} = \frac{50 \ mL}{20 \ min}$$

Because $\frac{50}{20} = 2.5$

$$\frac{50 \ mL}{20 \ min} = 2.5 \frac{mL}{min}$$

So, the IV flow rate is 2.5 mL/min, which means that the patient receives a volume of 2.5 mL of solution every minute.

(b) Because 300 mg of cimetidine must infuse in 20 minutes, the dosage rate is

$$\frac{\text{drug}}{\text{time}} = \frac{300 \ mg}{20 \ min}$$

Because $\frac{300}{20} = 15$

$$\frac{300 \ mg}{20 \ min} = 15 \frac{mg}{min}$$

So, the dosage rate is 15 mg/min, which means that the patient receives 15 mg of cimetidine every minute.

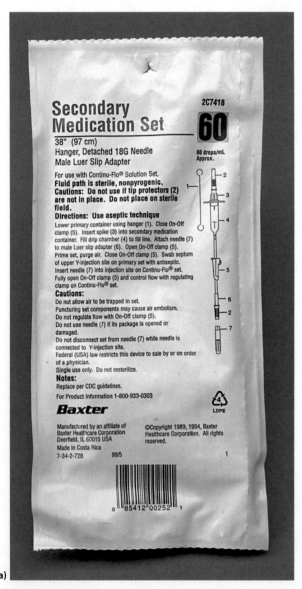

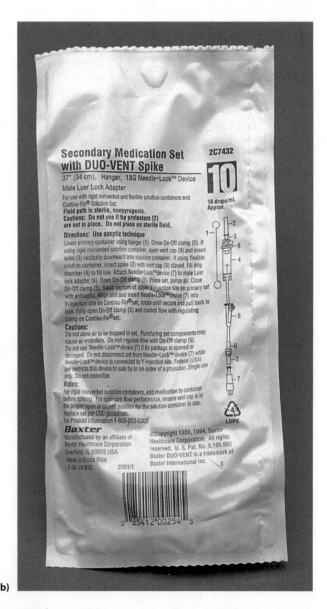

(a)   (b)

• **Figure 11.2**
Packages of secondary IV tubing: (a) 60 drops per mL, (b) 10 drops per mL.

(Courtesy of Baxter Healthcare Corporation. All rights reserved. Photos by Al Dodge.)

Converting IV Dosage Rates to Flow Rates

Each of the next four examples (11.2 through 11.5) converts rates from dosage rates (*amount of medication per time*) to IV flow rates (*volume of solution per time*).

> ## EXAMPLE 11.2
>
> Order: *cefoxitin 1 g IVPB q6h over 30 minutes*. Read the drug label in •Figure 11.3.
>
> (a) Find the dosage rate in *grams per hour*.
>
> (b) Change the dosage rate to the flow rate in *milliliters per hour*.
>
> (c) Change the flow rate from *mL/h* to *drops per minute* if the drop factor is 10 *gtt/mL*.

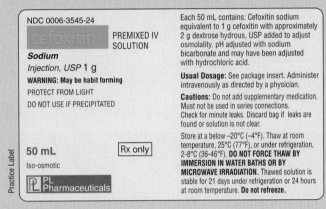

Practice Label

NDC 0006-3545-24	Each 50 mL contains: Cefoxitin sodium equivalent to 1 g cefoxitin with approximately 2 g dextrose hydrous, USP added to adjust osmolality. pH adjusted with sodium bicarbonate and may have been adjusted with hydrochloric acid.

cefoxitin   PREMIXED IV SOLUTION

Sodium
Injection, USP 1 g

WARNING: May be habit forming

PROTECT FROM LIGHT

DO NOT USE IF PRECIPITATED

Usual Dosage: See package insert. Administer intravenously as directed by a physician.

Cautions: Do not add supplementary medication. Must not be used in series connections. Check for minute leaks. Discard bag if leaks are found or solution is not clear.

Store at a below –20°C (–4°F). Thaw at room temperature, 25°C (77°F), or under refrigeration, 2-8°C (36-46°F). **DO NOT FORCE THAW BY IMMERSION IN WATER BATHS OR BY MICROWAVE IRRADIATION.** Thawed solution is stable for 21 days under refrigeration or 24 hours at room temperature. **Do not refreeze.**

50 mL   Rx only
Iso-osmotic

℞ PL Pharmaceuticals

•**Figure 11.3**
Drug label for cefoxitin.
(For educational purposes only)

DIMENSIONAL ANALYSIS

(a) Because 1 gram must infuse in 30 minutes, the dosage rate $\left(\dfrac{weight\ of\ drug}{time}\right)$ is $\dfrac{1\ g}{30\ min}$

$$\frac{1g}{30min} = ?\frac{g}{h}$$

To change the minutes to hours, use *1 h = 60 min*

$$\frac{1\ g}{30\ min} \times \frac{60\ min}{1\ h} = \frac{2\ g}{h}$$

So, the dosage rate is 2 *grams per hour*.

(b) $\dfrac{2\ g}{h} = ?\dfrac{mL}{h}$

Use the strength of the solution *50 mL = 1 g* to form the unit fraction.

$$\frac{2\ g}{h} \times \frac{50\ mL}{1\ g} = \frac{100\ mL}{h}$$

So, the flow rate is 100 *milliliters per hour*.

FC & PROPORTION

(a) The dosage rate in the order is $\dfrac{1g}{30\,min}$, and this rate must be changed to g/h. So the problem is

$$\frac{1g}{30\,min} = ?\frac{g}{h}$$

You can change 30 minutes to 1 hour by multiplying 30 min × 2 = 60 min = 1 *hour*.

Change $\dfrac{1g}{30\,min}$ to $\dfrac{g}{h}$ by multiplying by $\dfrac{2}{2}$ as follows:

$$\frac{1g}{30\,min} \times \frac{2}{2} = \frac{2g}{60\,min} = \frac{2g}{1h}$$

So, the dosage rate is 2 g/h.

(b) The dosage rate of 2 g/h must be changed to *mL/h*. So the problem is

$$2g = ?\,mL$$

(c) $\dfrac{100\ mL}{h} = ?\ \dfrac{gtt}{min}$

Use the drop factor of *10 gtt per mL.*

$$\frac{100\ \cancel{mL}}{\cancel{h}} \times \frac{1\ \cancel{h}}{60\ min} \times \frac{10\ gtt}{\cancel{mL}} = \frac{16.7\ gtt}{min}$$

Because the strength of the solution stated on the IV bag is *1 g = 50 mL,* you can use the proportion

$$\frac{2g}{x\ mL} = \frac{1g}{50\ mL}$$

$$x = 100$$

So, the IV flow rate is 100 mL/h.

(c) Now, change the rate 100 *mL/h* to gtt/min, using the FC method.

DF = 10 and $FC = \frac{60}{10} = 6$. You want Drops per minute, so Divide.

$$\frac{100}{6} \approx 16.7$$

Therefore,

$$100\ \frac{mL}{h} \approx 16.7\ \frac{gtt}{min}$$

So, the flow rate is 17 *drops per minute.*

EXAMPLE 11.3

The medication order reads: *Invanz (ertapenem sodium) 1g IVPB daily infuse over 30 min.* Read the label in • Figure 11.4. The directions indicate that the vial should be reconstituted with 10 mL of sterile water and then added to 50 mL NS. Calculate the flow rate for this beta-lactam antibiotic in

(a) mL/h

(b) gtt/min if the drop factor is 10 gtt/mL.

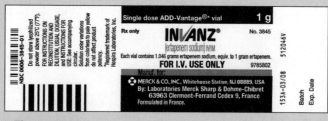

• **Figure 11.4**
Drug label for Invanz.

(a) First reconstitute by adding *10 mL* of sterile water to the vial. This yields an approximate concentration of *1 g/10 mL* in the vial. Because the order is *1 gram,* the entire contents of the 1-gram vial must be added to the *50 mL* bag of normal saline, and the bag will then contain *1 g* of Ivanz in *60 mL* (*50 mL + 10 mL*) of solution.

To obtain the flow rate (volume/time), divide the total volume of the infusion (*60 mL*) by the time of the infusion (*30 min*).

$$Flow\ Rate = \frac{volume}{time} = \frac{60\ mL}{30\ min} = ?\ \frac{mL}{h}$$

DIMENSIONAL ANALYSIS

You want to convert the flow rate from milliliters per minute to an equivalent flow rate in milliliters per hour, that is, convert the minutes to hours as follows:

$$\frac{60\,mL}{30\,\cancel{min}} \times \frac{\overset{2}{\cancel{60\,min}}}{h} = \frac{120\,mL}{h}$$

So, the flow rate is 120 mL/h.

(b) Now you must convert the flow rate from *120 mL/h* to an equivalent flow rate in *gtt/min*. Use the drop factor of *10 gtt = 1 mL* and

$$120\,\frac{\cancel{mL}}{\cancel{h}} \times \frac{1\,\cancel{h}}{60\,min} \times \frac{10\,gtt}{1\,\cancel{mL}} = 20\,\frac{gtt}{min}$$

So, the flow rate is *20 gtt/min*.

FC METHOD

Change $\frac{60\,mL}{30\,min}$ to $\frac{mL}{h}$ by multiplying by $\frac{2}{2}$ as follows:

$$\frac{60\,mL}{30\,min} \times \frac{2}{2} = \frac{120\,mL}{60\,min} = \frac{120\,mL}{1\,h}$$

So, the flow rate is 120 mL/h.

(b) Now, change the flow rate of 120 *mL/h* to *gtt/min*, using the FC technique.

DF = 10 and FC = $\frac{60}{10}$ = 6. You want Drops per minute, so Divide.

$$\frac{120}{6} = 20$$

Therefore,

$$120\,\frac{mL}{h} = 20\,\frac{gtt}{min}$$

EXAMPLE 11.4

The medication order reads: *heparin 1,250 units/hour IV*. The IV solution has 10,000 units of heparin in 1,000 mL of NS. Calculate the infusion rate in mL/h.

You want to convert the prescribed dosage rate of *1,250 units/hour* to a flow rate in *milliliters per hour*.

$$\frac{1,250\,units}{h} = ?\,\frac{mL}{h}$$

DIMENSIONAL ANALYSIS

Use the concentration of the IV bag (*10,000 units in 1,000 mL*) to make the unit fraction.

$$\frac{1,250\,units}{h} \times \frac{1,000\,mL}{10,000\,units} = \frac{125\,mL}{h}$$

RATIO & PROPORTION

In the numerator change 1,250 units to mL of solution.

Think:

$1,250\,units = x\,mL$

$10,000\,units = 1,000\,mL$ [strength of the solution]

Use the proportion

$$\frac{1,250\,units}{x\,mL} = \frac{10,000\,units}{1,000\,mL}$$

$$10,000x = 1,250,000$$

$$x = 125$$

This means that 1,250 units are contained in 125 mL and therefore,

$$\frac{1{,}250\,units}{1\,h} = \frac{125\,mL}{h}$$

So, the IV flow rate is *125 mL/h*.

EXAMPLE 11.5

The prescriber writes an order for 1,000 mL of 5% D/W with 10 units of Pitocin (oxytocin). Your patient must receive 3 mU of this drug per minute. Calculate the flow rate in microdrops per minute.

DIMENSIONAL ANALYSIS

Given dosage rate: 3 mU/min

Known equivalences: 10 units/1,000 mL (strength)

60 mcgtt/mL (standard microdrop drop factor)

1 unit = 1,000 mU

Flow rate you want to find: ? mcgtt/min

You want to change the dosage rate from milliunits per minute to a flow rate of microdrops per minute.

$$3\,\frac{mU}{min} = ?\,\frac{mcgtt}{min}$$

NOTE

1 unit = 1,000 milliunits (mU)

You want to cancel mU. To do this you must use a unit fraction containing mU in the denominator. Using the equivalence 1 mU = 1,000 units, this fraction will be $\dfrac{1\ unit}{1{,}000\ mU}$.

$$\frac{3\,\widebar{mU}}{min} \times \frac{1\,\widehat{unit}}{1{,}000\,\widebar{mU}} = ?\,\frac{mcgtt}{min}$$

Now, on the left side unit is in the numerator, and it must be cancelled. This will require a unit fraction with unit in the denominator. Using the strength, this fraction will be $\dfrac{1{,}000\ mL}{10\ units}$.

RATIO & PROPORTION

One way to do the problem is to first change the dosage rate to *mL/h*. The first problem is

$$\frac{3\,mU}{min} = ?\,\frac{mL}{h}$$

Multiply by $\dfrac{60}{60}$

$$\frac{3\,mU}{min} \times \frac{60}{60} = \frac{180\,mU}{60\,min} = \frac{180\,mU}{1\,h}$$

In the numerator change 180 mU to 0.18 units by moving the decimal point three places to the left. Now the problem becomes

$$\frac{0.18\,units}{min} = ?\,\frac{mL}{h}$$

To change 0.18 units of the drug to mL of solution, think:

$0.18\,units = x\,mL$

$10\,units = 1{,}000\,mL$ [strength of the solution]

Use the proportion

$$\frac{0.18\,units}{x\,mL} = \frac{10\,units}{1{,}000\,mL}$$

$$10\,x = 180$$

$$x = 18$$

So the flow rate is *18 mL/h*, which is the same as *18 mcgtt/min*.

$$\frac{3\,mU}{min} \times \frac{1\,unit}{1,000\,mU} \times \frac{1,000\,\boxed{mL}}{10\,units} = ?\,\frac{mcgtt}{min}$$

Now, on the left side mL is in the numerator, and it must be cancelled. This will require a unit fraction with mL in the denominator. Using the drop factor, this fraction will be $\frac{60\,mcgtt}{mL}$.

Now, cancel and multiply the numbers

$$\frac{3\,mU}{min} \times \frac{1\,unit}{1,000\,mU} \times \frac{1,000\,mL}{10\,units} \times \frac{60\,mcgtt}{mL}$$

$$= 18\,\frac{mcgtt}{min}$$

So, you will administer 18 mcgtt/min.

Converting IV Flow Rates to Dosage Rates

Each of the next three examples (11.6 through 11.8) converts infusion rates from IV flow rates (*volume of solution per time*) to dosage rates (*amount of medication per time*).

EXAMPLE 11.6

Calculate the number of units of Regular insulin a patient is receiving per hour if the order is *500 mL NS with 300 units of Regular insulin and it is infusing at the rate of 12.5 mL per hour via the pump.*

You want to convert the flow rate from mL per hour to the dosage rate in units per hour.

$$\frac{12.5\,mL}{h} \longrightarrow ?\,\frac{units}{h}$$

DIMENSIONAL ANALYSIS

Using the strength of the solution (300 units/500 mL) you do this in one line as follows:

$$\frac{12.5\,mL}{h} \times \frac{300\,units}{500\,mL} = \frac{37.5\,units}{5\,h}$$

$$\text{or}\quad 7.5\,\frac{units}{h}$$

RATIO & PROPORTION

In the numerator, change 12.5 mL of solution to units of insulin.

Think:

$12.5\,mL = x\,units$

$300\,mL = 500\,units = $ [strength of the solution]

Use the proportion

$$\frac{12.5\,mL}{x\,units} = \frac{500\,mL}{300\,units}$$

$$500x = 3,750$$

$$x = 7.5$$

This means that 7.5 units of insulin are contained in 12.5 mL of the solution.

So, the patient is receiving 7.5 units per hour.

EXAMPLE 11.7

An IV bag contains 1,000 mL of NS with 500 mg of a drug. It is infusing at 12 gtt/min. The drop factor is 10 gtt/mL.

(a) Find the dosage rate in *mg/min*.

(b) If the recommended dose is *0.5–2.5 mg/min*, is this infusion in the safe dose range?

DIMENSIONAL ANALYSIS

(a) The problem is to change the flow rate of *12 gtt/min* to a dosage rate in *mg/min*.

$$\frac{12 \; gtt}{min} = ? \; \frac{mg}{min}$$

The strength of the solution (*500 mg = 1,000 mL*) and the drop factor (*10 gtt = 1 mL*) will both be used to construct the necessary unit fractions.

$$\frac{12 \; \cancel{gtt}}{min} \times \frac{\cancel{mL}}{10 \; \cancel{gtt}} \times \frac{500 \; mg}{1,000 \; \cancel{mL}} = \frac{0.6 \; mg}{min}$$

FC & PROPORTION

Change the flow rate of 12 *gtt/min* to *mL/h*, using the FC technique.

$DF = 10$ and $FC = \dfrac{60}{10} = 6$. You want Milliliters per hour, so Multiply.

$$12 \times 6 = 72$$

Therefore,

$$12 \; \frac{gtt}{min} = 72 \; \frac{mL}{h}$$

Now, change 72 mL to mg. Because the strength of the solution is *500 mg/1,000 mL*, you can use the proportion

$$\frac{72 \; mL}{x \; mg} = \frac{1,000 \; mL}{500 \; mg}$$

$$1,000 \, x = 36,000$$

$$x = 36$$

So, the dosage rate is $\dfrac{36 \; mg}{1 \, h}$. Substituting 60 minutes for 1 hour, you obtain

$$\frac{36 \; mg}{1 \, h} = \frac{36 \; mg}{60 \; min} = 0.6 \; \frac{mg}{min}$$

So, the dosage rate is 0.6 *mg/min*.

(b) Because 0.6 is between 0.5 and 2.5, this infusion is in the safe dose range.

EXAMPLE 11.8

Order: *heparin 40,000 units continuous IV in 1,000 mL of D5W infuse at 30 mL/h.* Find the rate in units/day and determine if it is in the safe dose range—the normal heparinizing range is between 20,000 to 40,000 units per day.

You want to convert the flow rate from milliliters per hour to units per day.

$$\frac{30 \; mL}{1 \; h} \longrightarrow ? \; \frac{units}{day}$$

DIMENSIONAL ANALYSIS

Using the strength of the solution (40,000 units/1,000 mL) and that there are 24 hours in a day, you do this on one line as follows:

$$\frac{30\ \text{mL}}{\text{h}} \times \frac{40,000\ \text{units}}{1,000\ \text{mL}} \times \frac{24\ \text{h}}{\text{day}}$$

$$= 28,800\ \frac{\text{units}}{\text{day}}$$

RATIO & PROPORTION

In the numerator, change 30 mL of solution to units of heparin. A proportion may be used to do this by thinking:

$$30\,mL = x\,units$$
$$1,000\,mL = 40,000\,units = \text{(strength)}$$

Use the proportion

$$\frac{30\,mL}{x\,units} = \frac{1,000\,mL}{40,000\,units}$$

$$1,000x = 1,200,00$$
$$x = 1,200$$

This means that 1,200 units of heparin are contained in 30 mL of the solution and

$$\frac{30\,mL}{h} = \frac{1,200\,units}{h}$$

Change $1,200\,\frac{units}{h}$ to $\frac{units}{day}$ by multiplying by $\frac{24}{24}$

$$\frac{1,200\,units}{1h} \times \frac{24}{24} = \frac{28,800\,units}{24h}$$
$$= \frac{28,800\,units}{1\,day}$$

So, your patient is receiving 28,800 units of heparin per day. This rate is within the safe dosage range of 20,000 to 40,000 units per day.

IV Push

To infuse a small amount of medication in a short period of time, a syringe can be inserted directly into a vein, or a saline lock or heparin lock can be attached to an IV catheter. For patients who have a primary IV line, the medication should be administered through the port closest to the patient. The medication can then be "pushed" directly into the vein. This route of medication administration is referred to as **IV push (IVP)**. See •**Figure 11.5**.

Because the IVP flow rate is determined by the speed at which the plunger of the syringe is manually pushed, it is important to control that speed. It is difficult to maintain the desired flow rate over the entire infusion. Therefore, the infusion may be mentally divided into smaller segments or pieces to make the flow rate easier to control.

For example, suppose that 4 *mL* of solution must be infused IVP in 1 *minute* (60 *seconds*). Because the total infusion volume (4 *mL*) and duration (60 *sec*) are known, the flow rate is *4 mL/60 sec*. You may choose to divide numerator

An IV push generally involves medications administered over a short period of time. Be sure to verify the need for the drug, route, concentration, dose, expiration date, and clarity of the solution. It is also essential to verify the rate of injection with the package insert. Some medications (e.g., adenosine) require very rapid administration, whereas others (e.g., verapamil) are administered more slowly.

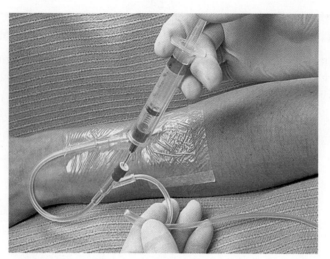

• **Figure 11.5**
IV push administration.

and denominator of this fraction by any convenient number. By doing so, you will make the numbers in the numerator and denominator smaller, and thereby obtain an equivalent infusion rate using the smaller quantities, as shown in the following:

- If you divide both the numerator and denominator of the flow rate of $\frac{4\ mL}{60\ sec}$ by 2, you obtain

$$\frac{4\ mL}{60\ sec} = \frac{4 \div 2\ mL}{60 \div 2\ sec} = \frac{2\ mL}{30\ sec}$$

  and the flow rate of $\frac{4\ mL}{60\ sec}$ is equivalent to $\frac{2\ mL}{30\ sec}$. So, you would push 2 *mL* every 30 *seconds* until the 4 *mL* of medication in the syringe are infused.

- On the other hand, if you divide both the numerator and denominator of the flow rate of $\frac{4\ mL}{60\ sec}$ by 4, you obtain

$$\frac{4\ mL}{60\ sec} = \frac{4 \div 4\ mL}{60 \div 4\ sec} = \frac{1\ mL}{15\ sec}$$

  and the flow rate of $\frac{4\ mL}{60\ sec}$ is equivalent to $\frac{1\ mL}{15\ sec}$. So, you would push 1 *mL* every 15 *seconds* until the 4 *mL* of medication in the syringe are infused.

EXAMPLE 11.9

750 mg of a drug is ordered IVP stat over 5 minutes, and the concentration of the drug is 75 mg/mL.

(a) Find the total number of milliliters you will administer.
(b) Determine the IVP flow rate if you divide the infusion into 5 equal segments.
(c) Determine the IVP flow rate if you divide the infusion into 10 equal segments.

DIMENSIONAL ANALYSIS	FORMULA METHOD

DIMENSIONAL ANALYSIS

(a) The problem is to change the dose of *750 mg* to the amount of the solution containing this dose measured in *mL*.

$$750 \ mg = ? \ mL$$

The strength of 75 *mg* = 1 *mL* will be used to form the unit fraction

$$\frac{750 \ \cancel{mg}}{1} \times \frac{1 \ mL}{75 \ \cancel{mg}} = 10 \ mL$$

FORMULA METHOD

(a)

D (desired dose) = 750 mg
H (dose on hand) = 75 mg
Q (dosage unit) = 1 mL
X (unknown) = ? mL

Fill in the formula $\dfrac{D}{H} \times Q = X$

$$\frac{750 \ mg}{75 \ mg} \times 1 \ mL = ? \ mL$$

Cancel

$$\frac{\overset{10}{\cancel{750 \ mg}}}{\underset{1}{\cancel{75 \ mg}}} \times 1 \ ml = 10 \ mL$$

So, you would administer 10 mL over the 5 minutes.

(b) In part (a), the rate of infusion is $\frac{10 \ mL}{5 \ min}$. Because you want to cut the infusion into 5 equal segments, divide both the numerator and denominator of the flow rate by 5.

$$\frac{10 \ mL \div 5}{5 \ min \div 5} = \frac{2 \ mL}{1 \ min}$$

So, 2 mL will be pushed during every 1 minute interval. If a 10 mL syringe is used, each tick represents 1 mL, and the plunger will move 2 ticks each minute.

(c) In part (a) the flow rate was determined to be 10 milliliters in 5 minutes. Because you want to cut the infusion into 10 equal segments, divide both the numerator and denominator of the flow rate by 10.

$$\frac{10 \ mL \div 10}{5 \ min \div 10} = \frac{1 \ mL}{0.5 \ min}$$

Substitute 30 seconds for 0.5 minutes to obtain

$$\frac{1 \ mL}{0.5 \ min} = \frac{1 \ mL}{30 \ sec}$$

So, each milliliter is administered in 30 seconds. If a 10 mL syringe is used, the plunger will move one tick on the syringe every 30 seconds.

EXAMPLE 11.10

Order: *Cefizox (ceftizoxime sodium) 1,500 mg IVP stat over 4 min.* The 2 g Cefizox vial has a strength of 1 g/10 *mL*.

(a) Find the total number of milliliters you will administer.

(b) Determine the number of mL you will push during each 30-second interval.

(c) Determine the number of seconds needed to deliver each 1 mL of the solution.

(a) The problem is to change the dose of 1,500 *mg* to a dose measured in *mL*.

$$1,500 \ mg = ? \ mL$$

DIMENSIONAL ANALYSIS

(a) The strength of *1 g = 10 mL* and the equivalence *1 g = 1,000 mg* will be used to form the unit fractions

$$\frac{1,500 \; \cancel{mg}}{1} \times \frac{1 \; \cancel{g}}{1,000 \; \cancel{mg}} \times \frac{10 \; mL}{1 \; \cancel{g}} = 15 \; mL$$

FORMULA METHOD

(a)

D (desired dose) = 1,500 mg

H (dose on hand) = 1 g

Q (dosage unit) = 10 mL

X (unknown) = ? mL

First change 1,500 mg to 1.5 g by moving the decimal point three places.

Fill in the formula $\dfrac{D}{H} \times Q = X$

$$\frac{1.5 \, g}{1 \, g} \times 10 \, mL = ? \, mL$$

Cancel $\quad\dfrac{1.5 \, \cancel{g}}{1 \, \cancel{g}} \times 10 \, ml = 15 \, mL$

So, you would administer a total of 15 mL of Cefizox over 4 minutes.

(b) In part (a), the rate of infusion is $\frac{15 \, mL}{4 \, min}$. Because $4 \, min = 240 \, sec$, the flow rate is $\frac{15 \, mL}{240 \, sec}$. You want to divide the 240 second infusion time into 30-second segments and

$$\frac{240 \, sec}{30 \, sec} = 8$$

So, divide both the numerator and the denominator of the flow rate by 8.

$$\frac{15 \, mL \div 8}{240 \, sec \div 8} = \frac{1.875 \, mL}{30 \, sec} \approx \frac{1.9 \, mL}{30 \, sec}$$

So, 1.9 mL of Cefizox should be pushed during every 30-second interval. This amount cannot be accurately measured on a 20 mL syringe; it is only a guideline. Because each tick on a 20 mL syringe represents 1 mL, the plunger will move about 2 ticks on the syringe each 30 seconds.

(c) In part (a) the flow rate was determined to be $\frac{15 \, mL}{240 \, sec}$

You want to divide the 15 mL into 1 mL pieces and

$$\frac{15 \, mL}{1 \, mL} = 15$$

So, both numerator and denominator of the IVP rate must be divided by 15.

$$\frac{15 \, mL \div 15}{240 \, sec \div 15} = \frac{1 \, mL}{16 \, sec}$$

So, 1 mL is administered each 16 seconds. If a 20 mL syringe is used, the plunger will move 1 tick on the syringe every 16 seconds.

Compound Rates

In Chapter 6, you calculated dosages based on the *size of the patient*, measured in either kilograms or meters squared. For example, if a patient weighing 100 *kg* has an order to receive a drug at the rate of *2 micrograms per kilogram (2 mcg/kg)*, the dose would be obtained by multiplying the size of the patient by the rate in the order, as follows:

$$\text{Size of the patient} \times \text{Order} = \text{Dose}$$

$$100 \text{ kg} \times \frac{2 \text{ mcg}}{kg} = 200 \text{ mcg}$$

So, the dose is 200 mcg, and the single unit of measurement (*100 kg*) was converted to another single unit of measurement (200 *mcg*).

In this chapter, some IV medications are prescribed not only based on the patient's size, but the amount of drug the patient receives also depends on *time*. For example, an order might indicate that a drug is to be administered at the rate of *2 micrograms per kilogram per minute (2 mcg/kg/min)*. This means that, *each minute*, the patient is to receive 2 mcg of the drug for every kg of body weight. Therefore, the amount of medication the patient receives depends on two things, body weight and time.

This new type of rate, called a **compound rate**, for computational purposes is written as follows:

$$\frac{2 \text{ mcg}}{kg \cdot min}$$

where the dot in the denominator stands for multiplication.

Suppose a patient weighing 100 *kg* has an order to receive a drug at the compound rate of *2 mcg/kg/min*. The dosage rate would be obtained by multiplying the size of the patient by the compound rate in the order as follows:

$$\text{Size of the patient} \times \text{Order} = \text{Dosage Rate}$$

$$100 \text{ kg} \times \frac{2 \text{ mcg}}{kg \cdot min} = \frac{200 \text{ mcg}}{min}$$

So, the dosage rate is 200 mcg/min, and the single unit of measurement (100 *kg*) was converted to a dosage rate (200 *mcg/min*).

EXAMPLE 11.11

The prescriber ordered: *250 mL 5% D/W with 60 mg of a drug 0.006 mg/kg/min IVPB daily.* The patient weighs 75 kg, and the drop factor is 20 gtt/mL. Calculate the flow rate for this drug in drops per minute.

Given:	75 kg (weight of the patient)
Known equivalences:	0.006 mg/kg/min (order)
	60 mg/250 mL (strength)
	20 gtt/mL (drop factor)
Find:	? gtt/min (flow rate)

As shown, multiplying the weight of the patient by the order will yield a rate based on *time*. This rate can then be converted to the desired flow rate (drops per minute). So you want to start with the weight of the patient (kilograms) and convert to drops per minute.

DIMENSIONAL ANALYSIS

$$75 \text{ kg} = \text{gtt/min}$$

You want to cancel kg. To do this you must use a fraction containing kg in the denominator. Using the order, this fraction will be $\dfrac{0.006 \text{ mg}}{\text{kg} \times \text{min}}$

$$75 \text{ kg} \times \frac{0.006 \text{ (mg)}}{\text{kg} \times \text{min}} = ? \frac{\text{gtt}}{\text{min}}$$

Now, on the left side mg is in the numerator, but you don't want mg. You need a fraction with mg in the denominator. Using the strength of the solution, the fraction is $\dfrac{250 \text{ mL}}{60 \text{ mg}}$

$$75 \text{ kg} \times \frac{0.006 \text{ mg}}{\text{kg} \times \text{min}} \times \frac{250 \text{ (mL)}}{60 \text{ mg}} = ? \frac{\text{gtt}}{\text{min}}$$

Now, on the left side mL is in the numerator, but you don't want mL. To cancel the mL you need a fraction with mL in the denominator. Using the drop factor, the fraction is $\dfrac{20 \text{ gtt}}{\text{mL}}$.

Now cancel and multiply the numbers.

$$75 \text{ kg} \times \frac{0.006 \text{ mg}}{\text{kg} \times \text{min}} \times \frac{250 \text{ mL}}{60 \text{ mg}} \times \frac{20 \text{ (gtt)}}{\text{mL}}$$

$$= 37.5 \frac{\text{gtt}}{\text{min}}$$

RATIO & PROPORTION AND FC

Notice that this order involves a compound rate 0.006 mg/kg/min. Multiply the size of the patient by the order as follows:

$$75 \text{ kg} \times \frac{0.006 \text{ mg}}{\text{kg} \cdot \text{min}} = \frac{0.45 \text{ mg}}{\text{min}}$$

This dosage rate of 0.45 mg/min must be changed to mL/h.

$$\frac{0.45 \text{ mg}}{\text{min}} = \frac{? \text{ mL}}{h}$$

In the numerator, change 0.45 mg to mL of solution.

Think:

$$0.45 \text{ mg} = x \text{ mL}$$
$$60 \text{ mg} = 250 \text{ mL} \quad \text{[strength of the solution]}$$

Use the proportion

$$\frac{0.45 \text{ mg}}{x \text{ mL}} = \frac{60 \text{ mg}}{250 \text{ mL}}$$

$$60x = 112.5$$
$$x = 1.875$$

This means that 0.45 mg of the drug are contained in 1.875 mL of the solution.

The problem becomes

$$\frac{1.875 \text{ mL}}{\text{min}} = \frac{? \text{ mL}}{h}$$

Change $1.875 \frac{mL}{min}$ to $\frac{mL}{h}$ by multiplying by $\frac{60}{60}$

$$\frac{1.875 \text{ mL}}{\text{min}} \times \frac{60}{60} = \frac{112.5 \text{ mL}}{60 \text{ min}} = \frac{112.5 \text{ mL}}{1 h}$$

Now, change the flow rate of 112.5 mL/h to gtt/min, using the FC technique.

$$DF = 20 \text{ and } FC = \frac{60}{20} = 3. \text{ You want } \underline{\text{Drops}}$$

per minute, so $\underline{\text{Divide}}$.

$$\frac{112.5}{3} = 37.5$$

So, the flow rate is 38 gtt/min.

EXAMPLE 11.12

The prescriber ordered: *Ifex (ifosfamide) 1.2 g/m²/d IVPB, infuse over 30 min. Repeat for 5 consecutive days.* The IV solution strength is 50 mg/mL. The patient has BSA of 1.50 m². Find the flow rate in mL/h.

Notice that the order contains the compound rate of *1.2 g/m²/d*. Multiply the size of the patient by this compound rate as follows:

$$1.50 \ m^2 \times \frac{1.2 \ g}{m^2 \cdot d} = \frac{1.8 \ g}{d}$$

This means that the patient should receive *1.8 g* of Ifex per day. Because the drug must be administered over 30 minutes, the dosage rate is $\frac{1.8 \ g}{30 \ min}$, and it must be changed to $\frac{mL}{h}$.

$$\frac{1.8 \ g}{30 \ min} = ? \frac{mL}{h}$$

DIMENSIONAL ANALYSIS

Use the concentration *50 mg/mL* to form a unit fraction.

$$\frac{1.8 \ g}{30 \ min} \times \frac{60 \ min}{h} \times \frac{1,000 \ mg}{1 \ g} \times \frac{mL}{50 \ mg}$$
$$= 72 \ \frac{mL}{h}$$

RATIO & PROPORTION

$$\frac{1.8 \ g}{30 \ min} = ? \frac{mL}{h}$$

Replace *1.8 g* with *1,800 mg*.

Change $\frac{1,800 \ mg}{30 \ min}$ to $\frac{mg}{h}$ by multiplying by $\frac{2}{2}$ as follows:

$$\frac{1,800 \ mg}{30 \ min} \times \frac{2}{2} = \frac{3,600 \ mg}{60 \ min} = \frac{3,600 \ mg}{1 \ h}$$

The problem becomes

$$\frac{3,600 \ mg}{h} = \frac{x \ mL}{h}$$

Think: 3,600 mg = x mL

50 mg = 1 mL   [strength of the solution in the bag]

Use the proportion

$$\frac{3,600 \ mg}{x \ mL} = \frac{50 \ mL}{1 \ mL}$$
$$50 \ x = 3,600$$
$$x = 72$$

Therefore

$$\frac{3,600 \ mg}{h} = \frac{72 \ mL}{h}$$

So, the flow rate is *72 mL/h*.

The next example, 11.13, shows how to determine the time it would take a patient to receive a given amount of drug when the dosage rate is known.

EXAMPLE 11.13

The patient weighs 80 kg and must receive a drug at the rate of 0.025 mg/kg/min.

(a) How many mg/min should the patient receive?

(b) How long will it take for the patient to receive 50 mg of the drug?

(a) Multiply the size of the patient by the order as follows:

$$80 \; kg \times \frac{0.025 \; mg}{kg \cdot min} = \frac{2 \; mg}{min}$$

So, the patient should receive the drug at the rate of 2 mg/min.

(b) The problem is to find the time (minutes) it will take for the patient to receive 50 mg of the drug.

DIMENSIONAL ANALYSIS	RATIO & PROPORTION
The problem is to change the dose of *50 mg* to time in *minutes*. Use the dosage rate of *2 mg = 1 min* to form the unit fraction.	Think:

DIMENSIONAL ANALYSIS

The problem is to change the dose of *50 mg* to time in *minutes*. Use the dosage rate of *2 mg = 1 min* to form the unit fraction.

$$50 \; mg = ? \; min$$

$$\frac{50 \; mg}{1} \times \frac{1 \; min}{2 \; mg} = \frac{25 \; min}{1}$$

RATIO & PROPORTION

Think:

$$50 \; mg = x \; min$$
$$2 \; mg = 1 \; min \; [dosage \; rate]$$

The proportion is

$$\frac{50 \; mg}{x \; min} = \frac{2 \; mg}{1 \; min}$$
$$2x = 50$$
$$x = 25$$

So, it will take 25 minutes for the patient to receive 50 mg of the drug.

Although premixed IVPB bags are generally supplied, sometimes the drug must be added to the bag at the time of administration. The next three examples (11.14–11.16) illustrate this.

EXAMPLE 11.14

A patient must receive a drug at the recommended rate of 15 mg/kg/d.

(a) If the patient weighs 100 kg, how many mg/d must the patient receive?

(b) The drug is to be administered IVPB in 200 mL D/5/W over 60 min. The vial contains 1.5 g of the drug in powdered form. This vial is used with a reconstitution device similar to that shown in •Figure 11.6. Find the IV flow rate in mL/h.

(c) How many mg/min will the patient receive?

(a) Multiply the size of the patient by this compound rate as follows:

$$100 \; kg \times \frac{15 \; mg}{kg \cdot d} = \frac{1,500 \; mg}{d}$$

This means that the patient should receive the dosage rate of 1,500 milligrams per day.

(b) Because the drug is dissolved in 200 mL and the infusion time is 60 minutes, the IV flow rate is

$$\frac{200\ mL}{60\ min}$$

Replace 60 minutes by 1 hour.

$$\frac{200\ mL}{60\ min} = \frac{200\ mL}{1\ h}$$

So, the IV flow rate is 200 mL/h.

(c) The problem is to find the dosage rate in mg/min.

Because the patient is receiving 1,500 mg in 60 min, the dosage rate is

$$\frac{1,500\ mg}{60\ min} = \frac{1,500}{60}\frac{mg}{min} = 25\frac{mg}{min}$$

So, the dosage rate is 25 mg/min.

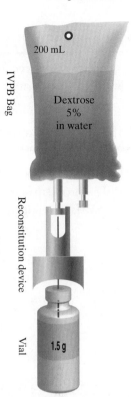

• **Figure 11.6**
Reconstitution system.

There are reconstitution systems that enable the healthcare provider to reconstitute a powdered drug and place it into an IVPB bag without using a syringe. One such device is shown in Figure 11.5. With this device, when the IVPB bag is squeezed, fluid is forced into the vial, dissolving the powder. The system is then placed in a vertical configuration with the vial on top and the IVPB bag on the bottom. The IVPB bag is then squeezed and released, thereby creating a negative pressure, which allows the newly reconstituted drug to flow into the IVPB bag.

Another reconstitution device is the ADD-Vantage system, which employs an IV bag containing intravenous fluid. The bag is designed with a special port, which will accept a vial of medication. When the vial is placed into this port, the contents of the vial and the fluid mix to form the desired solution. See • **Figure 11.7**.

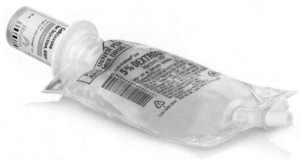

• **Figure 11.7**
ADD-Vantage System.

EXAMPLE 11.15

A patient is to receive 150 mg of a drug IVPB in 200 mL NS over 1 hour. The vial of medication indicates a strength of 75 mg/mL.

(a) How many milliliters must be withdrawn from the vial and added to the IV bag?

(b) At what rate in mL/h should the pump be set?

DIMENSIONAL ANALYSIS	RATIO & PROPORTION
(a) The problem is to change the dose of *150 mg* to *mL* of solution to be taken from the vial. $$150\ mg = ?\ mL$$ In the vial, the strength is *75 mg/mL*, use this to make the unit fraction. $$\frac{150\ \cancel{mg}}{1} \times \frac{1\ mL}{75\ \cancel{mg}} = \frac{2\ mL}{1}$$	(a) Think: $$150\ mg = ?\ mL\ \ [dose]$$ $$75\ mg = 1\ mL\ \ [strength\ in\ the\ vial]$$ Use the proportion $$\frac{150\ mg}{x\ mL} = \frac{75\ mg}{1\ mL}$$ $$75x = 150$$ $$x = 2$$

So, 2 mL of the drug must be withdrawn from the vial and added to the IV bag.

(b) *Method 1:* **Include** *the volume of drug added to the IV bag.*

After 2 mL of drug are withdrawn from the vial and added to the 200 mL of NS, the IVPB bag will then contain (200 + 2) 202 mL of solution. Because the infusion will last 1 hour, the pump rate would be set at 202 *mL/h*.

Method 2: **Do not include** *the volume of drug added to the IV bag.*

When the 2 mL of drug from the vial are added to the 200 mL of NS, the volume of the bag increases by $\left(\frac{Change}{Original} = \frac{2}{200}\right)1\%$. Because this increase in volume is relatively small, some institutional guidelines permit it to be excluded in IV flow rate calculation. If the increase in volume is excluded, the pump rate would be set at 200 *mL/h*.

Consult facility protocols to determine which calculation method to use. In the worked-out solutions to the Practice Sets, Method 1 will be used.

EXAMPLE 11.16

The order is: *a drug 100 mg/m² IVPB in 250 mL NS infuse over 3 h.* The patient's BSA is 1.65 m², and the drug is available in a vial labeled 60 mg/mL.

(a) How many milligrams of the drug must the patient receive?

(b) How many milliliters must be withdrawn from the vial and added to the IV bag?

(c) The order indicates that the drug should be added to 250 mL of NS. At what rate in mL/h should the pump be set?

(a) Multiply the size of the patient by the order.

$$1.65\ \cancel{m^2} \times \frac{100\ mg}{\cancel{m^2}} = 165\ mg$$

So, the patient should receive 165 mg of the drug.

(b) The problem is to change the dose of *165 mg* to *mL* of solution to be taken from the vial.

$$165 \, mg = ? \, mL$$

DIMENSIONAL ANALYSIS	**FORMULA**
Use the strength in the vial, *60 mg/mL,* to make the unit fraction	D (desired dose) = 165 mg
	H (dose on hand) = 60 mg
$$\frac{165 \, mg}{1} \times \frac{1 \, mL}{60 \, mg} = 2.75 \, mL$$	Q (dosage unit) = 1 mL
	X (unknown) = ? mL
	Fill in the formula $\dfrac{D}{H} \times Q = X$
	$$\frac{165 \, mg}{60 \, mg} \times 1 \, mL = ? \, mL$$
	Cancel $\dfrac{165 \, mg}{60 \, mg} \times 1 \, ml = 2.75 \, mL$

So, 2.8 *mL* of the drug must be withdrawn from the vial and added to the IV bag.

(c) If the additional volume of the drug is added to the volume of the IVPB bag, the bag will contain (250 + 2.8) 252.8 mL, and the pump rate would be set at $\frac{252.8 \, mL}{3 \, h} = 84.3 \, \frac{mL}{h}$. So, the pump would be set at the rate of 84 mL/h.

If only the volume of the IV solution (250 mL) is considered, the pump rate would be set at $\frac{250 \, mL}{3 \, h} \approx 83.3 \, \frac{mL}{h}$. So, the pump would be set at the rate of 83 mL/h.

EXAMPLE 11.17

A patient who weighs 55 kg is receiving a medication at the rate of 30 mL/h. The concentration of the medication is 400 mg in 500 mL of D5W. The recommended dose range for the drug is 2–5 mcg/kg/min. Is the patient receiving a safe dose?

First use the *minimum* recommended dose of *2 mcg/kg/h* to determine the minimum IV rate in mL/h that the patient may receive. Multiply the size of the patient by the order.

$$55 \, kg \times \frac{2 \, mcg}{kg \cdot min} = \frac{110 \, mcg}{min}$$

Change the dosage rate of 110 *mcg/min* to an IV rate in *mL/h.*

$$\frac{110 \, mcg}{1 \, min} = ? \frac{mL}{h}$$

DIMENSIONAL ANALYSIS

Use the strength of the solution (400 mg = 500 mL) to form a unit fraction.

$$\frac{110 \, \overline{mcg}}{1 \, \overline{min}} \times \frac{1 \, \overline{mg}}{1,000 \, \overline{mcg}} \times \frac{500 \, mL}{400 \, \overline{mg}} \times \frac{60 \, \overline{min}}{1 \, h}$$

$$= \frac{8.25 \, mL}{1 \, h}$$

So, the *minimum* IV flow rate is 8.25 mL/h.

Now use the *maximum* recommended dose of 5 mcg/kg/h to determine the *maximum* IV flow rate in *mL/h* that the patient should receive. It can be done in one line as follows:

$$\frac{55 \, kg}{1} \times \frac{5 \, \overline{mcg}}{kg \cdot \overline{min}} \times \frac{1 \, \overline{mg}}{1,000 \, \overline{mcg}} \times \frac{500 \, mL}{400 \, \overline{mg}}$$
$$\times \frac{60 \, \overline{min}}{1 \, h} = \frac{20.625 \, mL}{1 \, h}$$

RATIO & PROPORTION

Multiply $\frac{110 \, mcg}{1 \, min}$ by $\frac{60}{60}$ to change to mcg/h as follows:

$$\frac{110 \, mcg}{1 \, min} \times \frac{60}{60} = \frac{6,600 \, mcg}{60 \, min} = \frac{6,600 \, mcg}{1 \, h}$$

Convert 6,600 *mcg* to 6.6 *mg* by moving the decimal point 3 places to the left, and the problem becomes:

$$\frac{6.6 \, mg}{h} = ? \, \frac{mL}{h}$$

Think:

$$6.6 \, mg = x \, mL$$
$$400 \, mg = 500 \, mL \text{ [strength of the solution]}$$

Use the proportion

$$\frac{6.6 \, mg}{x \, mL} = \frac{400 \, mg}{500 \, mL}$$
$$400x = 3,300$$
$$x = 8.25$$

So, the *minimum IV flow rate* is 8 mL/h.

Now, use the *maximum* recommended dose of *5 mcg/kg/h* to determine the maximum IV rate in mL/h the patient should receive. You could follow a procedure similar to what was done for the minimum, but it is easier to use a single proportion, as follows:

Think:

| 2 mcg/kg/h | results in | 8.3 mL/h |
| 5 mcg/kg/h | results in | x mL/h |

Use the proportion

$$\frac{2 \, mcg/kg/ \min}{8.3 \, mL/h} = \frac{5 \, mcg/kg/ \min}{x \, mL/h}$$
$$41.5 = 2x$$
$$20.75 = x$$

So, the *maximum flow rate* is 21 mL/h.

The safe dose range of 2–5 mcg/kg/min is equivalent to the flow rate range of *8–21 mL/h* for this patient. The patient is receiving an IV rate of 30 mL/h. Because 30 mL/h is larger than the maximum allowable flow rate of 21 mL/h, the patient is not receiving a safe dose. The patient is receiving an overdose. Turn off the IV and contact the prescriber.

ALERT

Whenever your calculations indicate that the prescribed dose is not within the safe range, you must verify the order with the prescriber.

Titrated Medications

The process of adjusting the dosage of a medication based on patient response is called **titration**. Orders for titrated medications are often prescribed for critical-care patients. Such orders require that therapeutic effects, such as pain reduction, be monitored. The dose of the medication must be adjusted accordingly until the desired effect is achieved.

An order for a titrated medication generally includes a purpose for titrating and a maximum dose. If either the initial dose or directions for subsequent adjustments of the initial dose are not included in the order, the medication cannot be given, and you must contact the prescriber.

Dosage errors with titrated medications can quickly result in catastrophic consequences. Therefore, a thorough knowledge of the particular medication and its proper dosage adjustments is crucial. Dosage increment choices are medication-specific and depend on many factors that go beyond the scope of this book.

Suppose an order indicates that a certain drug must be administered with an initial dosage rate of 10 mcg/min, and that the rate should be increased by 5 mcg/min every 3–5 min for chest pain until response, up to a maximum rate of 30 mcg/min. The IV bag has a strength of 50 mg/250 mL.

To administer the drug, first determine the IV rate in *mL/h* for the initial dose rate of 10 *mcg/min*.

ALERT

Drugs that are titrated are administered according to protocol. Therefore, it is imperative to know the institution's protocols.

The problem is

$$\frac{10\ mcg}{min} = ?\frac{mL}{h}$$

DIMENSIONAL ANALYSIS

Use the strength of the solution (50 *mg* = 250 *mL*) to form a unit fraction

$$\frac{10\ \cancel{mcg}}{1\ \cancel{min}} \times \frac{1\ \cancel{mg}}{1,000\ \cancel{mcg}} \times \frac{250\ mL}{50\ \cancel{mg}} \times \frac{60\ \cancel{min}}{1\ h}$$

$$= \frac{3\ mL}{1\ h}$$

RATIO & PROPORTION

Change 10 mcg to 0.01 mg by moving the decimal 3 places to the left, and the problem becomes

$$\frac{0.01\ mg}{min} = ?\ \frac{mL}{h}$$

Multiplying $\frac{0.01\,mg}{min}$ by $\frac{60}{60}$ will convert the minutes to hours.

$$\frac{0.01\ mg}{min} \times \frac{60}{60} = \frac{0.6\ mg}{60\ min} = \frac{0.6\ mg}{1\ h}$$

The problem becomes

$$\frac{0.6\ mg}{h} = \frac{?\ mL}{h}$$

Now convert 0.6 mg in the numerator to mL. Think:

$$0.6\ mg = x\ mL$$

$$50\ mg = 250\ mL \quad \text{[strength of the solution]}$$

Use the porportion

$$\frac{0.6\,mg}{x\,mL} = \frac{50\,mg}{250\,mL}$$

$$50x = 150$$

$$x = 3$$

So, the initial IV rate is 3 mL/h.

After the initial dose is administered, the patient is monitored. If the desired response is not achieved, the order indicates to increase the dose rate by 5 mcg/min. This requires that you find the corresponding IV rate in mL/h for the new dosage rate. This titration may also require other dosage changes. Every time the dose rate is changed, recalculation of the corresponding IV rate is necessary. Rather than performing such calculations each time a dose is modified, it is useful to compile a *titration table* that will quickly provide the IV rate for any possible drug dosage rate choice.

Construction of the titration table for each incremental dose change of 5 mcg/min, up to the maximum rate of 30 mcg/min, could be accomplished by repeating a procedure similar to that which was used to determine the initial flow rate. Instead, however, the table can be quickly compiled by first finding the incremental IV flow rate for a dosage rate change of 5 mcg/min.

DIMENSIONAL ANALYSIS

$$5\,\frac{mcg}{min} = ?\,\frac{mL}{h}$$

Use the strength of the solution (50 mg = 250 mL) to form a unit fraction

$$\frac{5\,mcg}{1\,min} \times \frac{1\,mg}{1,000\,mcg} \times \frac{250\,mL}{50\,mg} \times \frac{60\,min}{1\,h}$$

$$= \frac{1.5\,mL}{1\,h}$$

RATIO & PROPORTION

Think:

$$10\,\frac{mcg}{min} = 3\,\frac{mL}{h} \quad [initial\ rate]$$

$$5\,\frac{mcg}{min} = x\,\frac{mL}{h} \quad [incremental\ rate]$$

The proportion is

$$\frac{10\,mcg/min}{3\,mL/h} = \frac{5\,mcg/min}{x\,mL/h}$$

$$10x = 15$$

$$x = 1.5$$

So, for each change of *5 mcg/min*, the incremental IV flow rate is *1.5 mL/h*.

Table 11.1 shows the titration table for the order. It contains the various dosage rates in mcg/min and their corresponding flow rates. As you move down the columns, the dosage rate increases in 5 mcg/min increments, whereas the corresponding flow rate increases in 1.5 mL/h increments.

Table 11.1 Titration Table

Dosage Rate (mcg/min)	Flow Rate (mL/h)
10 mcg/min (initial)	3 mL/h
15 mcg/min	4.5 mL/h
20 mcg/min	6 mL/h
25 mcg/min	7.5 mL/h
30 mcg/min (maximum)	9 mL/h

EXAMPLE 11.18

The order is: *Pitocin (oxytocin) start at 1 mU/min IV, may increase by 1 mU/min q 15 min to a max of 10 mU/min.* The IV strength is 10 mU/mL.

(a) Calculate the initial pump setting in mL/h.

(b) Construct a titration table for this order.

(a) Determine the flow rate in *mL/h* for the initial dosage rate of 1 *mU/min*.
The problem is

$$\frac{1\ mU}{min} = ?\frac{mL}{h}$$

DIMENSIONAL ANALYSIS

Use the strength of the solution (*10 mU = 1 mL*) to form a unit fraction

$$\frac{1\ \cancel{mU}}{1\ \cancel{min}} \times \frac{1\ mL}{10\ \cancel{mU}} \times \frac{60\ \cancel{min}}{1\ h} = \frac{6\ mL}{1\ h}$$

Therefore,

$$1\frac{mU}{min} = 6\frac{mL}{h}$$

and the initial flow rate is 6 mL/h.

RATIO & PROPORTION

Multiplying $\frac{1\,mU}{min}$ by $\frac{60}{60}$ will convert the minutes to hours.

$$\frac{1\,mU}{min} \times \frac{60}{60} = \frac{60\,mU}{60\ min} = \frac{60\,mU}{1\ h}$$

The problem becomes

$$\frac{60\,mU}{h} = \frac{?\,mL}{h}$$

Convert 60 mU in the numerator to mL using a proportion.

Think:

$$60\,mU = x\,mL$$
$$10\,mU = 1\,mL \quad [\text{strength}]$$

The proportion is

$$\frac{60\,mU}{x\,mL} = \frac{10\,mU}{1\,mL}$$
$$10x = 60$$
$$x = 6\,mL$$

Therefore,

$$1\frac{mU}{min} = 6\frac{mL}{h}$$

and the initial flow rate is 6 mL/h.

(b) The order indicates that the dosage rate may be changed in $1\frac{mU}{min}$ increments. Because in part (a) it was shown that $1\frac{mU}{min} = 6\frac{mL}{h}$, the flow rate increments are also 6 mL/h.

Table 11.2 shows the entire titration table. Notice that the dose rates increase in 1 mU/min increments, while the flow rates increase in 6 mL/h increments.

Table 11.2 **Titration Table for Example 11.18**	
Dosage Rate (mU/min)	**Flow Rate (mL/h)**
1 mU/min (initial)	6 mL/h
2 mU/min	12 mL/h
3 mU/min	18 mL/h
4 mU/min	24 mL/h
5 mU/min	30 mL/h
6 mU/min	36 mL/h
7 mU/min	42 mL/h
8 mU/min	48 mL/h
9 mU/min	54 mL/h
10 mU/min (maximum)	60 mL/h

Summary

In this chapter, the IV medication administration process was discussed. IVPB and IVP infusions were described, and orders based on body weight and body surface area were illustrated.

- A secondary line is referred to as an IV piggyback.
- IV push, or bolus, medications can be injected into a heplock/saline lock or directly into the vein.
- In a gravity system, the IV bag that is hung highest will infuse first.
- An order containing a compound rate of the form *mg/kg/min* directs that each minute, the

patient must receive the stated number of milligrams of medication for each kilogram of the patient's body weight.

- For calculation purposes, write mg/kg/min as $\frac{mg}{kg \cdot min}$.
- When the size of the patient is multiplied by a compound rate, the dosage rate is obtained.
- When titrating medications, the dose is adjusted until the desired therapeutic effect is achieved.

Case Study 11.1

Read the Case Study and answer the questions. Answers can be found in Appendix A.

A woman is admitted to the labor room with a diagnosis of preterm labor. She states that she has not seen a physician because this is her third baby and she "knows what to do while she is pregnant." Her initial workup indicates a gestational age of 32 weeks, and she tests positive for chlamydia and Strep-B. Her vital signs are: T 100°F; P 98; R 18; B/P 140/88; and the fetal heart rate is 140–150. The orders include the following:

- NPO
- IV fluids: D5/RL 1,000 mL q8h
- Continuous electronic fetal monitoring
- Vital signs q4h
- Dexamethasone 6 mg IM q12h for 2 doses
- Brethine (terbutaline sulfate) 0.25 mg subcutaneous q30 minutes for 2h

- Rocephin (ceftriaxone sodium) 250 mg IM stat
- Penicillin G 5 million units IVPB stat; then 2.5 million units q4h
- Zithromax (azithromycin) 500 mg IVPB stat and daily for 2 days

1. Calculate the rate of flow for the D5/RL in mL/h.

2. The label on the dexamethasone reads 8 mg/mL. How many milliliters will you administer?

3. The label on the terbutaline reads 1 mg/mL. How many milliliters will you administer?

4. The label on the ceftriaxone states to reconstitute the 1 g vial with 2.1 mL of sterile water for injection, which results in a strength of 350 mg/mL. How many milliliters will you administer?

5. The instructions state to reconstitute the penicillin G (use the minimum amount of diluent), add to 100 mL D5W, and infuse in one hour. The drop factor is 15. What is the rate of flow of the stat dose in gtts/min? See the label in • **Figure 11.8.**

6. The instructions for the azithromycin state to reconstitute the 500 mg vial with 4.8 mL until dissolved to yield a strength of 100 mg/mL, and add to 250 mL of D5W and administer over at least 60 minutes. What rate will you set the infusion pump if you choose to administer the medication over 90 minutes?

7. The patient continues to have uterine contractions, and a new order has been written: *magnesium sulfate 4g IV bolus over 20 minutes, then 1 g/h.*

   The label on the IV bag states magnesium sulfate 40 g in 1,000 mL.

   (a) What is the rate of flow in mL/h for the bolus dose?

   (b) What is the rate of flow in mL/h for the maintenance dose?

   The patient continues to have contractions and her membranes rupture. The following orders are written:

   - Discontinue the magnesium sulfate.
   - Pitocin (oxytocin) 10 units/1,000 mL RL, start at 0.5 mU/min increase by 1 mU/min q20 minutes.
   - Stadol (butorphanol tartrate) 1 mg IVP stat.

8. What is the rate of flow in mL/h for the initial dose of Pitocin?

9. The Pitocin is infusing at 9 mL/h. How many mU/h is the patient receiving?

10. The vial of butorphanol tartrate is labeled 2 mg/mL. How many milliliters will you administer?

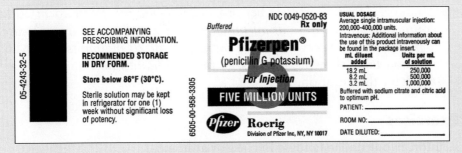

• **Figure 11.8**
Drug label for penicillin G.

(Reg. Trademark of Pfizer Inc. Reproduced with permission.)

Practice Sets

The answers to *Try These for Practice*, *Exercises*, and *Cumulative Review Exercises* are found in Appendix A. Ask your instructor for the answers to the *Additional Exercises.*

Workspace

Try These for Practice

Test your comprehension after reading the chapter.

1. Order: *ampicillin sodium 500 mg IVPB q6h infuse in 15 min*. Find the dosage rate of this antibiotic in *mg/min*.

2. Order: *Alimta 500 mg/m² IV on day 1 of a 21 day cycle infuse in 10 min*. Read the label in •**Figure 11.9**. The directions on the package insert of this antineoplastic drug states: "reconstitute the vial with *20 mL* NS and further dilute with NS for a total volume of 100 *mL*." The patient has BSA of 1 m². Find the

   (a) pump setting in mL/h.
   (b) dosage rate in mg/min.

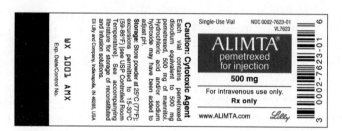

•**Figure 11.9**
Drug label for Alimta.

3. A patient with a systemic infection must receive *500 mg* of ampicillin sodium IV over 60 minutes. The concentration of the IV solution is 30 mg/mL. What is the flow rate of this antibiotic drug in mcgtt/min?

4. Order: *Ativan (lorazepam) 2 mg IVP 20 min preoperatively infuse in 1 minute*. The concentration of this anxiolytic drug is *2 mg/mL*. Every 15 seconds you will push
   (a) how many mg of Ativan?
   (b) how many mL of Ativan?

5. To induce labor, the prescriber orders *LR 1,000 mL IVc̄ Pitocin 20 units continuous drip. Infuse at an initial rate of 2 milliunits/min, increase by 2 milliunits/min every hour to a maximum of 20 milliunits/min*. Make a titration table showing the dosage rate (*milliunits/min*) and flow rate in *mL/h* for this titration.

Exercises

Reinforce your understanding in class or at home.

1. An IV is infusing at 80 mL/h. The concentration in the IV bag is 40 mg in 200 mL NS. What is the dosage rate in mg/min?

2. An IV is infusing at 0.5 mg/min. The concentration in the IV bag is 25 mg in 200 mL 0.9% NaCl. What is the pump setting in mL/h?

3. An IV is infusing at 15 gtt/min. The concentration in the IV bag is 40 mg in 250 mL NS. The drop factor is 10 gtt/mL. What is the dosage rate in mg/min?

4. An IV is infusing at 40 milliunits/min. The concentration in the IV bag is 10 units in 250 mL D5W. The drop factor is 10 gtt/mL. What is the drip rate in gtt/min?

5. Order: *Gemzar (gemcitabline HCl) 1,000 mg/m² IVPB add to 200 mL NS infuse in 30 min.* The BSA is 0.91 m². Read the label of this antineoplastic drug in •**Figure 11.10** and determine the

   (a) number of mL of diluent you would add to the Gemzar vial.

   (b) number of mL you would take from the Gemzar vial.

   (c) pump setting in mL/h.

   (d) dosage rate in mg/min.

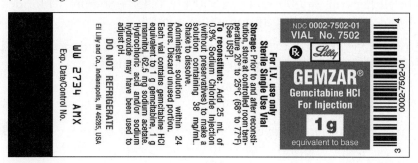

• **Figure 11.10**
Drug label for Gemzar.

6. The concentration in the IV bag is 150 mg in 200 mL. If the IV begins on Monday at 0800 hours, and it must infuse with a dosage rate of 1.5 mg/min, then

   (a) what should be the pump setting in mL/h?

   (b) when will the IV finish?

7. Order: *lidocaine drip 0.75 mg/kg IV in 500 mL D5W stat.* The patient weighs 169 pounds.

   (a) How many milliliters of lidocaine 2% will be added to prepare the IV solution?

   (b) Calculate the flow rate in *mL/h* in order for the patients to receive the dosage rate of 5 *mg/h*.

8. Order: *digoxin 0.75 mg IVP stat over 5 min.* The digoxin vial has a concentration of *0.1 mg/mL.* Find the

   (a) total number of milliliters you will administer.

   (b) number of mL you will push during each 30-second interval.

   (c) number of seconds needed to deliver each mL of the solution.

9. Order: *adenosine 140 mcg/kg/min IVP stat.* Read the label for this antiarrhythmic drug in •**Figure 11.11**. The patient weighs 43 kg.

   (a) Find the dosage rate in mg/min.

   (b) How many mL will you push every 15 seconds?

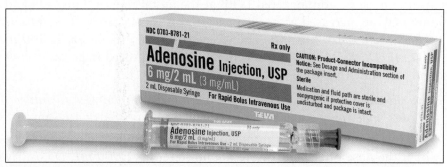

• **Figure 11.11**
Adenosine prefilled syringe.

Workspace

Workspace

10. The prescriber orders the cardiac stimulant dopamine hydrochloride at a rate of 3 mcg/kg/min. The patient weighs 155 lb. The pharmacist sends a solution of dopamine hydrochloride 200 mg in 250 mL of D5W.

    (a) How many mcg/min will the patient receive?
    (b) How many mL/h will the patient receive?

11. Order: *heparin 1,500 units/h via infusion pump stat.* The premixed IV bag is labeled heparin 25,000 units in 500 mL 0.45% Sodium Chloride. At what rate will you set the infusion pump in mL/h?

12. The prescriber ordered an insulin drip to run at 10 units per hour. The IV bag is labeled 100 units regular insulin in 250 mL NS.

    (a) At what rate will you set the infusion pump in mL/h?
    (b) How many hours will the IV run?

13. The prescriber ordered Covert (*ibutilide fumarate*) 0.01 mg/kg IVPB in 50 mL of 0.9% NaCl to infuse in 10 min stat. The vial label reads 1 *mg*/10 mL. The patient weighs 125 pounds.

    (a) How many milliliters of this antiarrhythmic drug will you need?
    (b) Calculate the flow rate in milliliters per minute.

14. Order: *desmopressin acetate 0.3 mcg/kg IVPB 30 minutes before surgery.* The vial label reads 4 mcg/mL and the patient weighs 80 kg.

    (a) Calculate the dose of this antidiuretic in mcg.
    (b) Add the dose to 50 mL 0.9% NaCl; and calculate the flow rate in milliliters/hour.

15. The physician orders *morphine sulfate 200 mg IVPB in NS 1,000 mL to be infused at a rate of 20 mcg/kg/h stat.* The patient weighs 134 kg.

    (a) How many mg/h of this narcotic analgesic will the patient receive?
    (b) How many mL/h of the solution will the patient receive?

16. Order: *Elspar (asparaginase) 200 units/kg/day IV over 60 min for 28 days.* Add 10,000 units to 100 mL of D5W. The patient weighs 196 lb. Calculate the dosage rate for this antineoplastic enzyme in units/day.

17. Order: *Humulin R 100 units IVPB in 500 mL NS infuse at 0.1 unit/kg/h stat.* The patient weighs 46 kg. How long will it take for the infusion of this U-100 insulin to complete?

18. Order: *amikacin sulfate 7.5 mg/kg IVPB q8h in 200 mL D5W to infuse in 30 min.* The vial reads 500 mg/2 mL. Calculate the flow rate of this aminoglycoxide antibiotic drug in *mL/h* for a patient whose weight is 144 lb.

19. A drug must be administered IVPB at the initial rate of *2 mg/min* and the rate may be increased as needed every hour thereafter by *3 mg/min* up to a maximum of *20 mg/min.* The strength of the IV solution is *300 mg* in *100 mL D5W.* Make a titration table showing the dosage rate (*mg/min*) and flow rate (*mL/h*).

20. The physician ordered *Platinol (cisplatin) 100 mg/m^2 IV to infuse over 6 hours once every 4 weeks* for a patient who has BSA of 1.66 m^2.

    (a) How many mg of this antineoplastic drug should the patient receive?
    (b) If the dose of cisplatin were administered in *1,000 mL D5 1/2 NS* at how many mL/h would the IV run?

Additional Exercises

Now, test yourself!

1. The patient is to receive 20 mEq of KCl (potassium chloride) in 100 mL of IV fluid at the rate of 10 mEq/h. What is the flow rate in microdrops per minute? _____

2. A maintenance dose of *Levophed (norepinephrine bitartrate) 2 mcg/min IVPB* has been ordered to infuse using 8 mg in 250 mL of D5W solution. What is the pump setting for this vasoconstrictor in mL/h? _____

3. The patient is receiving lidocaine at 40 mL/h. The concentration of this antiarrhythmic drug is 1 g per 500 mL of IV fluid. How many mg/min is the patient receiving? _____

4. Order: *dopamine 400 mg in 250 mL D5W at 3 mcg/kg/min IVPB.* Calculate the flow rate for this cardiac stimulant in mL/h for a patient who weighs 91 kg. _____

5. A drug is ordered 180 mg/m^2 in 500 mL NS to infuse over 90 minutes. The BSA is 1.38 m^2. What is the flow rate in mL/h? _____

6. How long will 550 mL of IV solution take to infuse at the rate of 25 mL/h? _____

7. The patient is receiving heparin at 1,000 units/hour. The IV has been prepared with 24,000 units of heparin per liter. Find the flow rate of this anticoagulant drug in mL/h. _____

8. Order: *Humulin R 50 units in 500 mL NS infuse at 1 mL/min IVPB.* How many units per hour is the patient receiving? _____

9. An IVPB of 50 mL is to infuse in 30 minutes. After 15 minutes, the IV bag contains 40 mL. If the drop factor is 20 gtt/mL, recalculate the flow rate in gtt/min. _____

10. A drug is ordered to start at a rate of 4 mcg/min IV. This rate may, depending on the patient's response, be increased by 2 mcg/min q 15 min to a max of 12 mcg/min. The IV strength is 5 mcg/mL.

    (a) Calculate the initial pump setting in mL/h. _____
    (b) Construct a titration table for this order. _____

11. Order: *digoxin 0.5 mg IVP stat over 5 min.* The digoxin vial has a concentration of 0.1 mg/mL. Find the
    (a) total number of milliliters you will administer. _____
    (b) number of mL you will push during each 30-second interval.

    _____

    (c) number of seconds needed to deliver each mL of the solution.

    _____

12. The patient is to receive Aldomet (methyldopa) 500 mg IVPB dissolved in 100 mL of IV fluid over 60 minutes. If the drop factor is 15 gtt/mL, determine the rate of flow in gtt/min of this antihypertensive drug. _____

13. The patient is to receive Isuprel (isoproterenol) at a rate of 4 mcg/min. The concentration of this antiarrhythmic drug is 2 mg per 500 mL of IV fluid. Find the pump setting in mL/h. _____

Workspace

Workspace

14. The patient is receiving aminophylline at the rate of 20 mL/h. The concentration of this bronchodilator is 500 mg/1,000 mL of IV fluid. How many mg/h is the patient receiving? _____

15. Nipride 3 mcg/kg/min has been ordered for a patient who weighs 82 kg. The solution has a strength of 50 mg in 250 mL of D5W. Calculate the flow rate of this antihypertensive in mL/h. _____

16. A medication is ordered at 75 mg/m^2 IVP. The patient has BSA of 2.33 m^2. How many milliliters of the medication will be administered if the vial is labeled 50 mg/mL? _____

17. A liter of D5/NS with 10 units of Regular insulin is started at 9:55 A.M. at a rate of 22 gtt/min. If the drop factor is 20 gtt/mL, when will the infusion finish? _____

18. Mefoxin (cefoxitin) 2 g in 100 mL NS IVPB. Infuse in 1 hour. After 30 minutes, 70 mL remain in the bag. Reset the flow rate of this cephalosporin antibiotic on the pump in mL/h. _____

19. Order: *heparin sodium 40,000 units IV in 500 mL of $\frac{1}{2}$ NS to infuse at 1,200 units/hour*. What is the flow rate in mL/h? _____

20. A patient who weighs 150 pounds is receiving medication at the rate of 100 mL/h. The concentration of the IVPB solution is 200 mg in 50 mL NS. The recommended dosage range is 0.05–0.1 mg/kg/min. Is the patient receiving a safe dose? _____

Cumulative Review Exercises

Review your mastery of earlier chapters.

1. What is the reading at the arrow on this scale in mL? _____

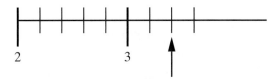

2. What is the weight in grams of an infant who weighs 7 lb 8 oz? _____

3. Read the label in • **Figure 11.12** and determine the total number of micrograms contained in two tablets of this antiplatelet drug. _____

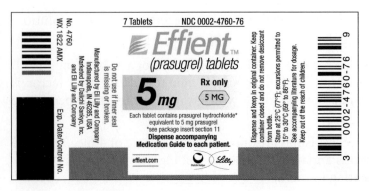

• **Figure 11.12**
Drug label for Effient.

4. What is the BSA of a person who is 155 cm and 90 kg? _____

5. The order is *carboplatin 360 mg/m² once q4wk*. How many mg of this antineoplastic drug would be prescribed for a patient who weighs 180 pounds and is 6 feet tall? _____

6. Order: *quinidine gluconate 7.5 mg/kg administer IVPB over 4 hours for 7 days*. The patient weighs 150 lb. See •**Figure 11.13**.

   (a) How many mg of this antimalarial drug would be prescribed for the patient? _____
   (b) How many mL would be needed from the vial? _____
   (c) Add the quinidine to 100 mL. What would be the pump setting in mL/h? _____
   (d) What would be the dosage rate in mg/min? _____

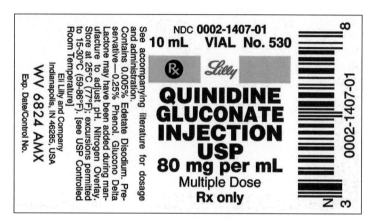

•**Figure 11.13**
Drug label for quinidine gluconate.

7. A wound has a diameter of 37 mm. What is the diameter in centimeters? _____

8. Two teaspoons equal how many milliliters? _____

9. Your calculations lead to a result of 2.75 mL.
   (a) Round off this calculation to one decimal place. _____
   (b) Round down this calculation to one decimal place. _____

10. Order: *Uniphyl (theophylline) 5 mg/kg po loading dose stat*. Read the label in •**Figure 11.14**. How many tablets of this bronchodilator would you administer to a patient who weighs 81 kg? _____

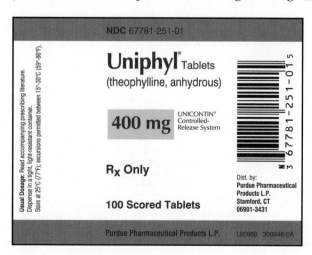

•**Figure 11.14**
Drug label for Uniphyl.

Workspace

11. How many grams of NaCl are contained in 500 mL of a 0.9% NaCl solution? _____

12. What is the strength as a percent of a lidocaine solution that has 20 mg of lidocaine in each mL of the solution? _____

13. An IV is infusing at 70 mL/h, what is this flow rate in mcgtt/min? _____

14. An IV is infusing at 25 mL/h. The concentration in the IV bag is 50 mg in 200 mL NS. What is the dosage rate in mg/min? _____

15. An IV is infusing at 125 milliunits/min. The concentration in the IV bag is 15 units in 300 mL D5W. The drop factor is 15 gtt/mL. What is the drip rate in gtt/min?_____

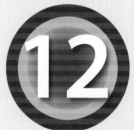

Pediatric Dosages

Learning Outcomes

After completing this chapter, you will be able to

1. Determine if a pediatric dose is within the safe dose range.
2. Calculate pediatric oral and parenteral dosages based on body weight.
3. Calculate pediatric oral and parenteral dosages based on body surface area.
4. Perform calculations necessary for administering medications using a volume control chamber.
5. Calculate daily fluid maintenance.

Because the metabolism and body mass of children are different from those of adults, children are at greater risk of experiencing adverse effects of medications. Therefore, with pediatric and high-risk medications, it is essential to *carefully calculate* the dose, determine if the dose is in the *safe dose range* for the patient, and *validate your calculations* with another healthcare professional. As always, before administering any medication it is imperative to know its *indications*, *uses*, *side effects*, and possible *adverse reactions*.

In this chapter, you will be applying many of the techniques that you have already learned in the previous chapters to the calculation of pediatric dosages.

Pediatric dosages are generally based on the weight of the child. It is important to *verify* that the dose ordered is safe for the particular child. Pediatric dosages are sometimes rounded down, instead of rounded off, because of the danger that overdose poses to infants and children. Consult your facility's policy on rounding pediatric dosages. In this chapter, dosages will be rounded down (rather than rounded off) to provide practice in rounding down.

Pediatric Drug Dosages

Most pediatric doses are based on body weight. Body surface area (BSA) is also used, especially in pediatric oncology and critical care. You must be able to determine whether the amount of a prescribed pediatric dosage is within the recommended range. To do this, you must compare the child's ordered dosage to the recommended safe dosage as found in a reputable drug resource. The recommended dose or dosage range found can be on the package insert, hospital formulary, *Physician's Desk Reference (PDR)*, *United States Pharmacopeia*, manufacturer's Web site prescribing information, or drug guide books.

Oral Medications

When prescribing medications for the pediatric population, the oral route is preferred. However, if a child cannot swallow, or the medication is ineffective when given orally, the parenteral route is used.

The developmental age of the child must be taken into consideration when determining the device needed to administer oral medication. For example, an older child may be able to swallow a pill or drink a liquid medication from a cup. Children younger than five years of age, however, generally are not able to swallow tablets and capsules. Therefore, most medications for these children are in the form of elixirs, syrups, or suspensions. An *oral syringe, calibrated dropper, or measuring spoon* can be selected when giving medication to an infant or younger child. An oral syringe is different from a parenteral syringe in two ways. Generally, an oral syringe does not have a Luer-Lok™ hub and has a cap on the tip that must be removed before administering a medication. Because a needle does not fit on an oral syringe, the chance of administering a medication via a wrong route is decreased. See •**Figures 12.1** and **12.2**.

> **NOTE**
>
> Many oral pediatric medications are suspensions. Remember to shake them well immediately before administering.

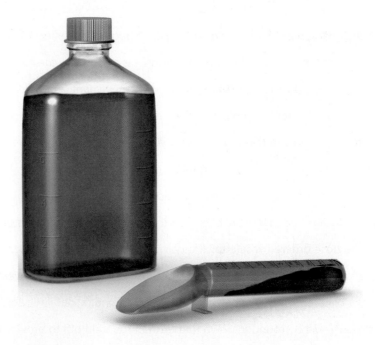

• **Figure 12.1**
A bottle of oral medication and a measuring spoon.

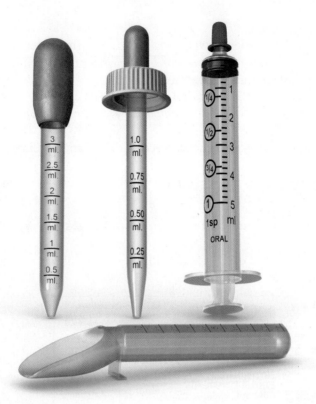

• **Figure 12.2**
Liquid medication administration devices: Two droppers, an oral syringe, and a measuring spoon.

Parenteral Medications

Subcutaneous or intramuscular routes may be necessary, depending on the type of medication to be administered. For example, many childhood immunizations are administered subcutaneously or intramuscularly. Intramuscular injections are rarely ordered on a routine basis for children because of: limited sites, developmental considerations, and the possibility of trauma. Because of the small muscle mass of children, usually not more than 2 mL is injected. You should consult a current pediatric text for the equipment, injection sites, and procedure.

Dosages Based on Body Size

Drug manufacturers can recommend pediatric dosages based on patient size, as measured by either body weight (kg) or body surface area (m^2). Body weight in particular is frequently used when prescribing drugs for infants and children.

Dosages Based on Body Weight

> **EXAMPLE 12.1**
>
> The order is for *Biaxin (clarithromycin) 7.5 mg/kg PO q12h*. How many milligrams of this antibiotic would you administer to a child who weights 25 kg?

The patient's weight is 25 kg, and the order is for 7.5 mg/kg. *Multiply the size of the patient by the order* to determine how many milligrams of Biaxin to give the patient.

$$25 \, kg \times \frac{7.5 \, mg}{kg} = 187.5 \, mg$$

So, the child should receive 187.5 mg of Biaxin.

EXAMPLE 12.2

The prescriber ordered *EES (erythromycin ethylsuccinate) oral suspension 10 mg/kg PO q8h* for a child who weighs 50 kg.
Read the label in •**Figure 12.3** and calculate the number of milliliters of this macrolide antibiotic you will administer to the child.

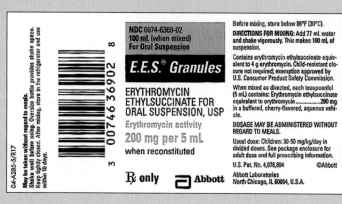

•**Figure 12.3**
Drug label for EES.

DIMENSIONAL ANALYSIS

You want to convert the body weight to the dose in milliliters.

$$50 \, kg \longrightarrow ? \, mL$$

Do this problem on one line as follows:

$$50 \, kg \times \frac{? \, mg}{? \, kg} \times \frac{? \, mL}{? \, mg} = ? \, mL$$

Because the order is 10 mg/kg, the first unit fraction is $\frac{10 \, mg}{1 \, kg}$
Because the strength is 200 mg/5 mL, the second unit fraction is $\frac{5 \, mL}{200 \, mg}$
You cancel the kilograms and milligrams and obtain the dose in milliliters

$$50 \, kg \times \frac{10 \, mg}{kg} \times \frac{5 \, mL}{200 \, mg} = 12.5 \, mL$$

FORMULA METHOD

The patient's weight is 50 kg, and the order is for 10 mg/kg. Multiply the *size of the patient by the order* to determine how many milligrams of E.E.S. to give the child.

$$50 \, kg \times \frac{10 \, mg}{kg} = 500 \, mg$$

Think: $500 \, mg = ? \, mL$
D (desired dose) = 500 mg
H (dose on hand) = 200 mg
Q (dosage unit) = 5 mL
X (unknown) = ? mL

Fill in the formula $\frac{D}{H} \times Q = X$

$$\frac{500 \, mg}{200 \, mg} \times 5 \, mL = ? \, mL$$

Cancel $\frac{\overset{5}{500 \, mg}}{\underset{2}{200 \, mg}} \times 5 \, mL = 12.5 \, mL$

So, you would administer 12.5 mL of EES to the child.

EXAMPLE 12.3

The prescriber ordered: *Zithromax (azithromycin) 10 mg/kg PO stat, then give 5 mg/kg/day for 4 days.* The child weighs 18 kg. Read the information on the label in •Figure 12.4 and determine the number of milliliters that would contain the stat dose.

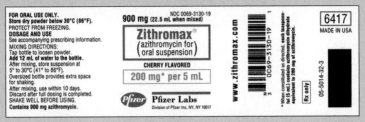

•Figure 12.4
Drug label for Zithromax.
(Reg. Trademark of Pfizer Inc. Reproduced with permission.)

DIMENSIONAL ANALYSIS

You want to convert the body weight to a dose in milliliters.

$$18\,kg \longrightarrow ?\,mL$$

Do this on one line as follows:

$$18\ kg \times \frac{?\ mg}{?\ kg} \times \frac{?\ mL}{?\ mg} = ?\ mL$$

Because the order is 10 mg/kg, the first unit fraction is $\dfrac{10\ mg}{kg}$

Because the strength is 200 mg per 5 mL, the second unit fraction is $\dfrac{5\ mL}{200\ mg}$

$$18\ kg \times \frac{10\ mg}{kg} \times \frac{5\ mL}{200\ mg} = 4.5\ mL$$

RATIO & PROPORTION

The patient's weight is 18 kg, and the stat dose is 10 mg/kg. Multiply the *size of the patient by the order* to determine how many milligrams of Zithromax to give the child.

$$18\ kg \times \frac{10\ mg}{kg} = 180\ mg$$

Think:

$$180\ mg = ?\ mL \quad \text{(dose)}$$
$$200\ mg = 5\ mL \quad \text{(strength)}$$

One way to set up the proportion is

$$\frac{180\ mg}{x\ mL} = \frac{200\ mg}{5\ mL}$$
$$200x = 900$$
$$x = 4.5$$

So, 4.5 mL would contain the stat dose.

EXAMPLE 12.4

The recommended dose for neonates receiving amikacin sulfate is 7.5 mg/kg IM q12h. If an infant weighs 2,600 grams, how many milligrams of amikacin would the neonate receive in one day?

DIMENSIONAL ANALYSIS

You want to convert the body weight to the dose in milligrams.

$$2{,}600\ g\ \text{(body weight)} \longrightarrow ?\ mg\ \text{(drug)}$$

FORMULA METHOD AND MOVING THE DECIMAL POINT

The patient's weight is 2,600 g. Convert this weight to kilograms by moving the decimal point *three places to the left*. Therefore, the

Do this problem on one line as follows:

$$2{,}600 \text{ g} \times \frac{?\,kg}{?\,g} \times \frac{?\,mg}{?\,kg} = ?\,mg$$

Because 1 kg = 1,000 g, the first unit fraction is $\dfrac{1\,kg}{1{,}000\,g}$

Because the recommended dose is 7.5 mg/kg, the second unit fraction is $\dfrac{7.5\,mg}{1\,kg}$

$$2{,}600 \text{ g} \times \frac{1\,kg}{1{,}000\,g} \times \frac{7.5\,mg}{kg} = 19.5 \text{ mg per dose}$$

neonate weighs 2.6 kg, and the order is for 7.5 mg/kg. Multiply the *size of the neonate by the order* to determine how many milligrams of amikacin sulfate needed.

$$2.6\,kg \times \frac{7.5\,mg}{kg} = 19.5\,mg\,per\,dose$$

Because the neonate receives two doses per day, the total daily dose is 39 mg.

Dosages Based on BSA

Pediatric dosages may also be based on body surface area (BSA). For example, antineoplastic agents used in the treatment of cancer are often ordered using the BSA. To calculate the BSA accurately, it is important that the *actual* height and weight be assessed, not just estimated. In most instances, the prescriber will calculate the BSA. However, it is the responsibility of the person who administers the drug to verify that the BSA is correct, and that the dose is within the safe dosage range.

EXAMPLE 12.5

A child who has BSA of 0.76 m^2 is to receive Cosmegen (dactinomycin) 2.5 mg/m^2 IVP daily for 5 days. Calculate the dose of this antineoplastic drug in milligrams.

The child's BSA is 0.76 m^2. Multiply the *BSA of the child by the order* to determine how many milligrams of Cosmegen are needed per day.

$$0.76\,m^2 \times \frac{2.5\,mg}{m^2} = 1.9\,mg$$

So, the child should receive 1.9 mg of Cosmegen daily.

EXAMPLE 12.6

Order: *methotrexate 15 mg/m^2 PO once every week.* The strength of the methotrexate is *2.5 mg/mL*. How many milliliters of this antineoplastic drug should a child who weighs 88 pounds and is 45 inches tall receive?

You want to find the body surface area and convert it to a dose in milliliters. Calculate the BSA using the formula:

$$\text{BSA} = \sqrt{\frac{88 \times 45}{3131}} \approx 1.12 \text{ m}^2$$

So, the child has a BSA of approximately 1.12 m^2.

DIMENSIONAL ANALYSIS	FORMULA METHOD
$$1.12\,m^2 \longrightarrow mL$$ $$m^2 \times \frac{?\,mg}{?\,m^2} \times \frac{?\,mL}{?\,mg} = ?\,mL$$ Because the strength is *2.5 mg/mL*, the second unit fraction is $\dfrac{1\,mL}{2.5\,mg}$ You cancel the square meters and milligrams to obtain the dose in milliliters $$1.12\,\cancel{m^2} \times \frac{15\,\cancel{mg}}{\cancel{m^2}} \times \frac{1\,mL}{2.5\,\cancel{mg}} = 6.72\ mL$$	Multiply the size of the patient by the order to obtain the dose. $$1.12\,m^2 \times \frac{15\,mg}{m^2} = 16.8\,mg$$ Think: $16.8\ mg = ?\,mL$ D (desired dose) = 16.8 mg H (dose on hand) = 2.5 mg Q (dosage unit) = 1 mL X (unknown) = ? mL Fill in the formula $\dfrac{D}{H} \times Q = X$ $$\frac{16.8\,mg}{2.5\,mg} \times 1\,mL = ?\,mL$$ Cancel $\dfrac{16.8\,\cancel{mg}}{2.5\,\cancel{mg}} \times 1\,mL = 6.72\,mL$

So, the child should receive 6.7 mL of methotrexate.

Determining Safe Dosage Range

The following example illustrates that pediatric dosage orders should always be compared with recommended dosages, as found in reputable drug references such as the *PDR* and drug package inserts.

EXAMPLE 12.7

> The order reads: *morphine sulfate 2 mg IM q4h*. The recommended dose is 0.1–0.2 mg/kg q4h (max 15 mg/dose). Is the ordered dose safe for the child who weighs 30 kg?
>
> Use the *minimum* recommended dose of *0.1 mg/kg* to determine the minimum number of milligrams the child should receive q4h.
>   Multiply the size of the patient by the minimum recommendation.
>
> $$30\,kg \times \frac{0.1\,mg}{kg} = 3\,mg$$
>
> So, the minimum safe dose is 3 mg q4h.
>   Now, use the *maximum* recommended dose of *0.2 mg/kg* to determine the maximum number of milligrams the child may receive q4h.
>   Multiply the size of the patient by the maximum recommendation.
>
> $$30\,kg \times \frac{0.2\,mg}{kg} = 6\,mg$$

ALERT

Both overdoses and underdoses are dangerous. Too much medication results in the risk of possible life-threatening effects, whereas too little medication risks suboptimal therapeutic effects.

So, the *maximum safe dose is 6 mg q4h.*

The safe dose range of *0.1–0.2 mg/kg q4h* is equivalent to a dose range of *3–6 mg q4h* for this child. The ordered dose of *2 mg* is smaller than the minimum recommended dose of 3 mg. Therefore, the ordered dose is not in the safe dose range, and it should not be administered. The healthcare provider must contact the prescriber.

EXAMPLE 12.8

The prescriber ordered *gentamicin 60 mg IM q8h* for a child who weighs 60 lb. The recommended dosage is 6–7.5 mg/kg/d in 3 divided doses.

(a) What is the recommended dosage in mg/day, and is the order safe?

(b) The strength on the vial is 80 mg/2 mL. Determine the number of milliliters you would administer.

DIMENSIONAL ANALYSIS

(a) You want to convert the body weight in pounds to kilograms, and then convert the body weight in kilograms to the recommended dose in milligrams of gentamicin per day.

$$60\,lb\,(body\ weight) \longrightarrow kg\,(body\ weight)$$
$$\longrightarrow mg\,(drug)$$

Do this on one line as follows:

$$\frac{60\ lb}{1} \times \frac{?\ kg}{?\ lb} \times \frac{?\ mg}{?\ kg \times d} = \frac{?\ mg}{d}$$

Because 1 kg = 2.2 lb, the first unit fraction is $\frac{1\ kg}{2.2\ lb}$

Because the *minimum recommended* dose is *6 mg/kg per day*, the second unit fraction is $\frac{6\ mg}{kg \times d}$

$$\frac{60\ lb}{1} \times \frac{1\ kg}{2.2\ lb} \times \frac{6\ mg}{kg \cdot d} = \frac{163.6\ mg}{d}$$

So, the minimum safe dose is 163.6 mg/d. Now, use the *maximum recommended* dose of 7.5 mg/kg to determine the maximum number of milligrams the child may receive. Because the *maximum recommended* dose is *7.5 mg/kg per day*, the second unit fraction is $\frac{7.5\ mg}{kg \times d}$

$$\frac{60\ lb}{1} \times \frac{1\ kg}{2.2\ lb} \times \frac{7.5\ mg}{kg \cdot d} = \frac{204.5\ mg}{d}$$

So, the maximum safe dose is 204.5 mg/d.

RATIO & PROPORTION

(a) The child's weight is 60 lb. Divide by 2.2 to convert this weight to kg.

$$\frac{60\,lb}{2.2} \approx 27.3\,kg$$

Multiply the *weight of the child* by the *minimum and maximum recommended doses* to determine the *safe dose range for this child in milligrams.*

$$27.3\,kg \times \frac{6\,mg}{kg \cdot d} \approx 164\,mg/d \quad \text{[min]}$$

$$27.3\,kg \times \frac{7.5\,mg}{kg \cdot d} \approx 205\,mg/d \quad \text{[max]}$$

The *safe dose range for this child is 164–205 mg/d*. Because the ordered dose of 60 mg three times a day (180 mg/d), the ordered dose is safe.

(b) Convert the ordered dose of 60 mg to milliliters.

Think:

$$60\,mg = ?\,mL$$
$$80\,mg = 2\,mL \quad \text{[strength on the label]}$$

One way to set up the proportion is

$$\frac{60\,mg}{x\,mL} = \frac{80\,mg}{2\,mL}$$

$$80x = 120$$

$$x = 1.5$$

The safe dose range of *6–7.5 mg/kg/d* is equivalent to a dose range of *163.6–204.5 mg/d* for this child.

The ordered dose of *60 mg q8h* is a total of *180 mg/d* and is within the recommended safe dose range.

(b) You want to convert the ordered dose in *milligrams* to *milliliters*.

$$mg\,(drug) \longrightarrow mL\,(drug)$$

Do this on one line as follows:

$$60\ mg \times \frac{?\ mL}{?\ mg} = ?\ mL$$

Because the strength of the gentamicin is *80 mg/2 mL*, the unit fraction is $\dfrac{2\ mL}{80\ mg}$

$$\frac{60\ \cancel{mg}}{1} \times \frac{2\ mL}{80\ \cancel{mg}} = 1.5\ mL$$

So, you would administer 1.5 mL of gentamicin IM q8h.

EXAMPLE 12.9

Valium (diazepam) 3.75 mg IVP stat was ordered for a child with status epilepticus. The package insert says that the recommended dose is 0.2–0.5 mg/kg/d IVP slowly. The child weighs 33 lbs, and the label on the vial reads 5 mg/mL.

(a) **Is the ordered dose within the safe range?**

(b) **How many milliliters would you administer?**

DIMENSIONAL ANALYSIS

(a) You want to convert the body weight in *pounds* to *kilograms*; then convert the body weight in *kilograms* to a recommended dose in *milligrams*.

$$33\,lb\,(body\ weight) \longrightarrow ?\,kg\,(body\ weight)$$
$$\longrightarrow ?\,mg\,(drug)$$

Do this on one line as follows:

$$33\ lb \times \frac{?\ kg}{?\ lb} \times \frac{?\ mg}{?\ kg} = ?\ mg$$

Because 1 kg = 2.2 lb, the first unit fraction is $\dfrac{1\ kg}{2.2\ lb}$

RATIO & PROPORTION

(a) The child's weight is 33 lb. Divide by 2.2 to convert this weight to kg.

$$\frac{33\,lb}{2.2} = 15\,kg$$

Multiply the *weight of the child* by the *minimum and maximum recommended doses* to determine the *safe dose range for this child in milligrams*.

$$15\,\cancel{kg} \times \frac{0.2\,mg}{\cancel{kg}} = 3\,mg \qquad [\text{min}]$$

$$15\,\cancel{kg} \times \frac{0.5\,mg}{\cancel{kg}} = 7.5\,mg \qquad [\text{max}]$$

Because the recommended dosage is 0.2 mg to 0.5 mg/kg per day, you need to find the minimum and the maximum recommended doses in milligrams for this patient. Use the unit fractions $\dfrac{0.2 \text{ mg}}{\text{kg}}$ and $\dfrac{0.5 \text{ mg}}{\text{kg}}$

$$\frac{33 \text{ lb}}{1} \times \frac{1 \text{ kg}}{2.2 \text{ lb}} \times \frac{0.2 \text{ mg}}{\text{kg}} = 3 \text{ mg}$$ 3 mg is the minimum dose

$$\frac{33 \text{ lb}}{1} \times \frac{1 \text{ kg}}{2.2 \text{ lb}} \times \frac{0.5 \text{ mg}}{\text{kg}} = 7.5 \text{ mg}$$ 7.5 mg is the maximum dose

The safe dose range for this patient is 3–7.5 mg.

Because the ordered dose of 3.75 mg is between 3 mg and 7.5 mg, it is a safe dose.

(b) You want to convert the ordered dosage in milligrams to the liquid daily dose in milliliters.

$$3.75 \text{ mg (drug)} \longrightarrow ? \text{ mL (drug)}$$

Do this on one line as follows:

$$3.75 \text{ mg} \times \frac{? \text{ mL}}{? \text{ mg}} = ? \text{ mL}$$

Because the vial label says that 5 mg/mL, the unit fraction is $\dfrac{1 \text{ mL}}{5 \text{ mg}}$

$$\frac{3.75 \text{ mg}}{1} \times \frac{1 \text{ mL}}{5 \text{ mg}} = 0.75 \text{ mL}$$

But 7.5 mg is above the recommended maximum of 5 mg as stated in the example, therefore the *safe dose range for this child is 3–5 mg.* Because the ordered dose of 3.75 mg is between 3 mg and 5 mg, the ordered dose is safe.

(b) Convert the ordered dose of 3.75 mg to milliliters.

Think:

$$3.75 \, mg = ? \, mL \quad \text{(dose)}$$
$$5 \, mg = 1 \, mL \quad \text{[strength on the label]}$$

One way to set up the proportion is

$$\frac{3.75 \, mg}{x \, mL} = \frac{5 \, mg}{1 \, mL}$$
$$5x = 3.75$$
$$x = 0.75$$

So, you would administer 0.75 mL of the Valium IVP slowly.

Intravenous Medications

When a child is NPO, needs pain relief, or needs a high concentration of a medication, the intravenous route is the most effective route to use. In addition, when the duration of the therapy is long term, or when gastrointestinal absorption is poor, the IV route is indicated.

Methods of intravenous infusions include peripheral intravenous catheters, peripherally inserted central catheters (PICC line), central lines, and long-term central venous access devices (VAD) or ports. The method chosen is based on the age and size of the child and the duration of therapy.

Most IV medications must be further diluted once the correct dose is calculated. Follow the directions precisely for the reconstitution process. An electronic infusion device and a volume control chamber should always be used to administer IV fluids and IVPB medications, especially high-alert drugs, to infants and children.

Using a Volume Control Chamber

To avoid fluid overload, pediatric intravenous medications are frequently administered using a volume control chamber (VCC) (burette, Volutrol, Buretrol, Soluset).

A VCC is calibrated in 1 mL increments and has a capacity of 100–150 mL. It can be used as a primary or secondary line. When administering IVPB medications, the medication is added to the top injection port of the VCC. Fluid is then added from the IV bag to further dilute the medication. After the infusion is complete, additional IV fluid is added to the VCC to flush any remaining medication left in the tubing. See •**Figure 12.5.**

ALERT

An excessively high concentration of an intravenous drug can cause irritation to the vein and have potentially life-threatening toxic effects. Read the manufacturer's directions very carefully.

NOTE

Know the facility's policy concerning the amount of fluid used to flush the VCC tubing.

Volume Control Chamber

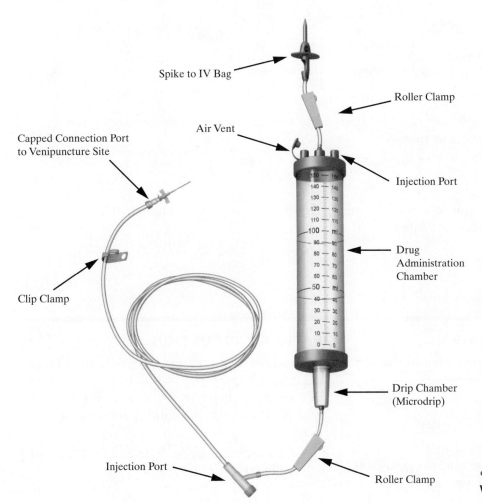

Spike to IV Bag

Roller Clamp

Air Vent

Capped Connection Port to Venipuncture Site

Injection Port

Drug Administration Chamber

Clip Clamp

Drip Chamber (Microdrip)

Injection Port

Roller Clamp

•**Figure 12.5**
Volume control chamber.

The following example illustrates the use of a VCC.

EXAMPLE 12.10

NOTE

In Example 12.10, following the infusing of the 100 mL, the tubing must be flushed; be sure to follow the institution's policy.

Order: *sulfamethoxazole and trimethoprim (SMZ-TMP) 75 mg in 100 mL D$_5$ W IVPB q6h. The recommended dose is 6–10 mg/kg/day every 6 hours.* The child weighs 40 kg.

(a) Is the prescribed dose in the safe range?

(b) Read the label in •Figure 12.6. The manufacturer directions state that "weight based doses are calculated on the TMP component." How many milliliters will you withdraw from the vial?

(c) Using a volume control chamber, how many milliliters of IV solution will you add?

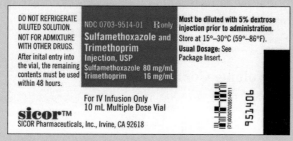

DO NOT REFRIGERATE DILUTED SOLUTION.
NOT FOR ADMIXTURE WITH OTHER DRUGS.
After inital entry into the vial, the remaining contents must be used within 48 hours.

NDC 0703-9514-01   R only
Sulfamethoxazole and **Trimethoprim** Injection, USP
Sulfamethoxazole 80 mg/mL
Trimethoprim   16 mg/mL

Must be diluted with 5% dextrose injection prior to administration.
Store at 15°–30°C (59°–86°F).
Usual Dosage: See Package Insert.

For IV Infusion Only
10 mL Multiple Dose Vial

sicor™
SICOR Pharmaceuticals, Inc., Irvine, CA 92618

951406

• Figure 12.6
Drug label for Sulfamethoxazole and Trimethoprim.

(a) Convert both the *safe dose range* and the *prescribed dose* to *mg/day.*

First, use the *minimum safe dose (6 mg/kg/day)* to determine how many mg/day the child should minimally receive as follows:

$$40 \text{ kg} \times \frac{6 \text{ mg}}{kg \cdot day} = 240 \frac{mg}{day} \quad \textit{Minimum}$$

Now, use the *maximum safe dose (10 mg/kg/day)* to determine how many mg/day the child should maximally receive as follows:

$$40 \text{ kg} \times \frac{10 \text{ mg}}{kg \cdot day} = 400 \frac{mg}{day} \quad \textit{Maximum}$$

So, the safe dose range for this child is *240–400 mg/day.*

DIMENSIONAL ANALYSIS

The ordered dose is 75 mg every 6 hours. Convert this to mg/day as follows:

$$\frac{75 \text{ mg}}{6 \text{ h}} \times \frac{24 \text{ h}}{day} = 300 \frac{mg}{day}$$

The ordered dose is equivalent to *300 mg/day.* This is within the safe dose range of 240–300 mg/day. So, the child is receiving a safe dose.

RATIO & PROPORTION

The ordered dose is *75 mg* every 6 hours (4 times per day). Therefore, the ordered dose is (75 × 4) *300 mg daily.* Because *300 mg/d* is in the range of *240–300 mg/d,* the child is receiving a safe dose.

(b) Convert the ordered dose of 75 mg to milliliters.

(b) You want to convert the order of 75 mg to mL.

$$75\,mg \longrightarrow ?\,mL$$

$$75\ mg \times \frac{?\,mL}{?\,mg} = ?\,mL$$

The directions state to use the trimethoprim (TMP) component. The strength of the TMP on the label is *16 mg/mL*. So, the unit fraction is $\dfrac{1\,mL}{16\,mg}$

$$\frac{75\ \cancel{mg}}{1} \times \frac{1\,mL}{16\,\cancel{mg}} = 4.6875\ mL$$

Think:

$$75\,mg = ?\,mL$$
$$16\,mg = 1\,mL \quad [\text{strength}]$$

One way to set up the proportion is

$$\frac{75\,mg}{x\,mL} = \frac{16\,mg}{1\,mL}$$

$$16x = 75$$
$$x = 4.6875$$

So, you would withdraw 4.6 mL of sulfamethoxazole and trimethoprim from the vial. Note that rounding *down* was used here.

(c) You would add *4.6 mL* of sulfamethoxazole and trimethoprim to the VCC, then add D5W to the *100 mL* mark.

Calculating Daily Fluid Maintenance

The administration of pediatric intravenous medication requires careful and exact calculations and procedures. Infants and severely ill children are not able to tolerate extreme levels of hydration and are quite susceptible to dehydration, and fluid overload. Therefore, you must closely monitor the amount of fluid a child receives. The fluid a child requires over a 24-hour period is referred to as *daily fluid maintenance needs*. Daily fluid maintenance includes both oral and parenteral fluids. The amount of maintenance fluid required depends on the weight of the patient (see the formula in Table 12.1). The daily maintenance fluid does not include body fluid losses through vomiting, diarrhea, or fever. Additional fluids referred to as *replacement fluids* (usually Lactated Ringer's or 0.9% NaCl) are utilized to replace fluid losses and are based on each child's condition (e.g., if 20 mL are lost, then 20 mL of replacement fluids are usually added to the daily maintenance).

Table 12.1 Daily Fluid Maintenance Formula

Pediatric Daily Fluid Maintenance Formula		
For the *first*	*10 kg* of body weight:	100 mL/kg
For the *next*	*10 kg* of body weight:	50 mL/kg
For *each kg above*	*20 kg* of body weight:	20 mL/kg

EXAMPLE 12.11

If the order is *half maintenance* for a child who weighs 35 kg, at what rate should the pump be set in mL/h?

Because the child weighs 35 kg, this weight would be divided into three portions following the formula in Table 12.1 as follows:

$$35 \text{ kg} = 10 \text{ kg} + 10 \text{ kg} + 15 \text{ kg}$$

For each of these three portions, the number of milliliters must be calculated. A table will be useful for organizing the calculations (Table 12.2). The daily "maintenance" was determined to be 1,800 mL. "Half maintenance" ($\frac{1}{2}$ of maintenance) is, therefore, $\frac{1}{2}$ of 1,800 mL, or 900 mL.

Now, you must change $\dfrac{900 \text{ } mL}{1 \text{ } day}$ to $\dfrac{mL}{h}$.

Replace 1 day with 24 hours to obtain

$$\frac{900 \text{ } mL}{1 \text{ } day} = \frac{900 \text{ } mL}{24 \text{ } h} = 37.5 \frac{mL}{h}$$

So, the pump would be set at the rate of 37 mL/h.

Table 12.2   Daily Fluid Maintenance Computations for Example 12.11

1st Portion	10 kg	×	$\dfrac{100 \text{ mL}}{\text{kg}}$	=	1,000 mL
2nd Portion	10 kg	×	$\dfrac{50 \text{ mL}}{\text{kg}}$	=	500 mL
3rd Portion	15 kg	×	$\dfrac{20 \text{ mL}}{\text{kg}}$	=	300 mL
Total	35 kg				1,800 mL

Summary

In this chapter, you learned to calculate oral and parenteral dosages for pediatric patients. Some dosages were based on the size of the patient: body weight (kg) or BSA (m²). The calculations needed for the use of the volume control chamber, as well as the method for determining daily fluid maintenance were explained.

- Taking shortcuts in pediatric medication administration can be fatal to the child.
- Always verify that the order is in the safe dose range.

- Consult a reliable source when in doubt about a pediatric medication order.
- Question the order or check your calculations if the ordered dose differs from the recommended dose.
- Pediatric dosages are sometimes rounded down (truncated) to avoid the danger of an overdose.
- Know your institution's policy on rounding.
- IV bags of no more than 500 mL should be hung for pediatric patients.

- No more than 2 mL should be given IM to a pediatric patient.
- Because accuracy is crucial in pediatric infusions, electronic control devices or volume control chambers should always be used.
- Minimal and maximal dilution volumes for some IV drugs are recommended to prevent fluid overload, minimize irritation to veins, and reduce toxic effects.
- When preparing IV drug solutions, the smallest added volume (minimal dilution) results in the strongest concentration; the largest added volume (maximal dilution), results in the weakest concentration.
- For a volume control chamber, a flush is always used to clear the tubing after the medication is infused.
- Know the facility policy regarding the inclusion of medication volume as part of the total infusion volume.
- Daily fluid maintenance depends on the weight of the child and includes both oral and parenteral fluids.

Case Study 12.1

Read the Case Study and answer the questions. Answers can be found in Appendix A.

An 8-year-old boy is admitted to the hospital with a diagnosis of sickle cell crisis and pneumonia. He complains of pain in his legs and abdomen, wheezing, and pain in his chest. He has a history of asthma, epilepsy, and is allergic to peanuts, tomatoes, and aspirin. He is 40 inches tall and weighs 55 pounds. Vital signs are: T 102° F; B/P 90/66; P 112; R 30. Chest x-ray confirms right upper lobe pneumonia, and the throat culture is positive for Group A streptococcus. His orders include the following:

- Bed Rest
- Diet as tolerated, encourage PO fluids
- IV D5 $\frac{1}{3}$ NS @ 110 mL/h
- morphine sulfate 0.025 mg/kg/h IV
- penicillin G 100,000 units/kg/day divided q6h, infuse via pump in 100 mL D5W, over one hour
- methylprednislone 1 mg/kg IM now, then 1 mg/kg PO daily in the A.M.
- Flovent HFA (fluticasone propionate) inhalation aerosol 2 puffs B.I.D.
- Folic Acid 1 mg PO daily
- Depakene (valproic acid) 30 mg/kg PO b.i.d.
- Tylenol (acetaminophen) 12 mg/kg PO q4h prn temp over 101°F
- montelukast 5 mg PO qhs
- albuterol 2 mg PO T.I.D.

Use the labels in • **Figure 12.7** to answer the following questions:

1. Calculate the child's 24-hour fluid requirement.
2. How many milliliters of diluent will you add to the Pfizerpen vial to obtain a strength of *250,000 units/mL*, and how many milliliters will you withdraw to obtain the prescribed dose?
3. What rate will you set the pump to infuse the Penicillin G?
4. The recommended dose for morphine is *0.05–0.1 mg/kg IV q4h*. Is the prescribed dose safe?
5. How many milliliters of methylprednisolone will you administer for the IM dose?
6. Select the correct label for valproic acid, and determine how many capsules you will administer.
7. The folic acid is available in 1-mg tablets. How many micrograms is the child receiving per day?
8. Select the correct label for montelukast and determine how many tablets you will administer.
9. The Tylenol available is labeled *160 mg/5 mL*. How many milliliters will the child receive for a temperature of 102°F?
10. Select the correct label for albuterol and determine how many milliliters you will administer.
11. The strength of the Flovent is *44 mcg/inhalation*. How many mcg is the patient receiving/day?

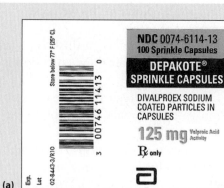

NDC 0074-6114-13
100 Sprinkle Capsules

DEPAKOTE®
SPRINKLE CAPSULES

DIVALPROEX SODIUM
COATED PARTICLES IN
CAPSULES

125 mg Valproic Acid
Activity

℞ only

Store below 77° F (25° C).

Exp.
Lot
02-8443-3/R10

6505-01-327-8510
Do not accept if seal over
bottle opening is broken or
missing.
Dispense in a USP tight,
light-resistant container.
Opaque white and blue
capsule bears THIS END UP
and DEPAKOTE® SPRINKLE
and 125 mg for product
identification.
Each capsule contains:
Divalproex sodium equivalent
to valproic acid.............125 mg
Capsule may be swallowed
whole or opened and contents
placed on food for
administration. See enclosure
for prescribing information.
U.S. Pat. No. 4,988,731
©Abbott
Abbott Laboratories
North Chicago, IL 60064 U.S.A.

(a)

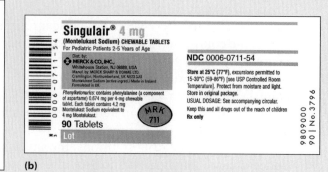

Singulair® 4 mg
(Montelukast Sodium) CHEWABLE TABLETS
For Pediatric Patients 2-5 Years of Age

Dist. by:
⊗ **MERCK & CO., INC.,**
Whitehouse Station, NJ 08889, USA
Manuf. by: MERCK SHARP & DOHME LTD.
Cramlington, Northumberland, UK NE23 3JU
Montelukast Sodium (active ingred.) Made in Ireland
Formulated in UK

Phenylketonurics: contains phenylalanine (a component
of aspartame) 0.674 mg per 4-mg chewable
tablet. Each tablet contains 4.2 mg
Montelukast Sodium equivalent to
4 mg Montelukast.

90 Tablets

Lot

MRK
711

NDC 0006-0711-54

Store at 25°C (77°F), excursions permitted to
15-30°C (59-86°F) [see USP Controlled Room
Temperature]. Protect from moisture and light.
Store in original package.
USUAL DOSAGE: See accompanying circular.
Keep this and all drugs out of the reach of children
℞ only

9809000
90 | No. 3796

(b)

(d)

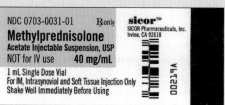

NDC 0703-0031-01   ℞ only

Methylprednisolone
Acetate Injectable Suspension, USP
NOT for IV use   **40 mg/mL**

1 mL Single Dose Vial
For IM, Intrasynovial and Soft Tissue Injection Only
Shake Well Immediately Before Using

sicor™
SICOR Pharmaceuticals, Inc.
Irvine, CA 92618

0021⁹A

(c)

Singulair® 5 mg
(Montelukast Sodium) CHEWABLE TABLETS
For Pediatric Patients 6-14 Years of Age

Dist. by:
⊗ **MERCK & CO., INC.,**
Whitehouse Station, NJ 08889, USA
Manuf. by: MERCK SHARP & DOHME LTD.
Cramlington, Northumberland, UK NE23 3JU
Montelukast Sodium (active ingred.) Made in Ireland
Formulated in UK

Phenylketonurics: contains phenylalanine
(a component of aspartame) 0.842 mg per
5-mg chewable tablet. Each tablet contains
5.2 mg Montelukast Sodium equivalent to
5 mg Montelukast.

90 Tablets

Lot

MRK
275

NDC 0006-0275-54

Store at 25°C (77°F), excursions permitted to 15-30°C
(59-86°F) [see USP Controlled Room Temperature].
Protect from moisture and light.
Store in original package.
USUAL DOSAGE: See accompanying circular.
Keep this and all drugs out of the reach of children
℞ only

9809200
90 | No. 3760

(e)

NDC 0093-6661-16
6505-01-256-4997

ALBUTEROL
SULFATE
Syrup
2 mg/5 mL

473 mL

TEVA

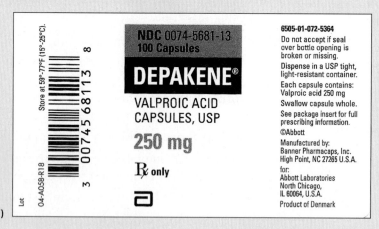

NDC 0074-5681-13
100 Capsules

DEPAKENE®

VALPROIC ACID
CAPSULES, USP

250 mg

℞ only

Store at 59°-77°F (15°-25°C).

Lot
04-A058-R18

6505-01-072-5364
Do not accept if seal
over bottle opening is
broken or missing.
Dispense in a USP tight,
light-resistant container.
Each capsule contains:
Valproic acid 250 mg
Swallow capsule whole.
See package insert for full
prescribing information.
©Abbott
Manufactured by:
Banner Pharmacaps, Inc.
High Point, NC 27265 U.S.A.
for:
Abbott Laboratories
North Chicago,
IL 60064, U.S.A.
Product of Denmark

(f)

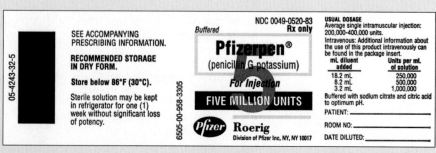

SEE ACCOMPANYING
PRESCRIBING INFORMATION.

RECOMMENDED STORAGE
IN DRY FORM.

Store below 86°F (30°C).

Sterile solution may be kept
in refrigerator for one (1)
week without significant loss
of potency.

05-4243-32-5

Buffered

Pfizerpen®
(penicillin G potassium)
For Injection

FIVE MILLION UNITS

Pfizer **Roerig**
Division of Pfizer Inc, NY, NY 10017

6505-00-958-3305

NDC 0049-0520-83
Rx only

USUAL DOSAGE
Average single intramuscular injection:
200,000-400,000 units.
Intravenous: Additional information about
the use of this product intravenously can
be found in the package insert.

mL diluent added	Units per mL of solution
18.2 mL	250,000
8.2 mL	500,000
3.2 mL	1,000,000

Buffered with sodium citrate and citric acid
to optimum pH.

PATIENT: _____

ROOM NO: _____

DATE DILUTED: _____

(g)

● **Figure 12.7**
Drug labels for Case Study.

Practice Sets

The answers to *Try These for Practice, Exercises,* and *Cumulative Review Exercises* are found in Appendix A. Ask your instructor for the answers to the *Additional Exercises.*

Try These for Practice

Test your comprehension after reading the chapter.

1. Order: *Omnicef (cefdinir) oral suspension 7 mg/kg q12h for 10 days.* Read the information on the label in •**Figure 12.8.** Calculate the number of milliliters of this cephalosporin antibiotic you would administer to a child who weighs 77 pounds.

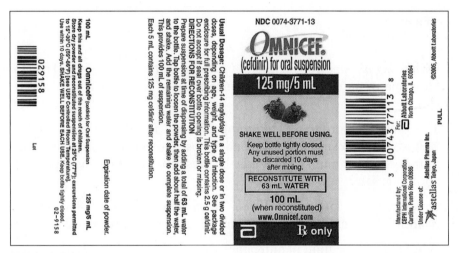

•**Figure 12.8**
Drug label for Omnicef.

2. Calculate the daily fluid maintenance and the hourly flow rate for a child who weighs 17 kg.

3. Order: *Tylenol (acetaminophen) 400 mg PO q4h prn for temp higher than 101°F.* The label on the vial reads 120 mg/5 mL. Calculate how many milliliters of this antipyretic drug the child would receive.

4. Order: *Cevi-Bid (vitamin C) 150 mg IM B.I.D.* The label on the vial reads 500 mg/mL. Calculate how many milliliters of vitamin C the child would receive.

5. Order: *Simulect (basiliximab) 12 mg/m^2 for 2 doses. Give 1st dose 2h before surgery, second dose four days after transplant.*

   Calculate the dose of this immunosuppressant drug for a child who weighs 22 pounds and is 28 inches long.

Exercises

Reinforce your understanding in class or at home.

1. The prescriber ordered *dicloaxacillin 75 mg oral suspension PO q6h* for a child who weighs 38 kg. The recommended dose for a child is 12.5–25 mg/kg/day in divided doses q6h. Is the prescribed dose of this penicillin antibiotic safe?

Workspace

2. Order: *Biaxin (clarithromycin) oral suspension 7.5 mg/kg PO q12h*. Read the label in • **Figure 12.9** and calculate the number of milliliters of this macrolide antibiotic you would administer to a child who weighs 18 pounds.

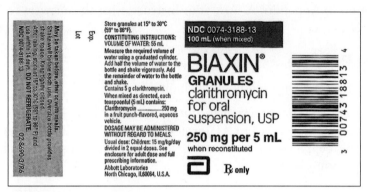

• **Figure 12.9**
Drug label for Biaxin.

3. Order: *theophylline 300 mg PO q6h*. The strength available is 150 mg/15 mL. How many milliliters of this bronchodilator will you administer to the child?

4. The prescriber ordered *cephradine 275 mg IVPB q6h* for a child who weighs 31 pounds. The recommended dose is 50–100 mg/kg/day divided in four doses (maximum 8 g/day). Is the prescribed dose of this cephalosporin antibiotic safe?

5. Order: *acyclovir 250 mg/m² IV q8h*. The child has a BSA of 0.8 m² and the vial is labeled "50 mg/mL". How many milliliters of this antiviral will you prepare?

6. What is the daily fluid maintenance for a child who weighs 82 pounds?

7. Order: *Humatrope (somatropin) 0.18 mg/kg/week subcut divided into equal doses give on Mon/Wed/Fri*. Read the label in • **Figure 12.10** and calculate how many milliliters of this growth hormone you will administer to a child who weighs 40 pounds. The package insert states to "reconstitute the 5 mg vial with 5 mL of diluent."

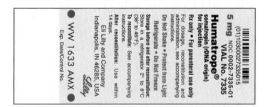

• **Figure 12.10**
Drug label for Humatrope.

8. Order: *Tavist (clemastine fumarate) 0.05 mg/kg/day PO divided into 2 doses*. The label states "0.67 mg/5 mL." Calculate how many milliliters of this antihistamine you will administer to a child who weighs 35 pounds.

9. Order: *Dilantin (phenytoin) 150 mg IVP stat*. The packages insert states give 1 mg/kg/min, and the label reads 250 mg/5 mL. Over how many minutes should you administer this anticonvulsant to a child who weighs 10 kg?

10. Order: *Cefadyl (cephaprin sodium) 40 mg/kg/day IVPB divided into 4 doses. Infuse in 50 mL D5W over 30 min*. The child weighs 20 kg and the directions

state to reconstitute the 500 mg vial with 1 ml of diluent, yielding 500 mg/ 1.2 mL. How many mL/h, of this cephalosporin antibiotic, will you infuse?

11. Order: *Zostavax (zoster vaccine live) 1 dose subcut now,* has been prescribed for a child. Read the information on the labels in •**Figure 12.11,** and use the diluent supplied to reconstitute the vaccine. Draw a line on the appropriate syringe, in •**Figure 12.12** indicating the number of milliliters of this reconstituted vaccine you will administer.

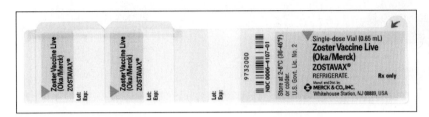

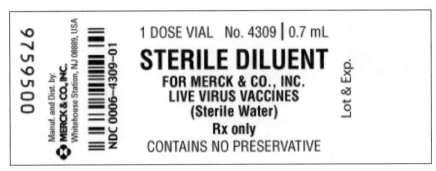

• **Figure 12.11**
Drug labels for Zostavax and Diluent.

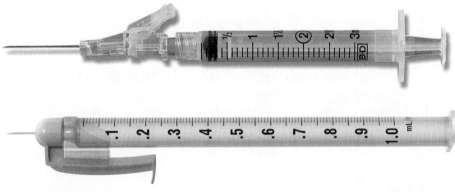

• **Figure 12.12**
Syringes for Question 11.

12. Order: *IV D5 $\frac{1}{3}$ NS, infuse at 40 mL/h.* What is the rate in microdrops per minute?

13. The prescriber ordered 1/3 maintenance for a child who weighs 10 kg. Calculate the rate at which the pump should be set in mL/h.

14. A child who weighs 33 pounds has diarrhea. To prevent dehydration, his fluid requirements are 100 mL/kg/day. The pediatrician tells the mom to give the child Pedialyte solution or "freezer pops." The label on the box states "62.5 mL per pop." What is the maximum number of Pedialyte freezer pops that the child may have in one hour?

15. Order: *albuterol sulfate syrup 3 mg PO T.I.D.* The recommended dose is 0.1–0.2 mg/kg T.I.D (max 4 mg/dose).
    (a) Is this a safe dose for a child who weighs 60 pounds?
    (b) If the dose is safe, read the label in •**Figure 12.13** and calculate the number of milliliters of this bronchodilator you would administer.

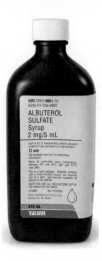

• **Figure 12.13**
Bottle of albuterol sulfate.

16. Order: *Children's Motrin (ibuprofen) 400 mg PO q4h prn temp over 101°F.* The recommended dose range is 5–10 mg/kg q4–6h up to 40 mg/kg/day. Is the ordered dose of this NSAID safe for a child who weighs 45 kg?

17. Order: *Cleocin (clindamycin phosphate) 600 mg IVPB q8h, infuse in 50 mL of D5W over 20 minutes.* At what rate in mL/h will you set the pump to infuse this cephalosporin antibiotic?

18. Order: *granisetron HCl 10 mcg/kg IVPB, 30 minutes before chemotherapy. Infuse in 20 mL of D5W over 15 minutes.* Read the information in •**Figure 12.14.**

    (a) Calculate how many milliliters of this antiemetic a child who weighs 10 kg will need.
    (b) At what rate will you set the infusion to run in mL/h?

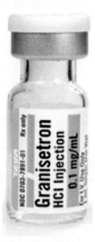

• **Figure 12.14**
Vial of granisetron HCl.

19. The prescriber ordered 2,000 units/m²/h IVPB of a drug. The solution is labeled 10,000 units in 100 ml D5W. Calculate the flow rate in mL/h for a child who has a BSA of 1.2 m².

20. Order: *150 units of regular insulin in 250 mL NS, infuse at 6 mL/h.* Calculate the number of units of insulin the child is receiving per hour.

Additional Exercises

Now, test yourself!

1. The prescriber ordered gentamicin 50 mg IVPB q8h for a child who weighs 40 lb. The recommended dosage is 6–7.5 mg/kg/day divided in three equal doses. Is the prescribed dose within the safe range? _____

2. The prescriber ordered Vancocin (vancomycin) 10 mg/kg q12h, IVPB for a neonate who weighs 4,000 g. What is the dose in milligrams? _____

3. The prescriber ordered methotrexate 2.9 mg PO weekly for a child who is 42 inches tall and weighs 50 pounds. The package insert states that the recommended dosage is 7.5–30 mg/m² q1–2 weeks. Is the order a safe dose? _____

4. Order: *Panadol (acetaminophen) 10 mg/kg PO q4h prn* for a child who weighs 32 kg. How many milligrams will you administer? _____

5. A manufacturer recommends giving from a minimum of 350 mg/m²/day to a maximum of 450 mg/m²/day for a certain drug. A child has a BSA of 1.2 m². Calculate the safe dose range (in milligrams per day) for this child. _____

6. Order: *Ceclor (cefaclor) suspension 30 mg/kg/day q8h.* The child weighs 77 pounds. The label reads 187 mg/mL. How many milliliters will you administer? _____

7. Order: *1,000 mL D5/RL infuse at 65 mL/h.* Calculate the infusion rate in microdrops per minute. _____

8. Order: *Zantac (ranitidine) 30 mg IV q8h.* The patient weighs 52 pounds. The package insert states that the recommended dose for pediatric patients is 2–4 mg/kg/day, to be divided and administered every 6 to 8 hours, up to a maximum of 50 mg per dose. Is the prescribed dose safe? _____

9. Order: Daily fluid maintenance IV D5/0.33% NS.
   (a) The child weighs 55 lb. If the child is NPO, what is the daily IV fluid maintenance? _____
   (b) What is the rate of flow in mL/h? _____

10. A child has a BSA of 0.82 m². The recommended dose of a drug is 2 million units/m². How many units will you administer? _____

11. Order: *Claforan (cefotamine sodium) 1.2 g IVPB q8h.* The safe dose range for the solution concentration is 20–60 mg/mL to infuse over 15 to 30 minutes. What is the minimal amount of IV fluid needed to safely dilute this dosage? [HINT: The minimal amount of IV fluid is the maximal safe concentration.] _____

Workspace

12. Calculate the daily fluid maintenance for an infant who weighs 7 lb. _____

13. Order: *Retrovir (zidovudine) 160 mg/m² q8h PO*. The child has a BSA of 1.1 m² and the strength of the Retrovir is 50 mg/5 mL. How many milliliters of this antiviral drug will you prepare? _____

14. Order: D5/$\frac{1}{2}$NS with KCl 20 mEq per liter, infuse at 30 mL/h. The child is 60 cm and weighs 9.1 kg.
    (a) How many mEq of KCl would you add to a 500 mL IV bag? _____
    (b) The label on the KCl vial reads 2 mEq/mL. How many milliliters will you add to the IV? _____
    (c) How many mEq/h will the child receive? _____

15. Order: *erythromycin estolate* 125 mg PO q4h. The child weighs 14.5 kg. The recommended dosage is 30–50 mg/kg/day in equally divided doses. The label reads 125 mg/mL.
    (a) Is the ordered dose safe? _____
    (b) How many milliliters would you administer? _____

16. Order: Vancocin (vancomycin) 40 mg/kg/d IVPB q6h to infuse over 90 minutes in 200 mL NS. The child weighs 41 kg. The Vancocin vial has a concentration of 50 mg/mL. At what rate in mL/h will you set the pump?

17. A medication of 100 mg in 1 mL is diluted to 15 mL and administered IVP over 20 minutes. How many mg/min is the patient receiving?

18. 40 mL of IV fluid is to infuse over 60 minutes. What is the rate of flow in microdrops per minute?

19. Order: *Pediaprophen (ibuprofen) 10 mg/kg PO q4h*. The label reads 100 mg/2.5 mL. The child weighs 35 pounds. How many milliliters will you administer?

20. Order: *ampicillin 125 mg PO q6h*. A child weighs 22 pounds. The package insert states that the recommended dose is 50 mg/kg/24 h. Is the prescribed dose safe?

Cumulative Review Exercises

Review your mastery of previous chapters.

1. Order: *1 unit (250 mL) packed red blood cells to infuse in 2 h*. At what rate in mL/h will you set the pump to complete this infusion on time? _____

2. Order: *NovoLog Mix 70/30 6 units subcut 15 minutes before breakfast and 10 units at bedtime*. Select the correct label shown in •**Figure 12.15** and place an arrow on the appropriate syringe for the evening dose. _____

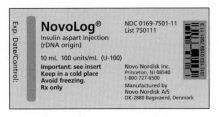
(a)

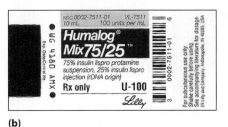
(b)

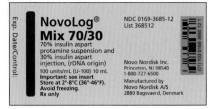
(c)

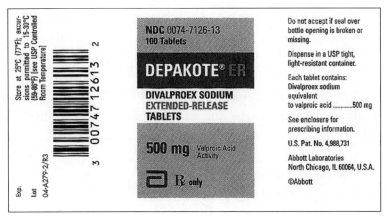

• **Figure 12.15**
Drug labels for question 2.

3. Order: *Depakote ER 500 mg PO daily for one week for migraine headache.* Use the information in •**Figure 12.16** to calculate the number of grams of this GABA inhibitor the patient will have taken in 5 days. _____

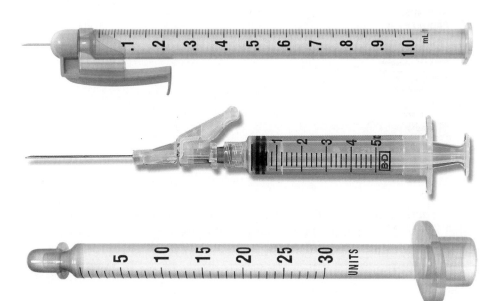

• **Figure 12.16**
Drug label for Depakote ER.

4. Order: *cephalexin oral suspension 375 mg PO q6h.* The recommended dosage range for this cephalosporin antibiotic for a child who has otitis media is 75–100 mg/kg/day.

(a) Read the information in •**Figure 12.17** and determine if this is a safe dose for a child who weighs 44 pounds. _____

Workspace

(b) If the dose is safe, how many milliliters would the child receive?
_____

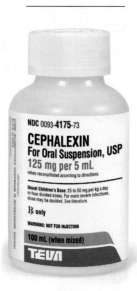

• **Figure 12.17**
Drug label for cephalexin.

5. Order: *activated charcoal 1 g/kg mixed in 6 ounces of water PO stat*. The label states 208 mg/mL. How many milliliters will you administer to a child who weighs 31 pounds? _____

6. Order: *Mandol (cefamandole nafate) 50 mg/kg IM 30 minutes before surgery*. The instructions for reconstitution state to add 3 mL of diluent yielding 285 mg/mL. How many milliliters will you administer to a child who weighs 10 kg? _____

7. Order: *Dynapen (dicloxacillin sodium) 125 mg PO q6h*. The recommended dosage range is 12.5–25 mg/kg/day in equally divided doses q6h (max 4 g/day). Is the ordered dose safe for a child who weighs 33 pounds? _____

8. Order: *azithromycin 500 mg IVPB daily for 2 days, infuse in 250 mL D5W over 1 hour*. Reconstitution directions are to add 4.8 mL of diluent to the 500 mg vial, yielding 100 mg/mL. How many milliliters of reconstituted azithromycin must be added to the 250 mL of D5W? _____

9. Order: *amoxicillin and clavulanate potassium 400/57 mg PO q8h*. Read the information in •**Figure 12.18** and calculate how many milligrams of clavulanate the patient will receive per day. _____

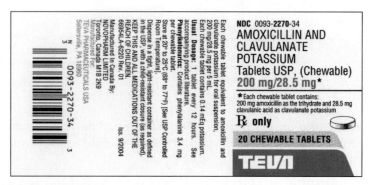

• **Figure 12.18**
Drug label for amoxicillin and clavulanate potassium.

10. What is the BSA of a person who is 63 inches tall and weighs 150 pounds? _____

11. Order: *Ticar (ticarcillin disodium) 1 g IVPB q6h, infuse in 50 mL D5W over 45 minutes*. The instructions for the 1 g vial state to reconstitute with 2 mL of sterile water for injection yielding 1g/2.6 mL. At what rate in mL/h will you set the pump? _____

12. Order: *morphine sulfate 3 mg IV stat*. The label reads 10 mg/ml. How many milliliters of this narcotic analgesic will you administer? _____

13. Order: *Videx (didanosine) 250 mg PO B.I.D.* The directions state to reconstitute the 4 g bottle, add 200 mL of water. How many milliliters of this antiretroviral will you administer? _____

14. Order: *Nalfon (fenoprofen calcium) 900 mg/m² PO daily in two divided doses*. How many milligrams of this analgesic would a child who weighs 23 kg and is 128 cm tall receive per day? _____

15. Which is the strongest solution? 1:1,000, 1:10,000; 1:15,000. _____

nursing.pearsonhighered.com
Prepare for success with animated examples, practice questions, challenge tests, and interactive assignments.

Workspace

Comprehensive
Self-Tests

Comprehensive Self-Test 1

Answers to *Comprehensive Self-Tests* 1–4 can be found in Appendix A at the back of the book.

1. Order: *Cardizem LA (dilitazem HCl) 180 mg PO daily*. Read the label in • **Figure S.1** and calculate how many grams are in the bottle.

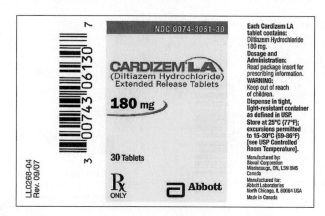

• **Figure S.1**
Drug label for Cardizem LA.

2. Order: *lactulose 2.5 g/d PO prn*. The strength on the label • **Figure S.2** is 10 g/15 mL. How many milliliters will you prepare?

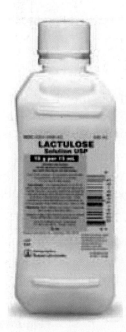

• **Figure S.2**
Bottle of lactulose.

3. Order: *Trandate (labetalol HCl) 20 mg IVP, give slowly over 2 min*. The label strength is 5 mg/mL.
   (a) How many milliliters will you prepare?
   (b) How many mL will you administer every 15 seconds?

4. Order: *Toradol (ketorolac tromethamine) 15 mg IM q6h prn pain*. The strength on the label is 30 mg/mL.
   (a) How many milliliters will you administer?
   (b) What size syringe will you use?

5. A newborn has an order for *Prostin VR (alprostadil) 0.15 micrograms IV per hour* to maintain patency of the ductus arteriosus. The pharmacy prepared a Prostin drip with 25 mcg alprostadil in 50 ml of D5W. What hourly rate is needed to deliver the dosage of medication as ordered?

6. Order: *Campral DR (acamprosate calcium) 666 mg PO T.I.D.* Read the label in • **Figure S.3** and calculate how many tablets the patient will receive each day.

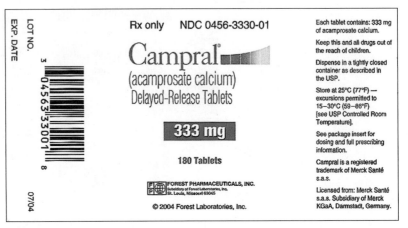

• **Figure S.3**
Drug label for Campral.

7. Order: *Dilaudid (hydromorphone HCl) 0.75 mg IM q4h prn moderate pain.* The strength on the vial is 1 mg/mL.
   (a) How many milliliters will you administer?
   (b) What size syringe will you use?

8. Order: *Camptosar (irinotecan HCl) 125 mg/m^2 IV, once a week for 4 weeks.* The strength on the label on the 5 mL multidose vial is 20 mg/mL. How many milliliters will you prepare for a patient who has a BSA of 0.8 m^2?

9. Order: *Levemir (insulin detemir) 0.2 units/kg subcut daily with dinner.* Read the information in • **Figure S.4** and calculate how many units you would administer to a patient who weighs 200 pounds.

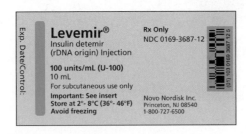

• **Figure S.4**
Drug label for Levemir.

10. Order: *Nexium (esomeprazole magnesium) 20 mg IVPB daily, infuse in 50 mL D5W over 20 minutes.* The reconstitution directions are to add 5 ml of NS. At what rate will you set the IV pump in mL/h?

11. Order: *Taxotere (docetaxel) 75 mg/m^2 IVPB in 250 mL D5W, infuse over 1 h.* The patient weighs 150 pounds and is 72 inches tall.
   (a) How many milligrams are required for the prescribed dose?
   (b) At what rate will you set the infusion pump

12. Order: *Mycamine (micafungin) 50 mg IVPB daily for 18 days. Infuse in 100 mL D5W over 1h.* How many mcgtt/min will the infusion run?

13. Order: *Lanoxicaps (digoxin solution in capsules) 0.1 mg PO daily.* The strength on the label is 50 mcg (0.05 mg)/cap. How many capsules will you administer?

14. Calculate the daily fluid maintenance for a child who weighs 44 pounds.

15. Order: *Acular (ketorolac tromethamine) 1 drop 0.5% ophthalmic solution to right eye Q.I.D. for 2 weeks.* The vial contains 10 mL. How many milligrams of Acular are in the vial?

16. A patient has an IV of 250 mL with 1 g of lidocaine infusing via pump at a rate of 10 mL/h.
    (a) What is the concentration of lidocaine measured in mg/mL?
    (b) How many milligrams of lidocaine is the patient receiving per hour?
    (c) How many milliliters per minute of the lidocaine solution is the patient receiving?

17. Order: *Motrin (ibuprofen) 10 mg/kg PO q8h.* The strength on the label is 100 mg/5 mL. How many milliliters will you prepare for a child who weighs 70 pounds?

18. Order: *hyoscyamine sulfate oral solution 0.025 mg PO 1h before meals and at bedtime.* The recommended dose for this anticholinergic drug is 0.0625–0.125 mg q4h prn (max: 0.75 mg/d).
    (a) Is the prescribed dose safe?
    (b) If the dose is safe, how many milliliters will you administer? The label reads 0.125 mg/mL (0.2 mL).

19. The prescriber ordered *Vitamin B_{12} alpha (hydroxocobalamin) 34 mcg IM/month* for a child who weighs 20 kg. The label reads 1000 mcg/mL.
    (a) How many milliliters will the child receive?
    (b) What size syringe will you use?

20. The prescriber ordered *Zanosar (streptozocin) 500 mg/m^2/d IV for 5 days.* Read the label in • **Figure S.5**.

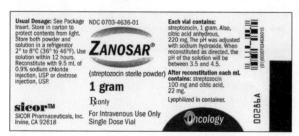

• **Figure S.5**
Drug label for Zanosar.

(a) How many grams will a patient who has a BSA of 1.8 m^2 receive in 5 days? The medication is to be infused in 250 mL of D5W over 50 minutes via pump.
(b) At what rate will you set the pump in mL/h?

21. Order: *Tegopen (cloxacillin) oral suspension 400 mg PO q6h.* The label reads 125 mg/5 mL, and the recommended dose is 12.5 mg–25 mg/kg/q6h (max: 4 g/d).
    (a) Is the prescribed dose safe for a child who weighs 66 pounds?
    (b) If the dose is safe how many milliliters will the child receive?

22. Order: *M-M-RII vaccine 1 dose subcut now.* Read the label in •**Figure S.6**. The vaccine must be reconstituted with 0.5 mL of diluent. Indicate the dose on the most appropriate syringe.

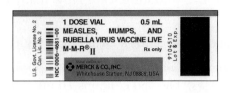

1 DOSE VIAL   **0.5 mL**
MEASLES, MUMPS, AND
RUBELLA VIRUS VACCINE LIVE
M-M-R® II   **Rx only**

NDC 0006-4681-00
U.S. Govt. License No. 2
Can. Lic. No. 2
9104510
Lot & Exp.

MERCK & CO., INC.
Whitehouse Station, NJ 08889, USA

• **Figure S.6**
Drug label for M-M-R II.

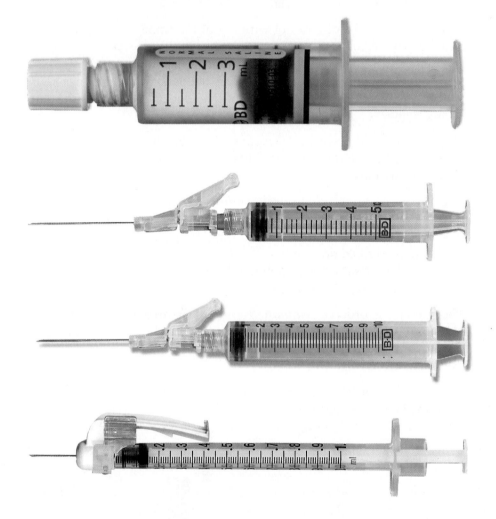

23. Order: *Prinvil (lisinopril) 0.07 mg/kg PO daily.* The label reads 1 mg/mL. Calculate the number of milliliters of this ACE inhibitor you will administer to a child who weighs 70 pounds.

24. Order: *Ativan (lorazepam) 3 mg IV push stat.* The strength on the vial is 4 mg/mL. The package insert recommends diluting the medication with an equal volume of compatible solution and to infuse slowly at a maximum rate of 2 mg/min.
    (a) How many milliliters of Ativan (lorazepam) will you prepare?
    (b) Over how many minutes will you administer the Ativan (lorazepam)?

25. Order: *heparin 1,000 units in 500 mL 0.9% NaCl, infuse at 100 mL/h.* How many units per hour is the patient receiving?

Comprehensive Self-Test 2

Answers to *Comprehensive Self-Tests* 1–4 can be found in Appendix A at the back of the book.

1. Order: *Lasix (furosemide) 40 mg via PEG tube daily*. Read the information in •**Figure S.7** and select the form and amount of this diuretic that you will administer.

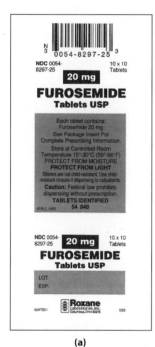

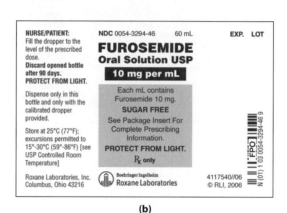

(a)   (b)

•**Figure S.7**
Drug labels for furosemide.

2. The prescriber ordered *Abilify (aripiprazole) 2 mg PO daily, increase to 5 mg after 2 days, and 10 mg after 2 more days*. How many milligrams of this antipsychotic medication will the patient have received in 1 week?

3. Order: *ascorbic acid (vitamin C) 350 mg IM daily for 4 weeks*. The strength on the label is 500 mg/mL. How many milliliters will you administer?

4. The prescriber ordered *Elspar (asparaginase) 6,000 International Units/m² IM three times per week*. The directions on the 10,000 unit vial state to reconstitute the powder with 2 mL for intramuscular injection or 5 mL for intravenous administration. How many milliliters of this antineoplastic drug will you administer for a patient who weighs 150 pounds and is 63 inches tall?

5. Order: *Atropair (atropine sulfate) 0.4 mg IVP 30 minutes before surgery*. The strength on the vial is 0.5 mg/ml. How many milliliters of this anticholinergic drug will you prepare?

6. Order: *Mepron (atovaquone) 750 mg oral suspension PO B.I.D for 21 days*. The label reads 750 mg/5 mL. How many grams of this antiprotozoal drug will the patient receive when the dose is completed?

7. The prescriber ordered *Zithromax (azithromycin) oral suspension 10 mg/kg PO on day 1, then 5 mg/kg for 4 more days*. The strength on the vial is

176 mg/5 mL. How many milliliters will a child who weighs 54 pounds receive on day 3?

8. Order: *naproxen oral suspension 12 mg/kg PO B.I.D.* The recommended maximum dosage is 1,000 mg/d.
   (a) Is this a safe dose for a child who weighs 80 pounds?
   (b) If the dose is safe, use the information on the label in • **Figure S.8** and calculate how many milliliters of this NSAID the child would receive.

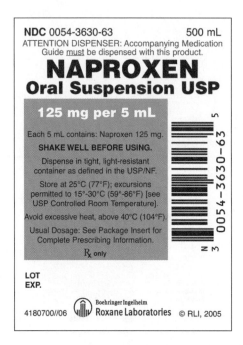

• **Figure S.8**
Drug label for naproxen.

9. Order: *Tysabri (natalizumab) 300 mg IV every week.* The strength on the vial is 300 mg/15 mL. The directions state to withdraw the 15 mL and add it to 100 mL of NS and infuse over 1h. At what rate in drops per min will you set the infusion if the drop factor is 10 gtt/mL?

10. Order: *Tarka (trandolapril/verapamil HCl ER) 2 mg/240 mg PO daily.* Read the information in • **Figure S.9** and calculate how many milligrams of verapamil the patient will receive in 1 week.

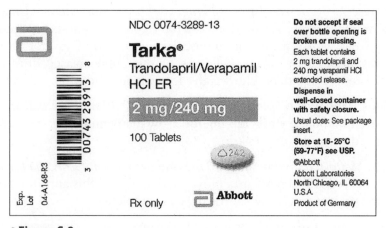

• **Figure S.9**
Drug label for Tarka.

11. Order: *Heparin 25,000 units IV in D5W 1,000 mL, infuse at 1,000 units/h.* What is the flow rate in mL/h?

12. Order: *magnesium sulfate 20 g IV in RL 1,000 mL, infuse at 2 g/h.* What is the flow rate in mL/h?

13. The prescriber ordered an *insulin drip of Humulin R Regular insulin 300 units IV in RL 150 mL, infuse at 10 mL/h.* How many units/h of insulin is the patient receiving?

14. The prescriber ordered *diazepam 10 mg IVP stat, give slowly 1 minute per 5 mg.* The strength on the label is 5 mg/mL.
    (a) How many milliliters are needed?
    (b) How many minutes will it take to administer the dose?
    (c) How many milliliters will be administered every 30 seconds?

15. Order: *vancomycin HCl 1500 mg IVPB q6h.* The recommended dosage is 40 mg/kg/d. Is the prescribed dose safe for a child who weighs 77 pounds?

16. Calculate the daily fluid maintenance requirements for a child who weighs 33 pounds.

17. The prescriber ordered *Azactam (aztreonam) 1 g IV q6h* for a child who has cystic fibrosis. The recommended dosage range is 50–200 mg/kg q6h (maximum 8 g/day). Is the prescribed dose safe for a child who weighs 70 pounds?

18. The prescriber ordered *dopamine 2 mcg/kg/min IV* for a patient who weighs 110 pounds. The label on the IV bag reads dopamine 200 mg/250 mL D5W. At what rate will you set the infusion pump in mL/h?

19. Order: *Solu-Cortef (hydrocortisone sodium succinate) 150 mg IM stat.* The strength on the label is 250 mg/2 mL. How many milliliters will the patient receive?

20. Order: *Dynapen (dicloxacillin sodium) mg 500 mg PO q6h.* The recommended dosage range for a child with a severe infection is 50–100 mg/kg/day divided into doses given q6h. Is the prescribed dose of this antibiotic safe for a child who weighs 77 pounds?

21. The prescriber ordered *Mannitol 12.5 g IVP stat.* The label on the 50-mL vial reads 25%. How many milliliters of this osmotic diuretic will you prepare?

22. Order: *Norvir (ritonavir) 250 mg/m^2 PO B.I.D.* How many milligrams are required for a child who weighs 15 kg and is 77 cm tall?

23. Order: *D5W 500 mL IV, infuse over 5 hours.* Calculate the flow rate in drops per minute. The drop factor is 15 gtt/mL.

24. The prescriber ordered *Synthroid (levothyroxine sodium) 0.05 mg PO daily.* The strength on the label is 25 mcg (0.025 mg)/tab. Calculate how many tablets you will administer.

25. Order: *heparin 8,000 units subcut q12h.* The strength on the vial is 10,000 units/mL. How many milliliters will you administer?

Comprehensive Self-Test 3

Answers to *Comprehensive Self-Tests* 1–4 can be found in Appendix A at the back of the book.

1. Calculate the dosage of calcium EDTA for a patient who has a BSA of 1.47 m^2. The recommended dose is 500 mg/m^2.

2. Order: *Tikosyn 1 mg PO q8h*. Read the label in •**Figure S.10** to determine how many capsules you will give the patient.

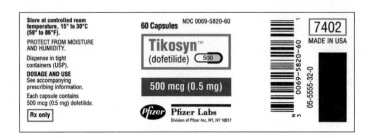

3. How would you prepare 400 mL of 10% Clorox solution from a 100% solution?

4. Kineret (anakinra) 100 mg subcut daily has been prescribed for a patient with rheumatoid arthritis. The prefilled syringe is labeled 100 mg/mL. Calculate the dose in grams.

5. An IV of 1,000 mL D5W is infusing at a rate of 40 gtt/min. How long will it take to finish if the drop factor is 20 gtt/mL?

6. Calculate the number of grams of dextrose in 250 mL of D5W.

7. Order: *Humulin Regular insulin U-100 6 units and Humulin NPH insulin 14 units subcutaneous ac breakfast*. Read the labels in •**Figure S.11** and place an arrow on the syringe indicating the total amount of insulin you will give.

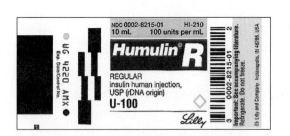
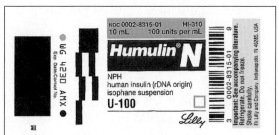

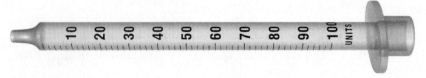

• **Figure S.11**
Drug label or Humulin R and Humulin N and syringe.

8. The prescriber ordered *Cordarone (amiodarone HCl) 400 mg PO b.i.d.* Each tablet contains 200 mg. How many tablets will you give the patient?

9. The prescriber ordered *Cefobid (cefoperazone) 1g IVPB q12h to infuse in 30 minutes*. The label on the 1-gram premixed IV bag reads cefoperazone 50 mL, 50 mg/mL.
   (a) Calculate the flow rate in milliliters per hour.
   (b) How many milligrams will the patient receive?

10. Your patient is to receive *morphine sulfate 5 mg subcutaneously stat*. The 20 mL multiple dose vial is labeled morphine 15 mg/mL. Calculate the dose in milliliters and place an arrow on the syringe indicating the dose.

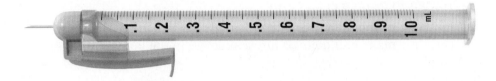

11. A dosage of 300 mcg has been ordered. The solution strength is 0.4 mg/mL. Calculate in milliliters the volume of medication needed.

12. A prescriber ordered a *premixed solution of nitroglycerine 25 mg in 250 mL D5W to be titrated at a rate of 5 mcg/min, increase q 5–10 min until pain subsides*. The medication is to be infused via pump. How many mL/h will you set the pump to begin the infusion?

13. Order: *Humulin R insulin 100 units in 100 mL NS, infuse at 0.1 unit/kg/h*. The patient weighs 68 kg. How many units per hour is the patient receiving?

14. The prescriber ordered *Claforan (cefotaxime) 750 mg IM q12h*. The 1-g vial of Claforan is in a powder form. The package insert states for IM injection, add 3 mL of sterile water for injection for an approximate volume of 3.4 mL containing 300 mg/mL. How many milliliters will you give the patient?

15. *Rebif (interferon beta-1a) 44 mcg subcutaneous three times a week* is prescribed for a patient with multiple sclerosis. How many milligrams will the patient receive in one week?

16. Order: *Lanoxin (digoxin) elixir 0.15 mg PO q12h*. The child weighs 70 lb and the recommended maintenance dose is 7–10 mcg/kg/day.
   (a) What is the minimum daily maintenance dosage in mg/day?
   (b) What is the maximum daily maintenance dosage in mg/day?
   (c) Is the dose ordered safe?

17. *Vibramycin (doxycycline hyclate) 4.4 mg/kg IVPB daily* is ordered for a child who weighs 80 pounds. The premixed IV solution bag is labeled Vibramycin 200 mg/250 mL D5W to infuse in 4 hours.
   (a) How many milligrams of Vibramycin will the patient receive?
   (b) Calculate the flow rate in mL/h.

18. Order: *Levaquin (levofloxacin) 500 mg in 100 mL D5W IVPB daily for 14 days to infuse in 1 h*. Calculate the flow rate in drops per minute if the drop factor is 15 gtt/mL.

19. Calculate the BSA of a child who is 44 inches and weighs 72 pounds.

20. Order: *heparin 5,000 units subcutaneous q12h.* The multidose vial label reads 10,000 units/mL. How many milliliters will you give the patient?

21. Order: *D10W 1,000 mL to infuse at 75 mL/h.* The drop factor is 20 gtt/mL.
    (a) What is the rate of flow in $\frac{mL}{min}$?
    (b) How many drops per minute will you set the IV to infuse?
    (c) How long will it take for the infusion to be complete?

22. Calculate the total daily fluid maintenance for a child who weighs 45 kg.

23. Order: *Keflex (cephalexin) oral suspension 50 mg/kg PO q6h.* The label reads 125 mg/5 mL. The patient weighs 33 pounds. How many milliliters will you give?

24. Read the label in •**Figure S.12**.
    (a) How many milligrams of furosemide are in 1 mL?
    (b) How many milliliters of furosemide are in the bottle?

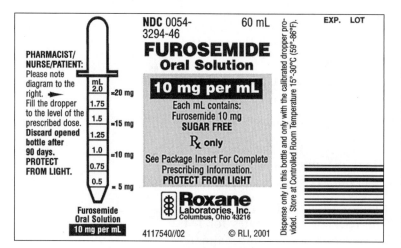
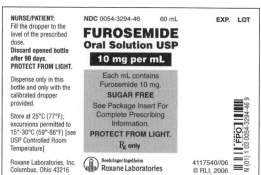

• **Figure S.12**
Drug label for furosemide.

(Courtesy of Roxane Laboratories inc.)

25. The prescriber ordered *ReoPro (abciximab) 0.125 mcg/kg/min IV* for a patient who weighs 75 kg. Calculate the dosage rate in micrograms per minute.

Comprehensive Self-Test 4

Answers to *Comprehensive Self-Tests* 1–4 can be found in Appendix A at the back of the book.

1. A patient has an IV of 250 mL D5RL with 25,000 units of heparin infusing at 20 mL/h. How many units of heparin is the patient receiving each hour?

2. Order: *Alkeran (melphalan HCl) 16 mg/m² 100 mL NSIV q2 weeks for four doses infuse in 20 min.* The package insert states to rapidly inject 10 mL of supplied diluent into a 50-mg vial and shake vigorously until a clear solution results (5 mg/mL). The patient has a BSA of 1.2 m².
    (a) How many milligrams contain the dose?
    (b) How many milliliters of Alkeran will you add to 100 mL of NS?
    (c) Determine the flow rate in mL/h.

3. A patient is receiving *Zantac (ranitidine HCl) 150-mg PO b.i.d.* The label reads 150-mg tablets. How many tablets will the patient receive in 24 hours?

4. Order: *Lanoxicaps (digoxin solution in capsules) 0.1 mg PO b.i.d.* The label on the bottle reads 50 mcg/capsule. How many capsules will you give the patient?

5. Order: *protamine sulfate 22 mg IVP over 10 min.* The label reads 50 mg/5 mL. Dilute with 20 mL of NS or D5W. How many milliliters of protamine sulfate will you prepare?

6. Order: *Garamycin (gentamicin sulfate) 9 mg IMq12h.* The package insert states that the recommended dose for neonates is 2.5 mg/kg q 12–24h. The label on the vial reads Pediatric Injectable Garamycin 10 mg/mL. The infant weighs 10 lb.
   (a) Is the dose safe?
   (b) How many milliliters will you give?

7. An IV of D5/NS (1,000 mL) is infusing at 50 mL/h. The infusion started at 1300h; what time will it finish?

8. The prescriber ordered *Dilantin (phenytoin sodium) 250 mg/m^2 per day in three divided doses* for a child who has a BSA of 1.25 m^2. The bottle is labeled 125 mg/5 mL oral suspension. How many milliliters will you give for each dose?

9. Order: *Lasix (furosemide) 20 mg IM stat.* The label reads 40 mg/4 mL.
   (a) How many milliliters will you give the patient?
   (b) Place an arrow on the syringe that indicates the dose.

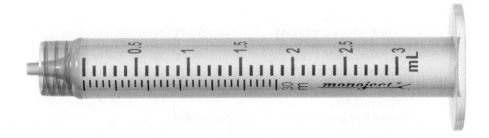

10. The recommended dose of Cleocin (clindamycin) pediatric oral solution is 8 to 25 mg/kg/day in three to four equally divided doses. A child weighs 60 pounds.
    (a) Calculate the minimum safe daily dose in mg/d.
    (b) Calculate the maximum safe daily dose in mg/d.

11. Calculate how many grams of sodium chloride are in 250 mL of a 0.9% NaCl solution.

12. A patient has an IV infusing at 25 gtt/min. How many mL/h is the patient receiving? The drop factor is 15 gtt/mL.

13. Calculate the total volume and hourly IV flow rate for a 10-pound infant who is receiving maintenance fluids.

14. Order: *nitroprusside sodium 50 mg in 250 mL D5W infuse at 1 mL/h.* The recommended dosage range is 0.1 to 5 mcg/kg/min. The patient weighs 154 pounds. Is this a safe dose?

15. A patient with aspiration pneumonia has an order for *aminophylline IVPB 250 mg in 250 mL D5W to Infuse at 0.5 mg/kg/h*. The patient weighs 80 kg. What is the flow rate in mL/h?

16. Your patient has an IV of Humulin R insulin 50 units in 500 mL of NS infusing at 12 units per hour. Calculate the flow rate in mL/h.

17. Order: *Ticar (ticarcillin disodium) 1 g IM q6h*. The package insert states to reconstitute each 1-g vial with 2 mL of sterile water for injection. Each 2.5 mL = 1g. How many milliliters will you administer?

18. Order: *Indocin SR (indomethacin) 150 mg PO t.i.d. for 7 days*. The label reads Indocin SR 75 mg capsules.
    (a) How many capsules will you give the patient for each dose?
    (b) Calculate the entire 7 day dosage in grams.

19. Order: *Colace (docusate sodium) syrup 100 mg via PEG t.i.d.* The label reads 50 mg/15 mL. How many mL will you give?

20. Order: *theophylline 0.8 mg/kg/h IV via pump*. The premixed IV bag is labeled theophylline 800 mg in 250 mL D5W. The patient weighs 185 pounds. How many mL/h will you set the pump?

21. Order: *cefazolin 1 g IVPB q6h, add to 50 mL D5W and infuse over 20 minutes*. Read the reconstitution information from the cefazolin label in •**Figure S.13**.
    (a) How many milliliters of diluent will you add to the vial, so that 1 gram of cefazolin is contained in 5 mL of the solution?
    (b) Based on the answer in part (a), calculate the flow rate in milliliters per minute.

Total Amount of Diluent	Approximate Concentration
45 mL	1 g/5 mL
96 mL	1 g/10 mL

•**Figure S.13**
Reconstitution information from the cefazolin label.

22. The nurse has prepared 7 mg of dexamethasone for IV administration. The label on the vial reads 10 mg/mL. How many milliliters did the nurse prepare?

23. Order: *Cogentin (benztropine mesylate) 2 mg IM stat and then 1 mg IM daily*. The label reads 2 mg/2 mL.
    (a) How many milliliters will you administer daily?
    (b) What size syringe will you use?

24. Order: $\frac{2}{3}$ *strength Sustacal 900 mL via PEG, give over 8h*. How will you prepare this solution?

25. An IV of 250 mL NS is infusing at 25 mL/h. The infusion began at 1800h. What time will it be completed?

Appendices

Appendix A

Diagnostic Test of Arithmetic

1. $\frac{3}{8}$ 2. 0.285   3. 6.5   4. 0.83

5. 3.2   6. 3.8   7. 0.0639   8. 500

9. 2   10. $\frac{1}{4}$ and 0.25   11. $2\frac{1}{3}$ 12. $\frac{1}{25}$

13. $\frac{9}{20}$ 14. 0.025   15. $\frac{18}{7}$ 16. 12

17. 7.6   18. 6   19. 0.4   20. $\frac{3}{4}$

Chapter 1

Try These for Practice

1. 0.875   2. 66.78 ≈ 66.8   3. 0.05 and $\frac{1}{20}$ 4. $\frac{5}{9}$ 5. $\frac{3}{10}$

Exercises

1. $\frac{13}{20}$ 2. $7\frac{1}{2}$ 3. 1   4. $\frac{3}{5}$

5. $23\frac{1}{13}$ 6. $8\frac{2}{5}$ 7. 5   8. 0.37

9. 0.64   10. 6.7   11. 0.015   12. 0.21

13. 0.457   14. 0.0228   15. 2.8   16. 0.8

17. 0.9   18. 0.0625   19. 0.009   20. 1.50

21. 0.47   22. 4.7   23. 2.6   24. 53.84

25. 0.5 $\frac{63}{125}$ 26. 17.3 $17\frac{1}{3}$ 27. $\frac{10}{49}$ 0.2   28. $6\frac{3}{7}$ 6.4

29. 0.1 $\frac{1}{8}$ 30. 0.4 $\frac{3}{8}$ 31. $\frac{1}{2}$ 32. $\frac{2}{3}$

33. $\frac{60}{100}$, 60   34. $\frac{6}{8}$, 6   35.   0.40   36. $2.0\overset{1}{6}\overset{1}{0}$
                                                      7.00 $-1.2\overset{1}{2}2$
                                                     +2.55   0.838
                                                      9.95

37. $\left.\begin{matrix} 0.70 \\ 0.24 \end{matrix}\right\}$ 0.7 is larger   38. 16   39. 25% increase   40. 30% decrease

Chapter 2

Try These for Practice

1. Cozaar   2. oral   3. adalimumab

4. Tarka   5. 5 micrograms/milliliter

Exercises

1. Intravenous

2. Tarka

3. 0.4 mL

4. 20 mg/0.4 mL

5. 240 mg

6. (a) Levemir and Darvocet N
   (b) 0800h & 2000h
   (c) eight
   (d) subcutaneous
   (e) Neurontin, Vantin, and Levemir

7. (a) Cipro (ciprofloxacin HCl)
   (b) digoxin, Crestor, Lasix
   (c) Two times a day
   (d) Intravenous
   (e) Up to a maximum of six times a day

8. (a) milnacipran HCl, tablets
   (b) fibromyalgia
   (c) 12.5 milligrams
   (d) No, Savella is not approved for use in pediatrics
   (e) 200 milligrams daily

9.

Standard Time	Military Time
7:30 A.M.	0730h
5:43 P.M.	1743h
12 midnight.	2400h
8:20 P.M.	2020h
12:57 P.M.	1257h
10:30 P.M.	2230h
3:32 P.M.	1532h
4:15 A.M.	0415h
12:04 A.M.	0004h
9:12 A.M.	0912h

10. (a) Administer Norvasc (amlodipine) ten milligrams by mouth daily. Do not administer if the systolic blood pressure is less than 100.

    (b) Administer morphine sulfate five milligrams subcutaneously every four hours as needed for moderate to severe pain.

    (c) Administer Methergine (methylergonovine maleate) two-tenths milligram intramuscularly immediately, then administer two-tenths milligram by mouth every six hours for six doses.

    (d) Administer Ceftin (cefuroxime axetil) one and five-tenths grams by intravenous piggyback thirty minutes before surgery, then administer seven hundred fifty milligrams by intravenous piggyback every eight hours for twenty-four hours.

    (e) Administer heparin five thousand units subcutaneously every twelve hours.

11. (a) Route
    (b) Frequency
    (c) Dose and frequency
    (d) Frequency
    (e) Dose and frequency

Chapter 3

Try These for Practice

1. 210 sec

2. 105 oz

3. 12 h

4. 90 qt/h

5. 24 in/min

Exercises

1. 15 min
2. 63 mon
3. 56 h
4. 40 oz

5. 45 min
6. $1\frac{1}{2}$ yr
7. 3 ft
8. $2\frac{1}{2}$ lb

9. 101 oz
10. 24 cups
11. $\frac{3}{8}$ h
12. 74 in

13. 1 wk
14. $4\frac{1}{2}$ ft
15. $2\frac{qt}{min}$
16. $120\frac{pt}{hr}$

17. $6\frac{qt}{h}$
18. 10 ft/h
19. $\frac{7}{8}\frac{lb}{wk}$
20. $6\frac{ft}{h}$

Chapter 4

Try These for Practice

1. (a) 1,000 mL
   (b) 1 cc
   (c) 1,000 cm^3
   (d) 1,000 g
   (e) 1,000 mg
   (f) 1,000 mcg
   (g) 10 mm
   (h) 2 pt
   (i) 2 cups
   (j) 8 oz
   (k) 8 oz
   (l) 2 T
   (m) 3 t
   (n) 12 in
   (o) 16 oz

2. 10,000 mcg
3. 0.84 g/wk
4. 1.4 L
5. 6 T

Exercises

1. 9,600 mcg
2. 60 mg
3. 0.04 g
4. 6,250 mL

5. 2.1 cm
6. 5 cups
7. 24 cc
8. 250 mg

9. 7 pt
10. 12 t
11. 16 oz
12. 350 g

13. 500,000 mcg
14. 0.1 g
15. 0.028 g
16. 3 T

17. 0.08 g
18. 0.4 g
19. 3,100 g

20. 1.7 mg is in the range of 1–2 mg. The order is safe.

Cumulative Review Exercises

1. 1,300 mg
2. 3 cups
3. 4,200 mL

4. 27 t
5. 0.9 L
6. 3 cups

7. 0.56 g
8. 2 oz
9. 400 mg

10. The route of administration
11. 80 mg
12. 80 mg

13. 40 mg
14. 2130 hours
15. 0100 h the next day

Chapter 5

Try These for Practice

1. (a) 1,000 mL
   (b) 1,000 g
   (c) 1,000 mg
   (d) 1,000 mcg
   (e) 10 mm
   (f) 2 pt
   (g) 2 cups
   (h) 8 oz
   (i) 8 oz
   (j) 2 T
   (k) 3 t
   (l) 16 oz
   (m) 12 in
   (n) 2.5 cm
   (o) 2.2 lb
   (p) 5 mL
   (q) 15 mL
   (r) 30 mL
   (s) 240 mL
   (t) 240 mL
   (u) 500 mL
   (v) 1,000 mL
   (w) 2, 6, 30
   (x) 2, 4, 32, 1,000

2. 1 t
3. 2 in
4. 0.9 L
5. 9 t

Exercises

1. 4,700 mcg
2. 0.4 L
3. 12 t
4. 60 mL
5. 22.7 kg
6. 110 lb
7. 56 oz
8. 2 oz
9. 3 in
10. 16 T
11. 172.5 cm
12. 3,182 g
13. 100 kg
14. $\frac{1}{5}$ t
15. $\frac{6\,T}{day}$
16. 0.36 g
17. 1,365 mL
18. 1 oz
19. 10 g
20. 24 doses

Cumulative Review Exercises

1. 600 mg
2. 10 T
3. 30 kg
4. 0.64 cm
5. 3 oz
6. 700 mg/wk
7. 2.8 g/wk
8. 3,000 mg
9. 1530 hours
10. 1.25 mg
11. 42.5 mm
12. 10 mL
13. 198 lb
14. 180 cm
15. 1 cup per hour

Chapter 6

Case Study

1. 1 tab [label c]
2. 2 cap
3. 4 tab
4. $8\frac{tab}{day}$
5. 4 tab
6. 0.075 g
7. 28 tab
8. 2 tab
9. 1 cap
10. $4\frac{cap}{day}$
11. 2.73 m^2

Practice Reading Labels

1. Strength: 25 mg/5 mL; 20 mL
2. Strength: 2.5 mg/tab; 4 tab
3. Strength: 2 mg/cap; 2 cap
4. Strength: 100 mg/5 mL; 20 mL
5. Strength: 600 mg/tab; 1 tab
6. Strength: 100 mg/tab; 2 tab

7. Strength: 2.5 mg/tab; 4 tab

8. Strength: 2.5 mg/tab; 2 tab

9. Strength: 10 mg/tab; 5 tab

10. Strength: 8 mg/tab; 2 tab

11. Strength: 25 mg/5 mL; 15 mL

12. Strength: 250 mg/5 mL; 7.5 mL

13. Strength: 500 mg/tab; 1 tab

14. Strength: 180 mg/tab; 1 tab

15. Strength: 125 mg/cap; 2 cap

16. Strength: 2 mg/240 mg/tab; 2 tab

17. Strength: 30 mg/tab; 2 tab

18. Strength: 2.5 mg/tab; 2 tab

19. Strength: 333 mg/tab; 2 tab

20. Strength: 20 mg/tab; 2 tab

21. Strength: 25 mcg/tab; 4 tab

22. Strength: 12.5 mg/tab; 4 tab

23. Strength: 18 mg/cap; 3 cap

24. Strength: 5 mg/tab; 4 tab

25. Strength: 10 mg/tab; 2 tab

26. Strength: 6 mg/50 mg/cap; 1 cap

27. Strength: 25 mg/cap; 2 cap

28. Strength: 10 mg/cap; 2 cap

29. Strength: 250 mg/cap; 2 cap

30. Strength: 50 mg/tab; 2 tab

31. Strength: 100 mg/cap; 4 cap

32. Strength: 400 mg/cap; 1 cap

33. Strength: 125 mg/cap; 3 cap

34. Strength: 100-25 mg/tab; 2 tab

35. Strength: 100-12.5 mg/tab; 4 tab

36. Strength: 400 mg/tab; 1 tab

37. Strength: 50 mg/500 mg/tab; 2 tab

38. Strength: 50 mg/1000 mg/tab; 3 tab

39. Strength: 20 mg/tab; 3 tab

40. Strength: 40 mg/tab; 1 tab

41. Strength: 5 mg/tab; 2 tab

42. Strength: 5 mg/tab; 4 tab

43. Strength: 20 mg/tab; 2 tab

44. Strength: 15 mg/tab; 2 tab

45. Strength: 30 mg/tab; 1 tab

46. Strength: 100 mg/tab; 2 tab

47. Strength: 200 mg/tab; 1 tab

48. Strength: 15 mg/tab; 3 tab

49. Strength: 60 mg/tab; 3 tab

50. Strength: 400 mg/tab; 1 tab

Try These for Practice

1. 1.92 m^2

2. Yes, the order of 200 mg/d is in the recommended range.

3. 2.4 g

4. $\dfrac{3 \text{ cap}}{\text{d}}$

5. 4 mg

Exercises

1. $1\dfrac{\text{cap}}{\text{dose}}$

2. 3 tab

3. 20 mL

4. 15 mL

5. 1 t

6. 4.5 mL

7. 2.97 m^2

8. 1.52 m^2

9. 2 tab

10. 53.6 mL

11. 1 tab

12. 10 mL

13. 1 tab

14. The order of 400 mg/d is not in the recommended range. It is not safe; it is an overdose.

15. 1 g

16. 1.58 m^2 (using metric formula), 1.59 m^2 (using household formula)

17. 36 mL

18. $70\dfrac{\text{mL}}{\text{wk}}$

19. 3 tab

20. 2 tab

Cumulative Review Exercises

1. 30 mL   2. 40 kg   3. 32 oz   4. 10 mm

5. 12.5 mL   6. 3 tab   7. 3 t   8. 6 tab

9. 1.79 m²   10. John   11. 511 mg   12. 3.3 mL

13. 30 mL/h   14. 2 tab   15. 2230 h

Chapter 7

Case Study 7.1

1. (a) 0.75 mL

   (b) the 1 mL syringe

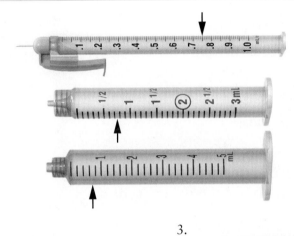

2. (a) 1 mL of Phenergan

   (b) 75 mg/mL because no calculation would be necessary

   (c)

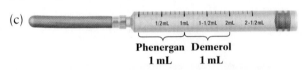

   Phenergan Demerol
     1 mL   1 mL

3.

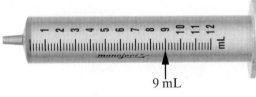

9 mL

4. 0.8 mL

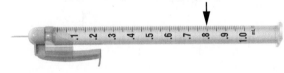

5. (a) 1 mL

   (b) 0.75 mL Demerol

   (c) Using a 3-mL syringe draw up 0.75 mL of Demerol and draw up 1 mL of
       Vistaril for a total volume of 1.75 mL.

   (d)

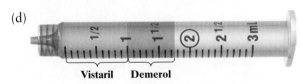

   Vistaril   Demerol

6. (a) 20 mL

   (b)

7. (a) 19 units

   (b)

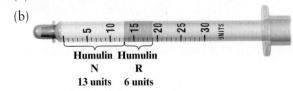

Humulin Humulin
   N   R
13 units 6 units

Try These for Practice

1. 1 mL tuberculin syringe; 0.91 mL

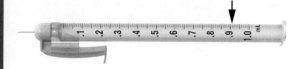

2. 12 mL syringe; 3.4 mL

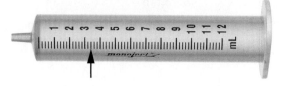

3. 3 mL syringe; 1.3 mL

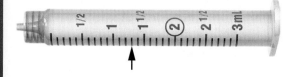

4. 5 mL syringe; 2.8 mL

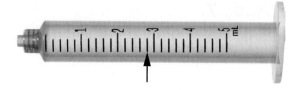

5. 1.5 mL using a 3 mL syringe

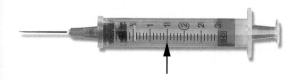

Exercises

1. 1 mL tuberculin syringe; 0.73 mL

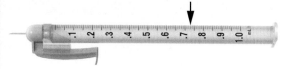

2. 30 unit Lo-Dose insulin syringe; 24 units

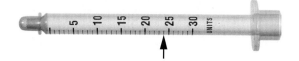

3. 5 mL syringe; 2.4 mL

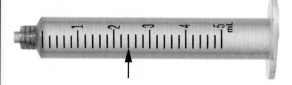

4. 3 mL syringe; 1.7 mL

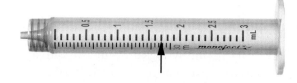

5. 35 mL syringe; 22 mL

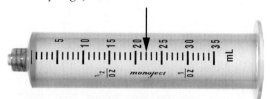

6. 12 mL syringe; 10.8 mL

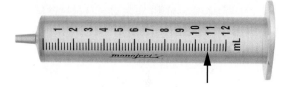

7. 50 unit Lo-Dose insulin syringe; 34 units

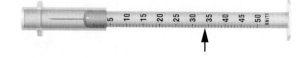

8. 100 unit insulin syringe; 78 units

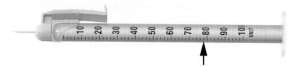

9. 0.5 mL syringe; 0.43 mL

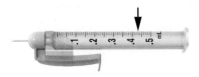

10. 100 unit insulin syringe; 81 units

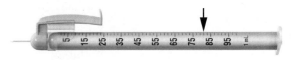

11. 12 mL syringe; 8.6 mL

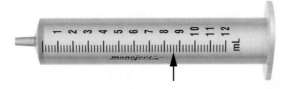

12. 1 mL tuberculin syringe; 0.56 mL

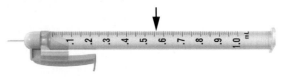

13. 12 mL syringe; 9.2 mL

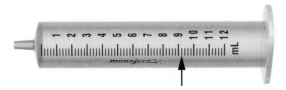

14. 35 mL syringe; 33 mL

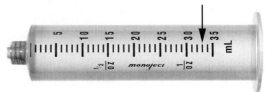

15. 1.5 mL

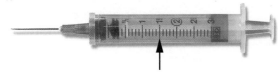

16. 50 units

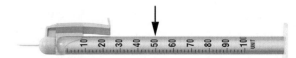

17. 2 mL

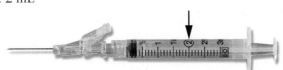

18. 0.4 mL

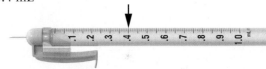

19. No, it is an overdose

20. 1.5 mL

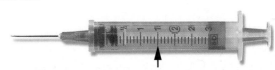

Cumulative Review Exercises

1. (a) no insulin   (b) 2 units   (c) 8 units

2. 40 mg   3. 20 mg   4. 1.4 g   5. $1\dfrac{oz}{h}$

6. 560 mcg   7. 148 cm   8. 70.5 kg   9. 25 mg/5 mL

10. 3 tab   11. 7 g   12. 1.64 m^2 13. 75 mg

14. 100 unit insulin syringe   15. 0.67 mL in a 1 mL tuberculin syringe

Chapter 8

Case Study 8.1

1. 0.5 mL—use 1 mL tuberculin syringe

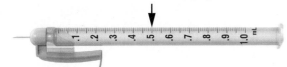

2. 180 mg = 120 mg + 60 mg

Use one 120 mg and one 60 mg tablet for each dose. Administer the two tablets daily.

3. 7.5 mL 4. Administer one 75 mg tablet. 5. 2 tab

6. Withdraw 10 units of Humulin R insulin, then into the same syringe withdraw 38 units of Humulin N insulin for a total of 48 units.

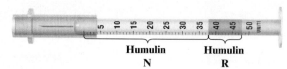

7. 9 g

Try These for Practice

1. Half-strength is stronger because $\frac{1}{2}$ strength is equivalent to 50%, whereas $\frac{1}{2}$% = 0.5%

2. 9:2,000   0.45% 3. 25 g 4. 2 L 5. 4 mL

Exercises

1. 1:20 & 5% 2. 1:5 & 20% 3. 1:5,000 & 0.02%

4. $\frac{1}{10}$ & 1:10 5. 2.5% 6. 1:10,000; 0.5%; $\frac{1}{3}$; 2 mg/mL

7.

Ratio	Fraction	Percent
1:5	$\frac{1}{5}$	20%
1:4	$\frac{1}{4}$	25%
1:10	$\frac{1}{10}$	10%
1:200	$\frac{1}{200}$	0.5%
9:1,000	$\frac{9}{1,000}$	0.9%

8. 140 mL 9. 0.4% should be 0.5%

10. 0.5 mL 11. 400 mg

12. 0.00005 g equals 0.005% 13. To 2 cans of Sustacal, add 2 cans of water

14. Take 250 g of boric acid crystals, dissolve, and dilute with water to 1 L

15. Take 8 tablets, dissolve, and dilute to 400 mL

16. 1,125 mg 17. 87 mg 18. Yes, they are equivalent.

19. (a) 8 mL (b) 25 mg 20. 0.07 mL

Cumulative Review Exercises

1. 400 mg 2. 6 T 3. 40 kg

4. 0.34 cm 5. $\frac{1}{2}$ oz 6. 350 $\frac{mg}{wk}$

7. (a) 4 servings   (b) 140 g   8. 0.56 g   9. 0400 hours Tuesday

10. 2 mL   11. 100 kg   12. 1/2 tab

13. 25 mL   14. 1,800 mg   15. 2,727 g

Chapter 9

Case Study 9.1

1. (a) 0.63 mL   2. (a) 1.5 mL
   (b) Use a 1 mL syringe   (b) Use a 3 mL syringe

3. (a) 15.9 mL   4. 2.5 mL
   (b) Use a 20 mL syringe

5. (a) Label j   6. (a) Label h   7. (a) Label g
   (b) 1 tablet   (b) 1 tablet   (b) 15 mL

8. (a) Label i   10. 60 mg/day
   (b) 4 tab   9. $\frac{1}{2}$ tab

Try These for Practice

1. (a) 0.5 mL
   (b) use a 1 mL syringe

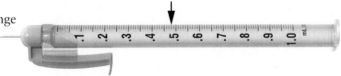

2. (a) 2.6 mL
   (b) use a 3 mL syringe

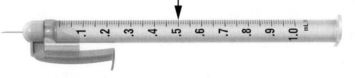

3. (a) 0.4 mL
   (b) use a 1 mL syringe

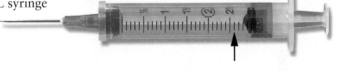

4. (a) 0.48 mL
   (b) use a 1 mL syringe

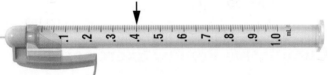

5. (a) Use the 2 g vial   (b) 5 mL   (c) 6 mL
   (d) 330 mg/mL   (e) 4.5 mL   (f) one

Exercises

1. 0.8 mL   2. 0.5 mL
3. (a) 0.8 mL   4. (a) 6.4 mL
   (b) 1 mL syringe   (b) 8 mL
                                    (c) 3 g/8 mL or 375 mg/mL
                                    (d) 5.3 mL (divided into two injections)

5. 2 mL

6. (a) yes, total of 270 mg/d is less than the maximum of 400 mg/d

   (b) 0.9 mL

   (c) 1 mL syringe

7. (a) 1.1 mL

   (b) 3 mL

8. (a) 2 g vial

   (b) 3.4 mL

   (c) two 3 mL syringes with 1.7 mL each

9. (a) 1.4 mL

   (b) 3 mL syringe

   (c) No, because 84 mg/d is more than 10 mg/d

10. (a) 1.5 mL

   (b) 3.3 doses/vial or 3 full doses

11. (a) 0.2 mL

   (b) 1 mL syringe

   (c) 14 doses/vial

12. (a) 8.2 mL

   (b) 250,000 units/mL

   (c) 5 million units

   (d) 1,000,000 units/mL

   (e) 2 mL

13. (a) 1 g

   (b) 0.75 mL

14. (a) 3 mL

   (b) 3 mL syringe

15. 2.6 mL

16. (a) 250 mg/1.5 mL

   (b) 3 mL

17. (a) 15 units

   (b) 300 units

18. 4 units

19. (a) 1.5 mg/d

   (b) 2 mg/d

20. (a) 0.25 mL

   (b) 1 mL syringe

   (c) 0.5 mL/30 min

Cumulative Review Exercises

1. Potassium Chloride

2. Oral, by mouth

3. Abbott

4. 10 mEq per dose

5. (a) 100 mL

   (b) 250 mg per 5 mL

   (c) 10 mL

   (d)

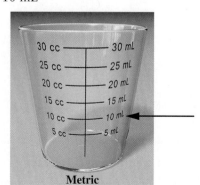

Metric

6. caspofungin acetate

7. intravenous

8. 10.8 mL

9. Two vials

10. (a) 0.65 mL

(b)

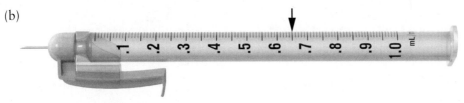

11. 200 g

12. 20 mL

13. 4 cap

14. Take 160 mL of Sustacal and add 80 mL of water.

15. (a) 0.75 mL

(b) 1 mL syringe

Chapter 10

Case Study 10.1

1. 10 mL of Cleocin

2. 83 mcgtt/min

3. 0.5 mL

4.

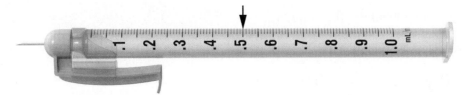

5. 10,000 units of heparin per day

6. 10 mL

7. 80 mL/h

8. Total enteral fluid in 24h = 610 mL

9. 1,992 mL

10. 1.175 mg

Try These for Practice

1. 42 mL/h

2. 28 gtt/min

3. 21 mcgtt/min

4. 16 h   0630h on Saturday

5. 75 mL (in)

Exercises

1. $167 \dfrac{mL}{h}$

2. 10 gtt/min

3. 135 mL

4. 6 h 40 min

5. 13 h 20 min 8:20 PM Tuesday

6. 225 mL

7. $133 \dfrac{mL}{h}$ is within the guidelines

8. 25 gtt/min

9. 33 gtt/min

10. 35 mcgtt/min

11. 150 mL (in)

12. 4 h   7:15 P.M. Monday

13. (a) 21 gtt/min

(b) 17 gtt/min

(c) Yes, the change (4 gtt/min) is within the guidelines

14. 13 gtt/min   15. 10h   9 A.M. Thursday   16. 23 gtt/min

17. 6 h   1300h the same day   18. 83 $\frac{mL}{h}$ 19. 50 mcgtt/min

20. 140 mL (in)

Cumulative Review Exercises

1. 0.4 in   2. 0.58 mL   3. 91 kg   4. 4.5 cm

5. 2 oz   6. 2,250 mg   7. 30 mL/h   8. 37 gtt/min

9. 1.41 m^2 10. 2 tab   11. 1 mL   12. 2 tab

13. 5 g   14. 150 mL   15. 1200h on Thursday

Chapter 11

Case Study 11.1

1. 125 mL/h   2. 0.75 mL   3. 0.25 mL

4. 0.71 mL   5. 26 gtt/min   6. 170 mL/h

7. (a) 300 mL/h   (b) 25 mL/h

8. 3 mL/h   9. 90 mU/h   10. 0.5 mL

Try These for Practice

1. 33 mg/min   2. (a) 600 mL/h   (b) 50 mg/min

3. 17 mcgtt/min   4. (a) $\frac{0.5\ mg}{15\ sec}$ (b) 0.25 mL

5.

Dosage Rate	Flow Rate
2 mU/min	6 mL/h
4 mU/min	12 mL/h
6 mU/min	18 mL/h
8 mU/min	24 mL/h
10 mU/min	30 mL/h
12 mU/min	36 mL/h
14 mU/min	42 mL/h
16 mU/min	48 mL/h
18 mU/min	54 mL/h
20 mU/min	60 mL/h

Exercises

1. 0.27 mg/min   2. 240 mL/h   3. 0.24 mg/min   4. 10 gtt/min

5. (a) 25 mL   6. (a) 120 mL/h   7. (a) 2.9 mL

   (b) 23.9 mL   (b) 1 h 40 min 0940 h   (b) 43 mL/h or 44 mL/h

   (c) 448 mL/h   the same day   (depending on

   (d) 30.3 mg/min   rounding)

8. (a) 7.5 mL

(b) 0.75 mL each
   30 seconds

(c) 40 sec for each mL

9. (a) 6.02 mg/min

(b) 0.5 mL every 15 sec

10. (a) 211 mcg/min

(b) 15.8 mL/h

11. 30 mL/h

12. (a) 25 mL/h

(b) 10 h

13. (a) 5.7 mL

(b) 5.6 mL/min

14. (a) 24 mcg

(b) 112 mL/h

15. (a) 2.68 mg/h

(b) 13.4 mL/h

16. 17,818 units

17. 21 h 44 min

18. 404 mL/h

19.

Dosage Rate	Flow Rate
2 mg/min	40 mL/h
5 mg/min	100 mL/h
8 mg/min	160 mL/h
11 mg/min	220 mL/h
14 mg/min	280 mL/h
17 mg/min	340 mL/h
20 mg/min	400 mL/h

20. (a) 166 mg

(b) 167 mL/h

Cumulative Review Exercises

1. 3.4 mL

2. 3,409 g

3. 10,000 mcg

4. 1.97 m^2

5. 732 mg

6. (a) 511 mg   (b) 6.4 mL   (c) 27 mL/h   (d) 2.1 mg/min

7. 3.7 cm

8. 10 mL

9. (a) 2.8 mL   (b) 2.7 mL

10. 1 tab

11. 4.5 g

12. 2%

13. 70 mcgtt/min

14. 0.1 mg/min

15. 38 gtt/min

Chapter 12

Case Study 12.1

1. 1,600 mL DFM

2. add 18.2 mL, give 2.5 mL

3. 103 mL/h

4. Yes, the dose is safe.

5. 0.62 mL (rounding down)

6. 3 cap   label (f)

7. 1,000 mcg

8. 1 tab   label (e)

9. 9.3 mL   (rounded down)

10. 5 mL   label (d)

11. 176 mcg/day

Try These for Practice

1. 9.8 mL

2. 56 mL/h

3. 16.6 mL   (rounded down)

4. 0.3 mL

5. 5.28 mg

Exercises

1. No, the dose is not safe (underdose).   2. 1.2 mL

3. 30 mL of theophylline   4. Yes, the dose is safe.

5. 4 mL of acyclovir   6. 1,844 mL DFM

7. 1 mL   (rounded down)   8. 2.9 mL   (rounded down)

9. 10 mg/min   15 min   10. 100 mL/h   (rounded down)

11. 0.65 mL

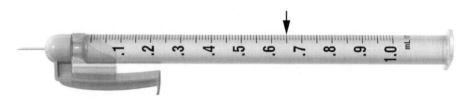

12. 40 mcgtts/min   13. $13.8 \dfrac{mL}{h}$ (rounded down)

14. 1 pop/h   15. (a) Yes, the dose is safe   (b) 7.5 mL

16. Yes, the dose is safe   17. 150 mL/h

18. (a) 1 mL   (b) 84 mL/h   19. 24 mL/h

20. 3.6 units/h

Cumulative Review Exercises

1. 125 mL/h

2. use label c 10 units

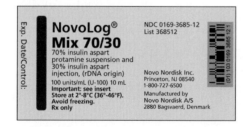

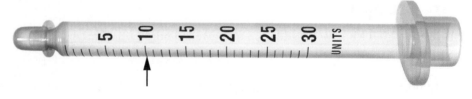

3. 2.5 g   4. (a) Yes, the dose is safe   (b) 15 mL

5. 67.7 mL   6. 1.7 mL (rounded down)   7. No

8. 5 mL   9. 171 mg   10. 1.74 m^2

11. 70 mL/h   12. 0.3 mL   13. 12.5 mL

14. 813 mg   15. 1:1,000

Answers to the Comprehensive Self-Tests

Comprehensive Self-Test 1

1. 5.4 g
2. 3.75 mL
3. (a) 4 mL   (b) 0.5 mL
4. (a) 0.5 mL   (b) 1 mL
5. 0.3 mL/h
6. 6 tab
7. (a) 0.75 mL   (b) 1 mL tuberculin syringe
8. 5 mL
9. 18 units
10. 150 mL/h
11. (a) 139 mg   (b) 250 mL/h
12. 100 mcgtt/min
13. 2 cap
14. 1,500 mL
15. 50 mg
16. (a) 4 mg/mL   (b) 40 mg/h   (c) 0.17 mg/min
17. 15.9 mL
18. (a) No the dose is not safe, it is not enough

    (b) Do not give the medication, contact the prescriber

19. (a) 0.03 mL   (b) 1 mL
20. (a) 4.5 g   (b) 311 mL/h
21. (a) Yes, the dose is safe, it is between the minimum dose of 375 mg and the maximum dose of 750 mg.

    (b) 16 mL

22.

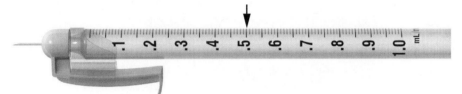

23. 2.2 mL
24. (a) 0.75 mL   (b) at least $1\frac{1}{2}$ minutes
25. 200 units/h

Comprehensive Self-Test 2

1. The form is oral solution (b) and the amount is 4 mL
2. 44 mg of Abilify (aripiprazole) in one week
3. Administer 0.7 mL of ascorbic acid (Vitamin C)
4. Administer 2.1 mL of Elspar (asparaginase)
5. Prepare 0.8 mL of Atropair (atropine sulfate)
6. The patient will receive 31.5 g of Mepron (atovaquone) when the dose is completed
7. 3.4 mL of Zithromax (azithromycin) on day 3
8. (a) Yes, the dose is safe   (b) 17.4 mL of naproxen oral suspension
9. 19 gtt/min
10. 1680 mg of Tarka (trandolapril/verapamil) in one week
11. 40 mL/h of heparin
12. 100 mL/h
13. 20 units/h
14. (a) 2 mL   (b) 2 minutes   (c) 0.5 mL/sec
15. No, the dose is not safe to administer, contact the prescriber
16. 1,250 mL
17. No, the dose is too low, contact the prescriber
18. 7.5 mL/h of dopamine
19. 1.2 mL of Solu-Cortef (hydrocortisone sodium succinate)
20. Yes, the prescribed dose is safe

21. 50 mL of Mannitol
22. 141.6 mg of Norvir (ritonavir)
23. 25 gtt/min of D5W
24. 2 tab of Synthroid (levothyroxine)
25. 0.8 mL of heparin

Comprehensive Self-Test 3

1. 735 mg   2. 2 cap

3. Take 40 mL of 100% Clorox solution and dilute to 400 mL

4. 0.1 g   5. 8 hours 20 min   6. 12.5 g

7.

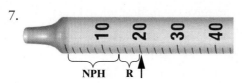

8. 2 tab   9. 100 mL/h, 1,000 mg

10.

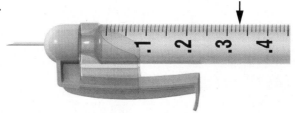

11. 0.75 mL   12. 3 mL/h   13. 6.8 units/h

14. 2.5 mL   15. 0.132 mgs

16. 0.22 mg/d, 0.32 mg/d, yes 17. 160 mg, 50 mL/h   18. 25 gtt/min

19. 1 m^2 20. 0.5 mL

21. 1.25 mL/min, 25 gtt/min, 13 hours 20 minutes

22. 2,000 mL   23. 30 mL

24. 10 mg, 60 mL   25. 21 mL/h

Comprehensive Self-Test 4

1. 2,000 units per hour

2. 19.2 mg, 3.8 mL, 311 mL/h

3. 2 tab   4. 2 cap   5. 2.2 mL

6. Yes, 0.9 mL   7. 0900 h the next day   8. 4.1 mL

9. 2 mL, arrow at 2 mL   10. 218 mg/d, 681 mg/d   11. 2.25 g

12. 100 mL/h   13. 454 mL/d, 18.9 mL/h   14. No

15. 40 mL/h   16. 120 mL/h   17. 2.5 mL

18. 2 cap, 3.15 g   19. 30 mL   20. 21 mL/h

21. 45 mL, 2.75 mL/h   22. 0.7 mL

23. 3 mL syringe   24. Take 600 mL of Sustacal and dilute to 900 mL

25. 0400 h the next day

FDA and ISMP Lists of
Look-Alike Drug Names with Recommended Tall Man Letters

The look-alike drug names in the Tables that follow have been modified using tall man (mixed case) letters to help draw attention to the dissimilarities in their names. Several studies have shown that highlighting sections of drug names using tall man letters can help distinguish similar drug names,[1] making them less prone to mix-ups.[2-3] ISMP, FDA, The Joint Commission, and other safety-conscious organizations have promoted the use of tall man letters as one means of reducing confusion between similar drug names.

Table 1 provides an alphabetized list of FDA-approved established drug names with recommended tall man letters, which were first identified during the FDA Name Differentiation Project (www.fda.gov/Drugs/DrugSafety/MedicationErrors/ucm164587.htm).

Table 2 provides an alphabetized list of additional drug names with recommendations from ISMP regarding the use and placement of tall man letters. This is not an official list approved by FDA. It is intended for voluntary use by healthcare practitioners and drug information vendors. Any product label changes by manufacturers require FDA approval.

One of the difficulties with the use of tall man letters includes inconsistent application in health settings and lack of standardization regarding which letters to present in uppercase. A new study by Gerrett[4] describes several ways to determine which of the dissimilar letters in each drug name should be highlighted. To promote standardi-zation, ISMP followed one of these tested methodologies whenever possible. Called the CD3 rule, the methodology suggests working from the left of the word first by capitalizing all the characters to the right once two or more dissimilar letters are encountered, and then, working from the right of the word back, returning two or more letters common to both words to lowercase letters. When the rule cannot be applied because there are no common letters on the right side of the word, the methodology suggests capitalizing the central part of the word only. ISMP suggests that the tall man lettering scheme provided in Tables 1 and 2 be followed when presenting these drug names to healthcare providers to promote consistency. At this time, scientific studies do not support the use of tall man letters when presenting drug names to patients.

References: 1) Filik R, Purdy K, Gale A, Gerrett D. Drug name confusion: evaluating the effectiveness of capital ("Tall Man") letters using eye movement data. *Social Science & Medicine* 2004;59(12):2597-2601. 2) Filik R, Purdy K, Gale A, Gerrett D. Labeling of medicines and patient safety: evaluating methods of reducing drug name confusion. *Human Factors* 2006;48(1):39-47. 3) Grasha A. Cognitive systems perspective on human performance in the pharmacy: implications for accuracy, effectiveness, and job satisfaction. Alexandria (VA): NACDS; 2000 Report No. 062100. 4) Gerrett D, Gale AG, Darker IT, Filik R, Purdy KJ. Tall man lettering. Final report of the use of tall man lettering to minimize selection errors of medicine names in computer prescribing and dispensing systems. Loughborough University Enterprises Ltd.; 2009 (www.connectingforhealth.nhs.uk/systemsandservices/eprescribing/refdocs/tallman.pdf).

Table 1. FDA-Approved List of Generic Drug Names with Tall Man Letters

Drug Name with Tall Man Letters	Confused with
aceta**ZOLAMIDE**	aceto**HEXAMIDE**
aceto**HEXAMIDE**	aceta**ZOLAMIDE**
bu**PROP**ion	bus**PIR**one
bus**PIR**one	bu**PROP**ion
chlorpro**MAZINE**	chlorpro**PAMIDE**
chlorpro**PAMIDE**	chlorpro**MAZINE**
clomi**PHENE**	clomi**PRAMINE**
clomi**PRAMINE**	clomi**PHENE**
cyclo**SERINE**	cyclo**SPORINE**
cyclo**SPORINE**	cyclo**SERINE**
DAUNOrubicin	**DOXO**rubicin
dimenhy**DRINATE**	diphenhydr**AMINE**
diphenhydr**AMINE**	dimenhy**DRINATE**
DOBUTamine	**DOP**amine
DOPamine	**DOBUT**amine

continued on next page

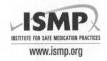

Table 1. FDA–Approved List of Generic Drug Names with Tall Man Letters (continued)

Drug Name with Tall Man Letters	Confused with
DOXOrubicin	DAUNOrubicin
glipiZIDE	glyBURIDE
glyBURIDE	glipiZIDE
hydrALAZINE	hydrOXYzine
hydrOXYzine	hydrALAZINE
medroxyPROGESTERone	methylPREDNISolone - methylTESTOSTERone
methylPREDNISolone	medroxyPROGESTERone - methylTESTOSTERone
methylTESTOSTERone	medroxyPROGESTERone - methylPREDNISolone
niCARdipine	NIFEdipine
NIFEdipine	niCARdipine
prednisoLONE	predniSONE
predniSONE	prednisoLONE
sulfADIAZINE	sulfiSOXAZOLE
sulfiSOXAZOLE	sulfADIAZINE
TOLAZamide	TOLBUTamide
TOLBUTamide	TOLAZamide
vinBLAStine	vinCRIStine
vinCRIStine	vinBLAStine

Table 2. ISMP List of Additional Drug Names with Tall Man Letters

Drug Name with Tall Man Letters	Confused with
ALPRAZolam	LORazepam
aMILoride	amLODIPine
amLODIPine	aMILoride
ARIPiprazole	RABEprazole
AVINza*	INVanz*
azaCITIDine	azaTHIOprine
azaTHIOprine	azaCITIDine
carBAMazepine	OXcarbazepine
CARBOplatin	CISplatin
ceFAZolin	cefoTEtan – cefOXitin – cefTAZidime – cefTRIAXone
cefoTEtan	ceFAZolin – cefOXitin – cefTAZidime – cefTRIAXone
cefOXitin	ceFAZolin – cefoTEtan – cefTAZidime – cefTRIAXone
cefTAZidime	ceFAZolin – cefoTEtan – cefOXitin – cefTRIAXone
cefTRIAXone	ceFAZolin - cefoTEtan – cefOXitin – cefTAZidime
CeleBREX*	CeleXA*
CeleXA*	CeleBREX*
chlordiazePOXIDE	chlorproMAZINE
chlorproMAZINE	chlordiazePOXIDE
CISplatin	CARBOplatin
clonazePAM	cloNIDine – cloZAPine – LORazepam

* Brand names always start with an uppercase letter. Some brand names incorporate tall man letters in initial characters and may not be readily recognized as brand names. An asterisk follows all brand names in Table 2.

continued on next page

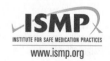

ISMP
INSTITUTE FOR SAFE MEDICATION PRACTICES
www.ismp.org

FDA and ISMP Lists of
Look-Alike Drug Names with Recommended Tall Man Letters (continued)

Table 2. ISMP List of Additional Drug Names with Tall Man Letters (continued)	
Drug Name with Tall Man Letters	**Confused with**
cloNIDine	clonazePAM – cloZAPine – KlonoPIN*
cloZAPine	clonazePAM – cloNIDine
DACTINomycin	DAPTOmycin
DAPTOmycin	DACTINomycin
DOCEtaxel	PACLitaxel
DOXOrubicin	IDArubicin
DULoxetine	FLUoxetine – PARoxetine
ePHEDrine	EPINEPHrine
EPINEPHrine	ePHEDrine
fentaNYL	SUFentanil
flavoxATE	fluvoxaMINE
FLUoxetine	DULoxetine – PARoxetine
fluPHENAZine	fluvoxaMINE
fluvoxaMINE	fluPHENAZine – flavoxATE
guaiFENesin	guanFACINE
guanFACINE	guaiFENesin
HumaLOG*	HumuLIN*
HumuLIN*	HumaLOG*
HYDROcodone	oxyCODONE
HYDROmorphone	morphine
IDArubicin	DOXOrubicin
inFLIXimab	riTUXimab
INVanz*	AVINza*
ISOtretinoin	tretinoin
KlonoPIN*	cloNIDine
LaMICtal*	LamISIL*
LamISIL*	LaMICtal*
lamiVUDine	lamoTRIgine
lamoTRIgine	lamiVUDine
levETIRAcetam	levOCARNitine
levOCARNitine	levETIRAcetam
LORazepam	ALPRAZolam – clonazePAM
metFORMIN	metroNIDAZOLE
metroNIDAZOLE	metFORMIN
mitoMYcin	mitoXANtrone
mitoXANtrone	mitoMYcin
NexAVAR*	NexIUM*
NexIUM*	NexAVAR*
niCARdipine	niMODipine – NIFEdipine
NIFEdipine	niMODipine – niCARdipine
niMODipine	NIFEdipine – niCARdipine
NovoLIN*	NovoLOG*

* Brand names always start with an uppercase letter. Some brand names incorporate tall man letters in initial characters and may not be readily recognized as brand names. An asterisk follows all brand names in Table 2.

continued on next page

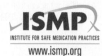

ISMP
INSTITUTE FOR SAFE MEDICATION PRACTICES
www.ismp.org

Table 2. ISMP List of Additional Drug Names with Tall Man Letters (continued)

Drug Name with Tall Man Letters	Confused with
NovoLOG*	NovoLIN*
OLANZapine	QUEtiapine
OXcarbazepine	carBAMazepine
oxyCODONE	HYDROcodone – OxyCONTIN*
OxyCONTIN*	oxyCODONE
PACLitaxel	DOCEtaxel
PARoxetine	FLUoxetine – DULoxetine
PEMEtrexed	PRALAtrexate
PENTobarbital	PHENobarbital
PHENobarbital	PENTobarbital
PRALAtrexate	PEMEtrexed
PriLOSEC*	PROzac*
PROzac*	PriLOSEC*
QUEtiapine	OLANZapine
quiNIDine	quiNINE
quiNINE	quiNIDine
RABEprazole	ARIPiprazole
RisperDAL*	rOPINIRole
risperiDONE	rOPINIRole
riTUXimab	inFLIXimab
romiDEPsin	romiPLOStim
romiPLOStim	romiDEPsin
rOPINIRole	RisperDAL* – risperiDONE
SandIMMUNE*	SandoSTATIN*
SandoSTATIN*	SandIMMUNE*
SEROquel*	SINEquan*
SINEquan*	SEROquel*
sitaGLIPtin	SUMAtriptan
Solu-CORTEF*	Solu-MEDROL*
Solu-MEDROL*	Solu-CORTEF*
SORAfenib	SUNItinib
SUFentanil	fentaNYL
sulfADIAZINE	sulfaSALAzine
sulfaSALAzine	sulfADIAZINE
SUMAtriptan	sitaGLIPtin – ZOLMitriptan
SUNItinib	SORAfenib
TEGretol*	TRENtal*
tiaGABine	tiZANidine
tiZANidine	tiaGABine
traMADol	traZODone
traZODone	traMADol

* Brand names always start with an uppercase letter. Some brand names incorporate tall man letters in initial characters and may not be readily recognized as brand names. An asterisk follows all brand names in Table 2.

continued on next page

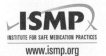

ISMP
INSTITUTE FOR SAFE MEDICATION PRACTICES
www.ismp.org

FDA and ISMP Lists of
Look-Alike Drug Names with Recommended Tall Man Letters (continued)

Table 2. ISMP List of Additional Drug Names with Tall Man Letters (continued)	
Drug Name with Tall Man Letters	**Confused with**
TRENtal*	TEGretol*
valACYclovir	valGANciclovir
valGANciclovir	valACYclovir
ZOLMitriptan	SUMAtriptan
ZyPREXA*	ZyrTEC*
ZyrTEC*	ZyPREXA*

* Brand names always start with an uppercase letter. Some brand names incorporate tall man letters in initial characters and may not be readily recognized as brand names. An asterisk follows all brand names in Table 2.

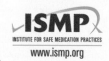

www.ismp.org

Appendix C

Commonly Used Abbreviations

To someone unfamiliar with prescription abbreviations, medication orders may look like a foreign language. To interpret prescriptive orders accurately and to administer drugs safely, a qualified person must have a thorough knowledge of common abbreviations. For instance, when the prescriber writes, "**hydromorphone 1.5 mg IM q4h prn,**" the healthcare professional knows how to interpret it as "hydromorphone, 1.5 milligrams, intramuscular, every four hours, whenever necessary." For measurement abbreviations, refer to Appendix D.

Abbreviation	Meaning	Abbreviation	Meaning
ā	before (*abante*)	gtt	drop
ac	before meals (*ante cibum*)	h, hr	hour
ad lib	as desired (*ad libitum*)	hs	hour of sleep; bedtime (*hora somni*)
A.M., am	morning	IC	intracardiac
amp	ampule	ID	intradermal
aq	aqueous water	IM	intramuscular; intramuscularly
b.i.d.	two times a day	IV	intravenous; intravenously
BP	blood pressure	USP	United States Pharmacopeia
c̄	with	IVP	intravenous push
C	Celsius; centigrade	IVPB	intravenous piggyback
cap	capsule	IVSS	IV Soluset
CBC	complete blood count	kg	kilogram
cc	cubic centimeter	KVO	keep vein open
CVP	central venous pressure	L	liter
d	day	LA	long acting
D/W	dextrose in water	lb	pound
D5W or D5/W or D$_5$W	5% dextrose in water	LIB	left in bag, left in bottle
daw	dispense as written	LOS	length of stay
dr	dram	MAR	medication administration record
Dx	diagnosis	mcg	microgram
elix	elixir	mcgtt	microdrop
ER	extended release	mEq	milliequivalent
F	Fahrenheit	mg	milligram
g	gram	min	minute
gr	grain	mL	milliliter
GT	gastrostomy tube	mU	milliunit

Abbreviation	Meaning	Abbreviation	Meaning
n, noct	night	q3h	every three hours
NDC	national drug code	q4h	every four hours
NGT	nasogastric tube	q6h	every six hours
NKA	no known allergies	q8h	every eight hours
NKDA	no known drug allergies	q12h	every 12 hours
NKFA	no known food allergies	q.i.d.	four times a day (*quarter in die*)
NPO	nothing by mouth (*per ora*)	qn	every night (*quaque noct*)
NS	normal saline	qs	quantity sufficient or sufficient amount (*quantitas sufficiens*)
NSAID	nonsteroidal anti-inflammatory drug		
OTC	over the counter	R	respiration
oz	ounce	R/O	rule out
p̄	after	Rx	prescription, treatment
PEG	percutaneous endoscopic gastrostomy tube	s̄	without (*sine*)
		SIG	directions to the patient
P	pulse	SL	sublingual
pc	after meals (*post cibum*)	SR	sustained release
PEJ	percutaneous endoscopic jejunostomy	stat	immediately (*statum*)
		subcut	subcutaneous
PICC	peripherally inserted central catheter	supp	suppository
P.M., pm	afternoon, evening	susp	suspension
PO	by mouth (*per os*)	T or tbs	tablespoon
POST-OP	after surgery	t or tsp	teaspoon
PR	by way of the rectum	T	temperature
PRE-OP	before surgery	t.i.d.	three times a day (*ter in die*)
prn	when required or whenever necessary		
Pt	patient	tab	tablet
pt	pint	TPN	total parenteral nutrition
q	every (*quaque*)	USP	United States Pharmacopeia
qh	every hour (*quaque hora*)	V/S	vital signs
q2h	every two hours	wt	weight

Appendix D

Units of Measurement in Metric and Household Systems

Abbreviations			
Volume			
Metric		**Household**	
milliliter	mL	microdrop	mcgtt
liter	L	drop	gtt
cubic centimeter	cc	teaspoon	t or tsp
		tablespoon	T or tbs
		fluid ounce	oz
		pint	pt
		quart	qt
Weight			
Metric		**Household**	
microgram	mcg	ounce	oz
milligram	mg	pound	lb
gram	g		
kilogram	kg		
Length			
Metric		**Household**	
millimeter	mm	inch	in
centimeter	cm	foot	ft
meter	m		
Area			
Metric			
square meter	m^2		

Appendix E

Celsius and Fahrenheit Temperature Conversions

Reading and recording a temperature is a crucial step in assessing a patient's health. Temperatures can be measured using either the Fahrenheit (F) scale or the Celsius or centigrade (C) scale. Celsius/Fahrenheit equivalency tables make it easy to convert Celsius to Fahrenheit, or vice versa. Still, it is useful to be able to make this conversion yourself.

You can use the following formulas to convert from one temperature scale to the other

$$C = \frac{F - 32}{1.8} \quad \text{and} \quad F = 1.8\,C + 32$$

For those unfamiliar with algebra, the following rules are equivalent to the algebraic formulas.

First rule: To convert to Celsius. Subtract 32 and then divide by 1.8.
Second rule: To convert to Fahrenheit. Multiply by 1.8 and then add 32.

NOTE

Temperatures are rounded to the nearest tenth.

EXAMPLE E.1

Convert 102.5°F to Celsius.

Using the first rule, you subtract 32.

$$\begin{array}{r} 102.5 \\ -32.0 \\ \hline 70.5 \end{array}$$

Then you divide by 1.8.

$$1.8\,)\overline{70.5000} \quad \rightarrow 39.17$$

So, 102.5°F equals 39.2°C.

EXAMPLE E.2

Convert 3°C to Fahrenheit.

Using the second rule, you first multiply by 1.8.

$$\begin{array}{r} 1.8 \\ \times 3 \\ \hline 5.4 \end{array}$$

Then you add 32.

$$
\begin{array}{r}
5.4 \\
+32.0 \\
\hline
37.4
\end{array}
$$

So, 3°C equals 37.4°F

For those unfamiliar with the Celsius system, the following rhyme might be useful:

Thirty is hot
Twenty is nice
Ten is chilly
Zero is ice

Appendix F

Diluting Stock Solutions

A stock solution is one in which a pure drug is already dissolved in a liquid. The strength of each stock solution is written on the label. If the order is for a stronger solution, you will need to prepare a new solution. However, if the order is for a weaker solution, you can dilute the stock solution to the prescribed strength. To find out how much stock solution to take, use the following formula.

$$\frac{\text{Amount prescribed} \times \text{Strength prescribed}}{\text{Strength of stock}} = \text{Amount of stock}$$

EXAMPLE F.1

How would you prepare 1 L of a 25% solution from a 50% stock solution? Because this example does not indicate whether the drug in the solution is a solid or a liquid in its pure form, you may choose either *grams* or *milliliters* for the amount of the pure drug, and the choice will have no effect on the answer. *Grams* are chosen in the following solution.

Given: Amount prescribed: 1,000 mL

        Strength prescribed: 25% or $\dfrac{25g}{100mL}$

        Strength of stock: 50% or $\dfrac{50g}{100mL}$

Find: Amount of stock: ? mL

$$\frac{\text{Amount prescribed} \times \text{Strength prescribed}}{\text{Strength of stock}} = \text{Amount of stock}$$

Substituting the given information into the formula, you get

$$\frac{1,000mL \times \dfrac{25g}{100mL}}{\dfrac{50g}{100\ mL}} = ?\ mL$$

This complex fraction may be written as a division problem as follows:

$$1,000\,mL \times \frac{25g}{100\ mL} \div \frac{50g}{100\ mL} = ?\ mL$$

This division problem may be changed to a multiplication problem by inverting the last fraction. Now, cancel and multiply.

$$1,000\,mL \times \frac{25g}{100mL} \times \frac{100mL}{50g} = 500\ mL$$

So, you would take 500 mL of the 50% stock solution and add water to the level of 1,000 mL.

EXAMPLE F.2

How would you prepare 2,500 mL of a 1:10 boric acid solution from a 40% stock solution of this antiseptic?

Given: Amount prescribed: 2,500 mL

Strength prescribed: 1:10 or $\dfrac{1 \text{ mL}}{10 \text{ mL}}$

Strength of stock: 40% or $\dfrac{40 \text{ mL}}{100 \text{ mL}}$

Find: Amount of stock: ? mL

$$\dfrac{2,500 \text{ mL} \times \dfrac{1 \text{ mL}}{10 \text{ mL}}}{\dfrac{40 \text{ mL}}{100 \text{ mL}}} = \text{Amount of stock}$$

$$2,500 \text{ mL} \times \dfrac{1}{10} \div \dfrac{40}{100} = ? \text{ mL}$$

$$\overset{250}{2,500} \times \dfrac{1}{\underset{1}{10}} \times \dfrac{100}{40} = 625 \text{ mL}$$

So, you would take 625 mL of the 40% stock solution of boric acid and add water to the level of 2,500 mL.

EXAMPLE F.3

How would you prepare 500 mL of a 1:25 solution from a 1:4 stock solution of the antiseptic Argyrol?

Given: Amount prescribed: 500 mL

Strength prescribed: 1:25 or $\dfrac{1 \text{ mL}}{25 \text{ mL}}$

Strength of stock: 1:4 or $\dfrac{1 \text{ mL}}{4 \text{ mL}}$

Find: Amount of stock: ? mL

$$\dfrac{500 \text{ mL} \times \dfrac{1 \text{ mL}}{25 \text{ mL}}}{\dfrac{1 \text{ mL}}{4 \text{ mL}}} = \text{Amount of stock}$$

$$500 \text{ mL} \times \dfrac{1}{25} \div \dfrac{1}{4} = ? \text{ mL}$$

$$\overset{20}{500} \text{ mL} \times \dfrac{1}{\underset{1}{25}} \times \dfrac{4}{1} = 80 \text{ mL}$$

So, you would take 80 mL of a 1:4 stock solution of Argyrol and add water to the level of 500 mL.

Exercises

1. How would you prepare 200 mL of a 5% solution from a 20% stock solution?

2. How would you prepare 500 mL of a 1:4 solution from a 1:3 stock solution?

3. How would you prepare 1 L of a 0.45% solution from a 0.9% stock solution?

4. How would you prepare 200 mL of a 25% solution from a 35% stock solution?

5. How would you prepare 2 L of a 1:5 solution from a $\frac{1}{2}$ strength stock solution?

Answers

1. Take 50 mL of the stock solution and add water to the level of 200 mL.

2. Take 375 mL of the stock solution and add water to the level of 500 mL.

3. Take 500 mL of the stock solution and add water to the level of 1 L.

4. Take 143 mL of the stock solution and add water to the level of 200 mL.

5. Take 800 mL of the stock solution and add water to the level of 2 L.

Appendix G

Apothecary System

The apothecary system is one of the oldest systems of drug measurement. Although the apothecary system was used in the past to write prescriptions, it has largely been replaced by the metric system. Apothecary units are rarely used on drug labels, but when they are, the metric equivalents are also provided.

NOTE

In the apothecary system, the abbreviation or symbol for the unit is placed before the quantity (as in drams 8). Ounces are used for liquid volume in both the household and apothecary systems. To avoid errors, the abbreviations dr and oz are preferred over the formerly used abbreviations ℥ and ʒ.

Liquid Volume in the Apothecary System

The equivalents for the units of measurement for liquid volume in the apothecary system are shown in Table G.1 along with their abbreviations.

Table G.1 Common Equivalents for Apothecary Liquid Volume Units
ounce (oz)1 = drams (dr)8
dram (dr)1 = minims 60

NOTE

Decimal numbers are never used in the apothecary system.

EXAMPLE G.1

How many minims would be equivalent to dr $\frac{1}{6}$?

Think:

$$dr\ \frac{1}{6} = minims\ ?$$

$$dr\ 1 = minims\ 60$$

Solve the proportion:

$$\frac{dr\ \frac{1}{6}}{minims\ x} = \frac{dr\ 1}{minims\ 60}$$

$$x = 10$$

So, minims 10 are equivalent to dr $\frac{1}{6}$.

EXAMPLE G.2

How many ounces would be equivalent to dr 4?

Think:

$$dr\ 4 = ounces\ ?$$

$$dr\ 8 = ounce\ 1$$

442

Solve the proportion:

$$\frac{dr\ 4}{ounces\ x} = \frac{dr\ 8}{ounce\ 1}$$
$$8x = 4$$
$$x = \frac{1}{2}$$

So, dr 4 is equivalent to oz $\frac{1}{2}$.

Weight in the Apothecary System

The grain (gr) is the only unit of weight in the apothecary system that is used in administering medications.

Roman Numerals

Dosages in the apothecary system are sometimes written using Roman numerals. Table G.2 shows Roman numerals.

Table G.2 Roman Numerals

	Roman Numerals		Roman Numerals		Roman Numerals
1	I	7	VII	$\frac{1}{2}$	ss
2	II	8	VIII	$1\frac{1}{2}$	iss
3	III	9	IX	$7\frac{1}{2}$	viiss
4	IV	10	X		
5	V	15	XV		
6	VI	20	XX		

Equivalents of Common Units of Measurement

Tables G.3 and G.4 list some common equivalent values for weight, volume, and length in the metric, household, and apothecary systems of measurement. Although these equivalents are considered standards, many of them are approximations.

NOTE

Here are some useful equivalents:

1 t = 5 mL = dr 1
2 T = 30 mL = oz 1 = dr 8

Table G.3 Equivalent Values for Units of Weight

Metric		Apothecary		Household
60 milligrams (mg)	=	grain (gr) 1		
1 gram (g)	=	grains (gr) 15		
1 kilogram (kg)			=	2.2 pounds (lb)

Table G.4 **Equivalent Values for Units of Volume**				
Metric		**Apothecary**		**Household**
1 milliliter (mL)	=	minims 15		
5 milliliters (mL)	=	dram (dr) 1	=	1 teaspoon (t)
15 milliliters (mL)	=	ounce (oz)$\frac{1}{2}$	=	1 tablespoon (T)
30 milliliters (mL)	=	ounce (oz) 1	=	2 tablespoons (T)
500 milliliters	=	ounces (oz) 16	=	1 pint (pt)
1,000 milliliters	=	ounces (oz) 32	=	1 quart (qt)

Metric–Apothecary Conversions

EXAMPLE G.3

Convert 40 milligrams to grains.

Think:

$$40 \; mg = gr \; ?$$
$$60 \; mg = gr \; 1$$

Solve the proportion:

$$\frac{40 \; mg}{gr \; x} = \frac{60 \; mg}{gr \; 1}$$
$$60x = 40$$
$$x = \frac{2}{3}$$

So, 40 milligrams are equivalent to grain $\frac{2}{3}$.

EXAMPLE G.4

Convert 0.12 milligrams to grains.

Think:

$$0.12 \; mg = gr \; ?$$
$$60 \; mg = gr \; 1$$

Solve the proportion:

$$\frac{0.12 \; mg}{gr \; x} = \frac{60 \; mg}{gr \; 1}$$
$$60x = 0.12$$
$$x = 0.002$$

A decimal number cannot be used in the apothecary system. Therefore, 0.002 must be written in fractional form.

$$0.002 = \frac{2}{1,000} = \frac{1}{500}$$

So, 0.12 milligrams are equivalent to grain $\frac{1}{500}$.

EXAMPLE G.5

Convert 1.5 grams to an equivalent weight in grains.

Think:

$$1.5\ g = gr\ ?$$
$$1\ g = gr\ 15$$

Solve the proportion:

$$\frac{1.5\ g}{gr\ x} = \frac{1\ g}{gr\ 15}$$
$$x = 22.5$$

A decimal number cannot be used in the apothecary system. Therefore, 22.5 must be written in fractional form as $22\frac{1}{2}$.

So, 1.5 grams are equivalent to grains $22\frac{1}{2}$.

NOTE

Grains are apothecary units and are expressed as fractions or whole numbers. Therefore, grains 22.5 should be expressed as grains $22\frac{1}{2}$.

EXAMPLE G.6

Convert grain $\frac{1}{300}$ to milligrams.

Think:

$$gr\ \frac{1}{300} = ?\ mg$$
$$gr\ 1 = 60\ mg$$

Solve the proportion:

$$\frac{gr\ \frac{1}{300}}{x\ mg} = \frac{gr\ 1}{60\ mg}$$
$$x = 0.2$$

So, *grain* $\frac{1}{300}$ is equivalent to 0.2 milligrams.

EXAMPLE G.7

Convert grains $7\frac{1}{2}$ to grams.

Think:

$$gr\ 7\frac{1}{2} = ?\ g$$
$$gr\ 15 = 1\ g$$

Solve the proportion:

$$\frac{gr\ 7\frac{1}{2}}{x\ mg} = \frac{gr\ 15}{1\ g}$$

$$15x = 7\frac{1}{2}$$

$$x = \frac{1}{2}$$

So, *grains* $7\frac{1}{2}$ are equivalent to 0.5 gram.

Household–Apothecary Conversions

EXAMPLE G.8

Convert ounces 2 to tablespoons.

Think:

$$oz\ 2 = ?\ T$$
$$oz\ 1 = 2\ T$$

Solve the proportion:

$$\frac{oz\ 2}{x\ T} = \frac{oz\ 1}{2\ T}$$

$$x = 4$$

So, *ounces* 2 is equivalent to 4 tablespoons.

Exercises

1. oz 1 = dr ?
2. dr 1 = minims ?
3. dr 12 = oz ?
4. dr $1\frac{1}{2}$ = minims ?
5. oz 64 = dr ?
6. dr 1 = ? t = minims ? = ? mL
7. oz 1 = ? T = dr ? = ? mL
8. 1 cup = ? glass = oz ? = ? pt
9. gr 1 = ? mg
10. 1 g = gr ?
11. 0.006 mg = gr ?
12. gr $3\frac{3}{4}$ = ? mg

Answers

1. dr 8
2. minims 60
3. oz $1\frac{1}{2}$
4. minims 90
5. dr 512
6. dr 1 = 1 t = minims 60 = 5 mL
7. oz 1 = 2 T = dr 8 = 30 mL
8. 1 cup = 1 glass = oz 8 = $\frac{1}{2}$ pt
9. 60 mg
10. gr 15
11. gr $\frac{1}{10,000}$
12. 225 mg

Index